1991-1992 GREEN INDEX

1991-1992 GREEN INDEX

A State-By-State Guide to the Nation's Environmental Health

**BOB HALL AND
MARY LEE KERR**

ISLAND PRESS

Washington, D.C. Covelo, California

ABOUT ISLAND PRESS

Island Press, a nonprofit organization, publishes, markets, and distributes the most advanced thinking on the conservation of our natural resources—books about soil, land, water, forests, wildlife, and hazardous and toxic wastes. These books are practical tools used by public officials, business and industry leaders, natural resource managers, and concerned citizens working to solve both local and global resource problems.

Founded in 1978, Island Press reorganized in 1984 to meet the increasing demand for substantive books on all resource-related issues. Island Press publishes and distributes under its own imprint and offers these services to other nonprofit organizations.

Support for Island Press is provided by Apple Computer, Inc., Mary Reynolds Babcock Foundation, Geraldine R. Dodge Foundation, The Charles Engelhard Foundation, The Ford Foundation, Glen Eagles Foundation, The George Gund Foundation, William and Flora Hewlett Foundation, The Joyce Foundation, The John D. and Catherine T. MacArthur Foundation, The Andrew W. Mellon Foundation, The Joyce Mertz-Gilmore Foundation, The New-Land Foundation, The J. N. Pew, Jr. Charitable Trust, Alida Rockefeller, The Rockefeller Brothers Fund, The Florence and John Schumann Foundation, The Tides Foundation, and individual donors.

© 1991 Institute for Southern Studies

All rights reserved. No part of this book may be reproduced in any form or by any means without permission in writing from the publisher: Island Press, Suite 300, 1718 Connecticut Avenue NW, Washington, D.C. 20009.

Text, map, and cover design by Jacob Roquet

ISSN 1055-9396
ISBN 1-55963-115-5 (cloth)
1-55963-114-7 (paper)

Printed on recycled, acid-free paper

Manufactured in the United States of America

10 9 8 7 6 5 4 3 2 1

TABLE OF CONTENTS

vii .... **ACKNOWLEDGMENTS**
1 .... **A USER'S GUIDE TO THE GREEN INDEX**
3 .... **GREEN INDEX FINAL RANKINGS**

CHAPTER 1
7 .... **ENVIRONMENTAL SCALES**
11 .... **WHERE EACH STATE EXCELS — AND FAILS**

CHAPTER 2
15 .... **AIR SICKNESS**
22 .... 18 Indicators and Sources

CHAPTER 3
27 .... **WATER POLLUTION**
35 .... 24 Indicators and Sources

CHAPTER 4
42 .... **ENERGY USE AND AUTO ABUSE**
51 .... 38 Indicators and Sources

CHAPTER 5
62 .... **TOXIC, HAZARDOUS, AND SOLID WASTE**
72 .... 30 Indicators and Sources

CHAPTER 6
82 .... **COMMUNITY AND WORKPLACE HEALTH**
89 .... 23 Indicators and Sources

CHAPTER 7
97 .... **FARMS, FORESTS, FISH, AND FUN**
105 .... 46 Indicators and Sources

CHAPTER 8
117 .... **CONGRESSIONAL LEADERSHIP**
125 .... 4 Indicators and Sources

CHAPTER 9
134 .... **STATE POLICY INITIATIVES**
142 .... 73 Indicators and Sources
157 .... **INDEX**

Acknowledgments

The Green Index began in late 1989 as an assessment of environmental conditions and policies in the South. But like many of our projects, it soon took on a life of its own; by Spring, it had blossomed into an analysis of all 50 states. The Institute for Southern Studies, where we work, released our initial results just prior to Earth Day 1990. Using 35 indicators to rank each state's environmental health, the Index received immediate and extensive media attention, including more than 100 front-page stories in the nation's newspapers.

We issued two more reports later that Spring, adding 45 indicators for environmental conditions, 45 for state policies, and a scorebox for each state's Congressional leadership. By teaming up with the imaginative and supportive staff of Island Press, we have now expanded the scope of the Index to more than 250 indicators that emphasize the interrelationships between the natural ecosystem, built environment, and human health.

The Institute has a longstanding interest in the links between environmental and economic justice. In 1972, it successfully challenged the wasteful and discriminatory pricing system of electric utilities, which gave radical discounts to their largest customers. Other Institute projects have produced pioneering work on nuclear energy, hazardous waste, land ownership, and occupational health issues. Many of these ventures are tied to local or regional organizing efforts; some yield special reports, such as our recent book, *Environmental Politics: Lessons from the Grassroots*. For nearly 20 years, the chief outlet for Institute research has been its quarterly journal, *Southern Exposure*. In 1990, *Southern Exposure* published the original Green Index and also won the National Magazine Award for an expose of the workplace and consumer health hazards resulting from the fast-paced, poorly regulated poultry industry.

In addition to the Institute, we are grateful for the assistance of many organizations whose reports provided statistics, case studies, and analyses for the Green Index. Renew America's series of "State of the States" reports offered a treasure chest of detailed data and served as a valuable model, along with the annual "Development Report Card" issued by the Corporation for Enterprise Development. Rick Piltz and Sheila Machado, former Renew America staff members, and Chris

Nichols, author of the group's report on drinking water, were especially helpful in setting us on the right course. Jeff Tryens, Rich Schrader, and Eugene Lee of the Center for Policy Alternatives impressed us with the innovative role of state lawmakers, then supplied us with chapter and verse of model legislation, a service we commend to others. The League of Conservation Voters and Common Cause kindly furnished the fruits of their evaluations of Congressional voting records and PAC contributions, which became the core for our chapter on Congressional leadership.

The address for each of the these Washington-based organizations is included in the "Source" listings, along with those for dozens of other private groups. The Council of State Governments, Environmental Law Institute, *BioCycle* magazine, and National Governors' Association conduct their own surveys to produce valuable reports on the status, cost, and comparative strength of state environmental programs. Most of the other groups depend heavily on data collected by various federal agencies. Having experienced the frustration of slogging through the bureaucracies to find a friendly source, we greatly appreciate the labor of these organizations.

The hard labor for this book was carried out by a bevy of generous volunteers and interns — Robin Donovan, David Goetzl, Krista Horstman, Betty Meeler, Max Moehs, Laura Neish, Loli Oates, Sarah Post, Derek Rodriguez, Al Sawyer, Margie Stude, and Shawn Thompson. From data entry to proofreading, original research to editorial guidance, each person made a wonderful contribution to the final product and helped stretch our limited resources. Graphic designer and McMapmaker Jacob Roquet neatly transformed the results to camera-ready copy, and Chuck Israel expertly fashioned the index. Following a timely lead grant from the Beldon Fund, financial support came in chunks and dribbles from the Jessie Smith Noyes Foundation, Mary Reynolds Babcock Foundation, Towncreek Foundation, Munson Foundation, Tides Foundation, Rockefeller Family & Associates, and the Wray Trust. We applaud these good friends; they deserve the credit if you find the Green Index useful. We accept the blame if you find it wanting in some way.

Finally, we pitch thanks to our families and colleagues at the Institute who endured our grouchy attitudes, piles of printouts, and erratic devotion to deadlines. We can't make up for the abuse of our past work, but we do promise not to get swallowed up by another massive project for at least four months.

—Bob Hall, Mary Lee Kerr
Durham, North Carolina
April 1991

1991-1992 GREEN INDEX

A User's Guide to the Green Index

WHAT IS THE GREEN INDEX?

The Green Index is a set of 256 indicators that measure and rank each state's environmental health. Taken together, these indicators describe the condition of things as they are, as well as the policies and political leadership in place to make things better. Unlike many studies, the Green Index adopts a broad view of environmental quality by choosing indicators that evaluate the different consequences of how people, machines, and nature interact across the nation.

Nobody wants to live in the most polluted town in America, especially if it means their children's lives will be cut short by poisons in the water or air. This book doesn't identify the worst town by name, but it does give a set of criteria to use in evaluating the environmental health of any community.

By using these criteria, or indicators, we do identify the worst state — Alabama — and the best — Oregon — because the data we used is collected on a statewide basis. Finding comparable data for each of thousands of cities is impossible. Yet the characteristics that make Alabama rank 50th are also the ones that should raise a red flag if you find them in your town or in the city you're moving to: public water systems that violate the Safe Drinking Water Act; acidic rain; groundwater contaminated by pesticides; large paper-pulp mills that dump toxic chemicals in the air and water; military bases or industrial sites with substantial hazardous waste; workplaces with high injury rates; politicians who vote against environmental protection; and weak regulatory agencies.

The purpose of the Green Index is not to pick on Alabama or praise Oregon. As the chart on page 11 illustrates, every state has something to be proud of and many more areas needing improvement. Rather than focus on the composite or final rankings, we recommend that you study how a state performs on each indicator, then see what states offer a better model.

HOW ARE THE STATES RANKED?

Throughout this book, a rank of 50 is the worst and rank 1 is best. Each indicator includes a set of numbers for the 50 states, such as pounds per capita (per person) of toxic chemical air emissions; those numbers are then ranked based on our judgment about whether less or more is better for the overall environmental health. For example, less toxic pollution is better, so the state with the smallest number gets ranked 1st, the best possible. On the other hand, more is better when it comes to funds spent to control air pollution, so the largest dollar figure gets the best ranking.

To minimize the difference in the sizes or populations of the states, we generally converted the raw data to a per-capita, per-acre, or similar ratio. We also included a wide range of indicators to balance those that inherently favor rural versus urban states, rich versus poor, industrial versus agricultural, and so forth.

In addition to the ranks for individual indicators, the Green Index features several composite rankings. These are derived by adding together the ranks a state receives for each indicator in a subset, such as water pollution, to produce a "composite" or "summary" score. The composite scores are then ranked with the lowest total receiving the best "composite rank."

Using a similar method, the final Green Index score is the sum of the state's ranks for all 256 indicators, with each indicator carrying equal weight and an appropriate multiplier to compensate for any missing items (Alaska and Hawaii, for example, lack data for pesticide-related indicators). The final scores are then ranked, yielding the best and worst states overall.

HOW IS THIS BOOK ORGANIZED?

Following the introduction, the indicators are grouped together in eight chapters. The first six chapters focus on environmental conditions, while the last two address federal and state policies. Each chapter has three parts:

• A *narrative essay* describes the relevance of a set of indicators, highlights their consequences for the environment, and provides numerous examples from specific states. Often regional patterns or groupings of states (for example, the energy-producing states) emerge with common problems. Some indicators also overlap or reinforce one another, such as traffic density and air pollution; accompanying maps help dramatize these connections.

• A *series of tables* presents the data for the indicators and ranks how well each state does compared to the other 49. Occasionally, background data is included for an item that is not ranked, such as the state's 1990 population. The U.S. totals generally represent a national average, such as per-capita fertilizer use, but they sometimes include data for Washington, DC or Puerto Rico not on the state charts.

• The *sources for the indicators* follow the tables, and include a longer description of what they measure and the basis used for their rankings. An address and telephone number are provided the first time a private group appears; we encourage you to contact these sources for copies of their studies, possible updates, and related reports.

WHERE IS MY STATE DISCUSSED?

The index at the end of the book will guide you to all references in the text for a particular state or an environmental issue. Check under the state's region (Farmbelt, New England, etc.) for additional citations. The indicators, and the tables where they appear, are listed in bold typeface. Since every state is on every table, we don't include references for those pages in the index. The overall scores and rankings for each state appear in Chapter 1, but we recommend that you take a closer look at how it performs on the individual indicators at the end of the other chapters.

IS MORE DATA AVAILABLE?

For the true connoisseur of numbers, we can generate a printout of the original data used to produce each indicator (for example, the total volume of fertilizer used by state rather than the per-capita number used as the indicator.) We can also provide the tables in a series of Lotus 1-2-3 spreadsheets or ASCII files. Please contact us at the Institute for Southern Studies (P.O. Box 531, Durham, NC 27702; telephone 919-688-8167) about fees and details for ordering this material.

GREEN INDEX FINAL RANKINGS

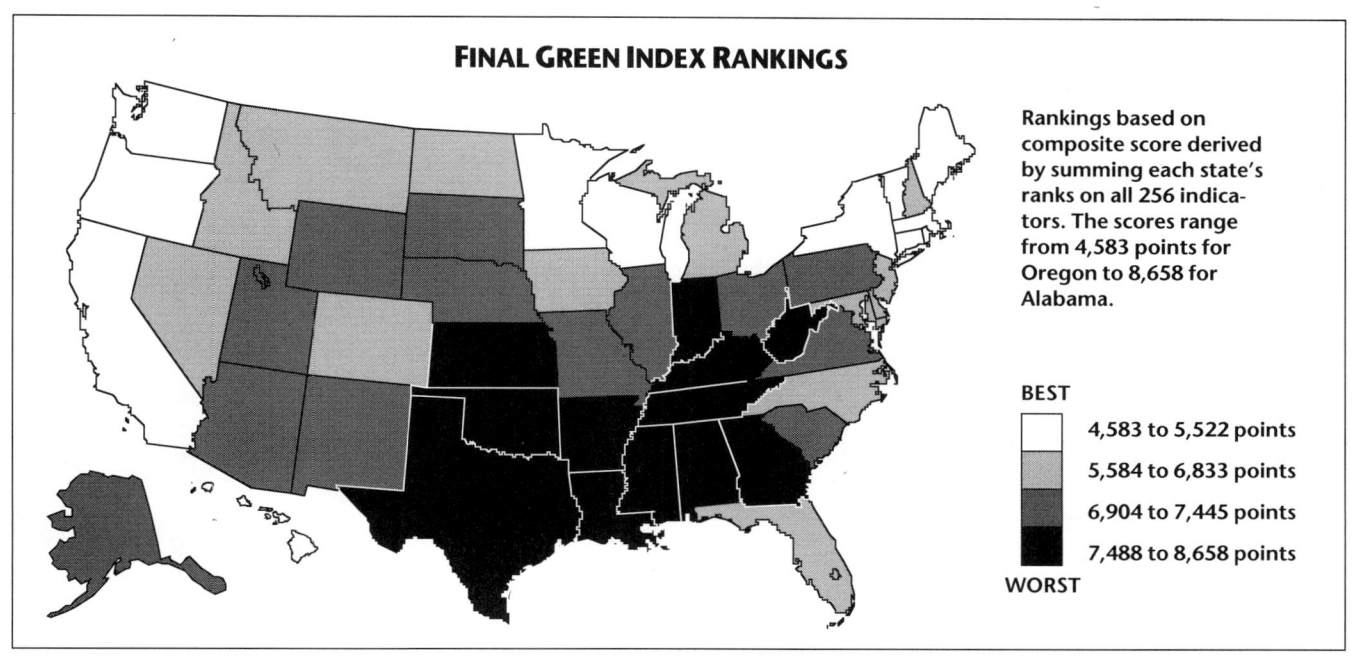

THE BEST AND WORST

State	FINAL GREEN INDEX 256 INDICATORS RANK	GREEN CONDITIONS 179 INDICATORS RANK	GREEN POLICIES 77 INDICATORS RANK	State	FINAL GREEN INDEX 256 INDICATORS RANK	GREEN CONDITIONS 179 INDICATORS RANK	GREEN POLICIES 77 INDICATORS RANK
Oregon	1	3	2	Pennsylvania	26	34	21
Maine	2	4	5	South Dakota	27	12	48
Vermont	3	2	12	New Mexico	28	20	38
California	4	19	1	Nebraska	29	24	30
Minnesota	5	5	7	Missouri	30	33	23
Massachusetts	6	6	9	Illinois	31	42	17
Rhode Island	7	7	10	Virginia	32	36	22
New York	8	17	8	Utah	33	22	41
Washington	9	13	14	Alaska	34	18	47
Wisconsin	10	21	6	Arizona	35	26	39
Connecticut	11	23	4	South Carolina	36	35	32
Hawaii	12	1	24	Ohio	37	46	19
Maryland	13	14	15	Wyoming	38	25	44
New Jersey	14	28	3	Georgia	39	38	29
New Hampshire	15	8	20	Oklahoma	40	31	42
Colorado	16	10	26	Kentucky	41	39	33
Michigan	17	32	11	Kansas	42	43	28
Florida	18	30	13	Indiana	43	49	27
Idaho	19	11	36	West Virginia	44	41	45
Iowa	20	29	16	Tennessee	45	45	40
Montana	21	15	31	Texas	46	48	35
Nevada	22	9	43	Mississippi	47	44	46
North Carolina	23	37	18	Arkansas	48	40	50
Delaware	24	27	25	Louisiana	49	50	34
North Dakota	25	16	37	Alabama	50	47	49

COMPOSITE RANKINGS FOR SETS OF INDICATORS

State	AIR POLLUTION (18 Indicators) Rank	WATER POLLUTION (24 Indicators) Rank	ENERGY USE & PRODUCTION (28) Rank	TRANSPORTATION EFFICIENCY (10) Rank	TOXIC CHEMICAL WASTE (13) Rank	HAZARDOUS & SOLID WASTE (17) Rank	COMMUNITY HEALTH (12) Rank	WORKPLACE HEALTH (11) Rank	AGRICULTURAL POLLUTION (14) Rank
Alabama	47	38	44	39	36	46	48	46	11
Alaska	7	30	42	22	5	27	45	22	48
Arizona	16	19	26	24	21	28	31	27	50
Arkansas	32	41	45	44	28	36	42	38	25
California	19	27	16	3	22	13	9	20	49
Colorado	12	2	20	19	8	4	10	25	42
Connecticut	40	17	11	8	39	10	3	8	9
Delaware	38	22	12	18	29	26	26	23	39
Florida	18	50	28	27	27	2	24	28	30
Georgia	42	29	21	28	32	42	39	40	28
Hawaii	2	16	4	6	2	17	2	4	34
Idaho	1	25	1	45	10	21	30	44	45
Illinois	41	46	46	13	40	16	34	7	41
Indiana	50	49	33	17	50	39	28	36	27
Iowa	23	34	36	39	18	33	7	19	43
Kansas	17	43	49	46	30	40	6	26	44
Kentucky	35	34	32	41	41	32	46	30	8
Louisiana	22	44	50	36	46	31	49	50	38
Maine	14	8	9	29	14	19	20	17	4
Maryland	24	12	17	4	18	15	16	5	15
Massachusetts	43	20	3	2	25	9	4	1	7
Michigan	33	31	25	14	47	35	21	12	22
Minnesota	21	21	15	7	20	3	1	6	47
Mississippi	27	32	39	35	34	41	50	49	36
Missouri	39	26	34	33	38	11	37	32	12
Montana	8	11	19	42	13	23	27	37	26
Nebraska	15	24	41	38	9	14	11	31	46
Nevada	3	1	7	37	6	34	44	24	20
New Hampshire	34	5	5	30	16	8	14	16	3
New Jersey	28	40	23	5	43	29	12	9	28
New Mexico	9	6	35	47	7	22	35	34	16
New York	30	15	18	1	24	5	22	2	30
North Carolina	44	28	27	25	42	30	40	21	19
North Dakota	11	4	38	48	1	7	18	42	30
Ohio	49	45	37	15	49	25	29	14	18
Oklahoma	20	14	43	32	16	47	36	43	12
Oregon	5	23	6	21	11	1	25	13	10
Pennsylvania	46	37	31	9	44	38	19	11	14
Rhode Island	26	8	2	11	23	6	17	3	17
South Carolina	29	18	29	20	33	50	43	33	21
South Dakota	6	10	10	49	3	24	41	45	33
Tennessee	48	47	24	43	48	43	38	35	6
Texas	24	36	48	26	45	48	33	48	35
Utah	30	3	22	16	26	49	5	47	24
Vermont	4	7	8	30	4	18	13	15	4
Virginia	37	42	30	23	37	44	32	29	2
Washington	13	33	13	10	12	12	15	18	40
West Virginia	45	48	40	34	35	45	47	39	1
Wisconsin	36	39	13	12	31	20	8	10	22
Wyoming	10	13	47	50	15	37	23	41	37

COMPOSITE RANKINGS FOR SETS OF INDICATORS

State	FORESTRY AND FISH (13 Indicators) Rank	FUN & LIFE QUALITY (19) Rank	GREEN CONDITIONS (179 Indicators) Score	GREEN CONDITIONS Rank	STATE POLICY INITIATIVES (73) Rank	LEADERSHIP IN CONGRESS (4) Rank	GREEN POLICIES (77 Indicators) Score	GREEN POLICIES Rank	TOTAL GREEN INDEX (256 Indicators) Score	TOTAL GREEN INDEX Rank
Alabama	27	43	5,446	47	48	46	3,212	49	8,658	50
Alaska	1	1	4,130	18	46	47	3,043	47	7,173	34
Arizona	12	27	4,540	26	38	44	2,802	39	7,342	35
Arkansas	19	16	5,123	40	50	34	3,230	50	8,353	48
California	48	22	4,167	19	1	16	764	1	4,931	4
Colorado	25	17	3,780	10	26	27	2,330	26	6,110	16
Connecticut	45	49	4,258	23	4	8	1,225	4	5,483	11
Delaware	48	19	4,560	27	25	7	2,261	25	6,821	24
Florida	23	24	4,716	30	11	28	1,604	13	6,320	18
Georgia	28	36	4,983	38	30	36	2,505	29	7,488	39
Hawaii	44	25	3,283	1	24	15	2,239	24	5,522	12
Idaho	2	13	3,805	11	36	49	2,708	36	6,513	19
Illinois	39	46	5,187	42	18	21	1,865	17	7,052	31
Indiana	36	50	5,607	49	27	26	2,332	27	7,939	43
Iowa	33	33	4,700	29	17	19	1,841	16	6,541	20
Kansas	41	44	5,254	43	29	32	2,478	28	7,732	42
Kentucky	25	30	5,069	39	34	38	2,625	33	7,694	41
Louisiana	37	34	5,739	50	33	45	2,644	34	8,383	49
Maine	17	7	3,646	4	6	3	1,246	5	4,892	2
Maryland	28	35	3,925	14	15	10	1,660	15	5,585	13
Massachusetts	24	41	3,699	6	9	1	1,377	9	5,076	6
Michigan	35	31	4,745	32	12	11	1,552	11	6,297	17
Minnesota	16	3	3,695	5	7	9	1,305	7	5,000	5
Mississippi	22	32	5,283	44	45	50	3,016	46	8,299	47
Missouri	34	21	4,824	33	23	29	2,182	23	7,006	30
Montana	7	6	4,013	15	32	20	2,533	31	6,546	21
Nebraska	40	20	4,491	24	28	43	2,510	30	7,001	29
Nevada	30	9	3,753	9	44	35	2,917	43	6,670	22
New Hampshire	15	38	3,749	8	21	17	2,054	20	5,803	15
New Jersey	47	40	4,640	28	3	6	1,150	3	5,790	14
New Mexico	10	14	4,200	20	37	42	2,798	38	6,998	28
New York	42	39	4,073	17	8	12	1,346	8	5,419	8
North Carolina	20	28	4,899	37	16	33	1,873	18	6,772	23
North Dakota	38	10	4,071	16	39	25	2,762	37	6,833	25
Ohio	50	48	5,401	46	19	24	2,010	19	7,411	37
Oklahoma	46	18	4,731	31	42	40	2,913	42	7,644	40
Oregon	14	5	3,487	3	2	13	1,096	2	4,583	1
Pennsylvania	32	42	4,847	34	20	22	2,058	21	6,905	26
Rhode Island	21	45	3,721	7	10	2	1,384	10	5,105	7
South Carolina	18	26	4,870	35	31	30	2,537	32	7,407	36
South Dakota	3	2	3,811	12	49	23	3,154	48	6,965	27
Tennessee	31	23	5,308	45	41	31	2,843	40	8,151	45
Texas	43	47	5,538	48	35	37	2,659	35	8,197	46
Utah	5	11	4,234	22	40	48	2,888	41	7,122	33
Vermont	13	12	3,343	2	14	4	1,578	12	4,921	3
Virginia	6	37	4,874	36	22	39	2,181	22	7,055	32
Washington	8	8	3,867	13	13	14	1,606	14	5,473	9
West Virginia	4	29	5,166	41	47	18	2,951	45	8,117	44
Wisconsin	8	15	4,217	21	5	5	1,261	6	5,478	10
Wyoming	11	4	4,521	25	43	41	2,924	44	7,445	38

THE GREEN INDEX: A NATIONAL OVERVIEW

People per square mile, 1970: 57.2
People per square mile, 1990: 70.1
Motor vehicles per square mile: 53.2
Vehicle miles driven per square mile: 571,400
Average miles per gallon of gas: 15.6
Spending on mass transit per $1 spent on highways: 14.7 cents
Percent of population breathing excessive carbon monoxide: 32.4
Toxic chemicals released into the air, pounds per square mile: 678
Pounds of toxic chemicals pumped to surface water or public sewers: 883.3 million
River and stream miles not meeting designated use: 30.4 percent
Investment needed for adequate sewage systems, per capita: $332
Percent of households relying on septic tanks: 26
Percent of population with water systems violating Safe Drinking Water Act: 14.5
Percent of groundwater likely contaminated with pesticides: 14.9
Pesticide use, pounds per capita of active ingredients: 3.9
Fertilizer use, tons per capita: 18.5
Annual loss of soil from cropland erosion, pounds per acre: 14,200
Percent of nation owned by U.S. government: 30
Percent of nation in forests: 32
Number of paper, cardboard, and pulp mills: 954
Daily discharge of toxic chemicals by paper industry: 1 million pounds
Oil and related spills in state waters, gallons in 1984-86: 44.8 million
Number of pipelines failing to meet safety standards: 13,490
Number of oil and gas injection wells: 155,967
Acid rain-making emissions from electric utilities, pounds per capita: 192
Percent growth in per-capita energy consumption, 1960-1975: 37
Percent growth in per-capita energy consumption, 1975-1987: -5
Percent of low-income homes weatherized: 18
Per-capita cost of decommissioning nuclear power plants: $89
Number of safety citations at nuclear power plants, 1989-1990: 1,976
Municipal solid waste generated per capita: 2,170 pounds
Hazardous waste generated per capita: 2,276 pounds
Number of accidents during transport of hazardous materials: 12,288
Damage cost from hazardous material transport accidents: $43.2 billion
Hazardous sites on military bases: 14,401
Toxic chemicals released to environment, pounds per square mile: 1,739
Chemicals released that cause birth defects, pounds per capita: 5.4
Cancer-causing chemicals released, pounds per capita: 2
Cancer deaths, per 100,000 people: 171
Workplace deaths, per 100,000 workers: 7.9
Percent of population without any health insurance: 15.7
Personal income derived from chemical industry, per capita: $180
State spending for environmental programs and natural resources, per capita: $30
Visitors to state parks, per 100 people: 294
Number of fishing licenses, per 100 people: 13
Annual landings of commercial fish: 8.5 billion pounds
Number of boats, per 100 people: 4
Number of vehicles per 100 people: 75
Gallons of gasoline consumed for every man, woman, and child: 502

CHAPTER 1

Environmental Scales: The Best & Worst

There's much to be said for picking up the trash. And for planting a tree, recycling our newspapers, and avoiding styrofoam. From the first Earth Day in 1970 to the media hoopla surrounding its 20th anniversary, we've heard a great deal about what we can do, each one of us, to make the planet a safer, healthier habitat. After all, we're either part of the problem or part of the solution.

But there's also something to be said for scale. Your trash and mine pale in comparison to the surge of garbage spewed from corporate polluters like the Union Carbide refinery in Texas City, Texas. In a single day, the plant pours 300,000 pounds of chemicals into the air, making it number 121 on the Environmental Protection Agency's list of the nation's biggest toxic polluters.

"I call this Toxic City," says Rita Carlson, a Texas City native who lives 12 blocks from Carbide. "We have eight plants like this one here, and 29 lined up along Galveston Bay to Houston. We're told that what they make — the plastics, pesticides, oil products — is essential to the nation, and that we shouldn't worry," she continues. "But I say this is a national sacrifice zone. If people don't wake up to what's happening along the Texas and Louisiana coast with all these chemicals, we're going to lose the nation. The air we all breathe comes from the ocean, and that's where this waste is going."

Union Carbide has an environmental conscience, too. As you approach the gate of its Texas City plant, a large sign boasts, "Adopt A Highway, Litter Control, Next Two Miles, Carbide Volunteers." Give Carlson a few minutes and she will put the "Litter Control" sign into proper perspective. A pool of groundwater tainted by 35 chemicals has left the plant and is headed for parts unknown, she points out. At another site, Texas officials estimate that Carbide has contaminated water supplies with more than 700,000 barrels of poisons.

Carlson rattles off a few more horror stories, then pauses. She points to one of the company's slick bulletins proclaiming its "good neighbor" policy, as if picking up highway litter was the best measure of its commitment to protecting the planet's environment. "We've got to stop this nonsense and start getting to the nitty gritty," she says. "There could be a 90-percent reduction of what these companies discharge, using methods already available if they would make the commitment."

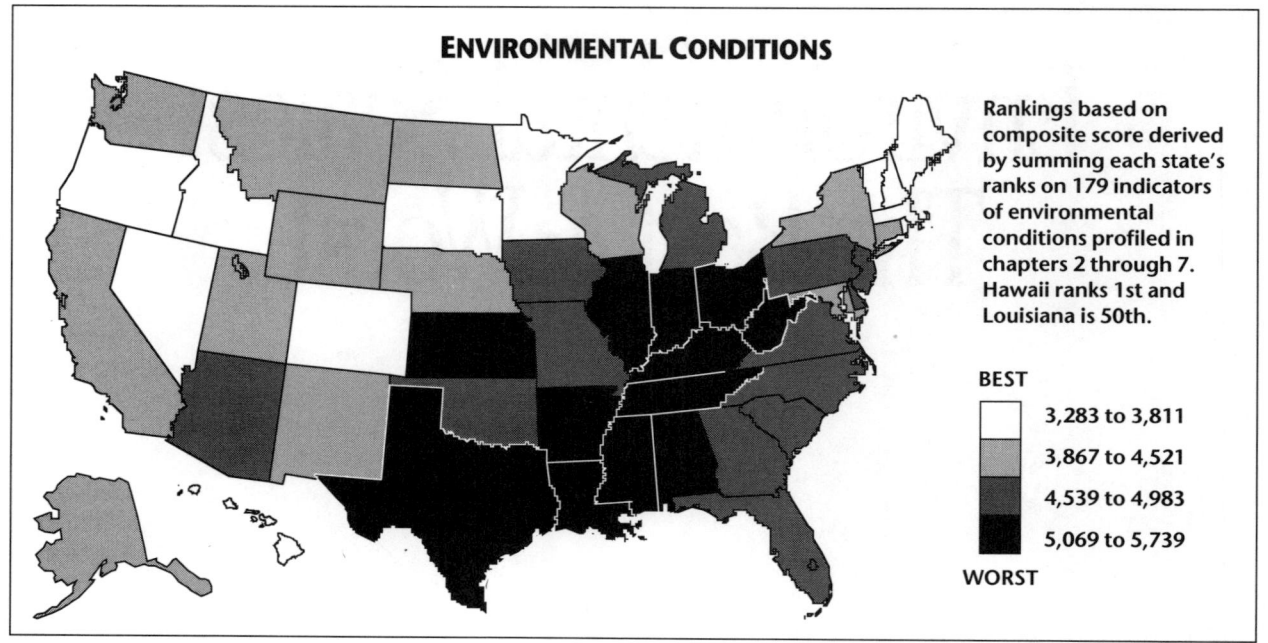

ENVIRONMENTAL CONDITIONS

Rankings based on composite score derived by summing each state's ranks on 179 indicators of environmental conditions profiled in chapters 2 through 7. Hawaii ranks 1st and Louisiana is 50th.

BEST
- 3,283 to 3,811
- 3,867 to 4,521
- 4,539 to 4,983
- 5,069 to 5,739

WORST

STRANGE BLOOD

For Carlson, environmental action is more than a choice of personal lifestyles. She's fighting on a larger scale. Her family's health is intimately tied to the fate of a multinational business; the personal and corporate, the global and local, it all operates together. Measuring the quality of Carlson's environment likewise requires a different approach than the traditional focus on trash, smog, and endangered species of fish.

What about measuring the concentration of toxic emissions and hazardous waste produced by firms like Union Carbide? Or counting their political contributions and the voting records of lawmakers who get their money? What about evaluating the health of Rita Carlson's children, who doctors say have abnormal lymph glands and a "strange" blood disorder? Or let's look at the health of the workers in the petrochemical industry, who are being killed and maimed at an alarming rate. And what about the fate of the poor, black, brown, or red communities that too often hug the edge of America's toxic factories and waste dumps? Shouldn't public policy count their destiny as important as the dwindling number of snail darters or spotted owls?

Fortunately, ordinary citizens like Carlson have made the connections between disappearing birds and the health of their children. Because of their efforts — often belittled as a "not in my backyard" psychosis — new energy is flowing into the environmental movement. It now has the capacity to link the concerns of farmers and mothers, birdwatchers and firefighters, factory workers and the jobless, lovers of our coasts and dwellers in our toxic slums.

To reinforce these links, the Green Index examines the relative rank of the 50 states using a comprehensive approach to environmental health. It recognizes, as do the Greens in Europe, that vital connections exist between economic justice, public health, and environmental integrity. A society that sacrifices one of these risks losing them all. Public and private policymakers who undervalue one ultimately jeopardize the others.

Nowhere are the interrelations more plainly visible than in the South. The reason has less to do with the fact that the region is poor than with the legacy of policymakers who promote the proposition that everything in the South is cheap — available for the taking, no questions asked. This century-old economic development strategy has produced a devastated environment, inequitable tax structure, and undervalued, unhealthy people — as well as a brand of homegrown resistance that offers enormous potential for change.

REGIONAL OVERVIEW

The South is not the only region with serious environmental problems. The 1991-92 Green Index shows that many of the states in the Northeast and Great Lakes regions rank even worse on indicators

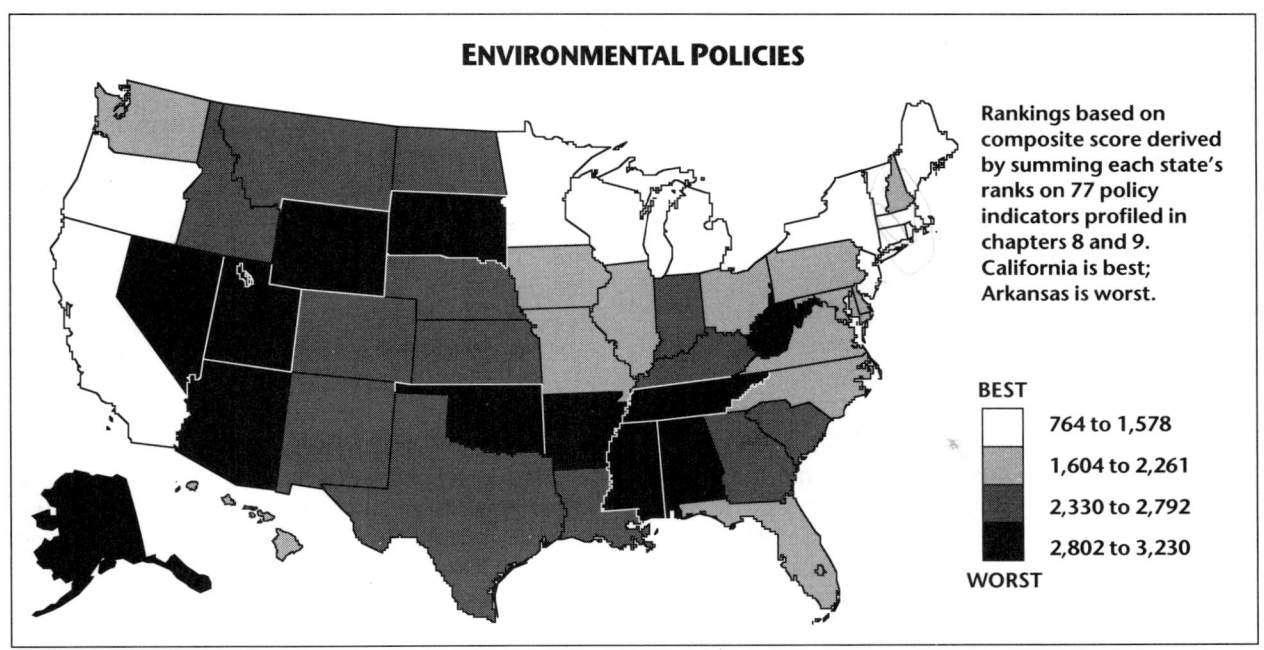

of air quality, water pollution, and toxic waste. But many of these same states have abandoned development strategies that sell themselves short. Relying on a relatively educated population and a higher standard of public accountability, they have taken aggressive actions to address their problems. As a result, they score much better on the indicators that evaluate innovative policies and energetic political leadership. Their records also demonstrate a greater commitment to energy efficiency and mass transit than most states. And they perform well on our Community and Workplace Health Index, which includes several indicators of state laws promoting health care for workers, the poor, children, and ordinary citizens.

By comparison, states in the Rocky Mountain region score very poorly in nearly all areas related to government initiative and planning, holding fast to the frontier belief that the less regulation, the better. Fortunately for them, they don't have the pollution levels of other regions, although their renewed reliance on mining and other resource-based industries promises escalating trouble. Several states already face serious air pollution and hazardous waste problems. Their workplace injury and death rates are well above the U.S. average, but they can point to fewer cancer deaths and other diseases as evidence of a healthier lifestyle. For now, the region's people still enjoy, and depend on, their natural habitat far more than most Americans.

The Farmbelt also relies heavily on its natural beauty and bounty. But decades of chemical assault on the land has left the region with some of the most contaminated groundwater, a dwindling farm population in the grip of agribusiness firms, and worsening public health conditions. Lawmakers in some of the states — most notably Iowa — have begun recognizing that even rural areas can have major environmental headaches. In fact, beyond groundwater pollution and pesticides, most of the region's states perform poorly on such indicators as impaired rivers, open landfills, safe drinking water, and energy efficiency.

The Far West has its problems, too — the nation's worst smog, serious water quality problems, military hazardous waste sites, substantial toxic emissions, ruined wetlands, and devastated forests. Perhaps because of these problems, this is also the region where environmentalism first took hold, and each state continues to experiment with new remedies. Largely because of the durable political support for innovation and conservation, the three states — Oregon, California, and Washington — rank 1st, 5th, and 9th on the 1991-92 Green Index.

Of all the regions, only the South maintains a backward resistance to positive policies in the face of extraordinary levels of poisons. On our final Green Index, Southern states occupy the seven worst positions. The region has 9 of the 17 states infected with the highest per-capita amounts of toxic chemical pollution, 9 of the 12 producing the most hazardous waste, and 108 of the 179 facilities that pose the greatest risk of cancer to their neighbors.

The South also has 10 of the 12 states with the highest rates of premature deaths, yet 8 of the 12 with the lowest rates of health insurance protection. Eleven of the South's 13 states experience above-average incident rates of job-related deaths, yet 11 also provide fewer statutory protections for worker rights and safety.

The numbers should make anyone question the wisdom of the region's traditional approach to economic development. Yet *Site Selection* magazine still brims with ads from government-funded recruiters enticing manufacturers to take advantage of Florida's "overabundance of land and virtually non-unionized labor force," Mississippi's "old-fashioned work ethic and refreshing spirit of cooperation," Georgia's "one-stop environmental permitting convenience," and Kentucky's "low land costs and tax incentives."

BROWN IS BEAUTIFUL

In a political climate that so shamelessly peddles its environment to major manufacturers, industry has no incentive to search for cleaner alternatives. Take the case of the paper-pulp mills, which not only dot the Southern landscape but are among the most dangerous polluters from Washington to Wisconsin, Michigan to Maine. These huge firms produce dioxin — one of the deadliest chemicals in the world — as they turn wood pulp into bleached white paper.

With its vast resources, the papermaking industry could easily adopt techniques already used in parts of Europe to reduce dioxin. Better yet, it could simply drop the bleaching and start marketing brown milk cartons, envelopes, paper plates, and toilet paper under the slogan, "Brown is Beautiful." Instead, International Paper, Weyerhaeuser, Georgia Pacific, and others are crisscrossing the nation, pressuring state regulators to relax what meager dioxin standards they have.

Faced with such gigantic adversaries, backyard environmental pioneers have much to fight — and much to offer the rest of the nation. The challenge remains one of scale. Like Rita Carlson, they must push beyond small-minded solutions for misnamed problems. They are making the connections between pollution and disease, between poisons and poverty, between racism and the politics of siting dangerous factories and toxic dumps. They keep working in their communities, but must knit their local protest groups into a collective enterprise capable of reshaping the environmental debate and tipping the scales in their favor.

In a society dominated by large-scale enterprises, it's not enough to simply clean up the mess — "waste management" and "litter control" won't solve the problem. Positive action requires stopping the mess before it happens, a radical change in production and marketing, thinking and doing. The Green Index can help pinpoint the areas needing serious attention in your state, and the states already doing a better job. Certainly we must pick up after ourselves, but let's also promote bold programs and insist that public officials apply tough standards to protect the public interest. By putting a high value on our health and environment, we will be giving our children a future they too can treasure.

Where Each State Excels — and Fails

A Sampling of the Best and Worst Indicators

State	BEST INDICATORS (RANKING AMONG 50 STATES)	WORST INDICATORS (RANKING AMONG 50 STATES)
Alabama	Water systems in significant noncompliance (4th) Impaired rivers and streams (5th)	Laws for worker safety (50th) Infant mortality (49th) Shellfishing waters limited (47th) Citations of nuclear power plants (48th)
Alaska	Percent of wetlands lost (1st) Commercial fish landings (1st)	Cancer death rate (49th) Energy consumption per capita (50th) Workplace deaths (50th) Safe Drinking Water Act violations (50th)
Arizona	Toxics injected underground per capita (1st) Solar collection systems (3d)	Population with SDWA violations (49th) Cropland irrigated (50th) Total toxics released to land (48th) Pipelines in noncompliance (48th)
Arkansas	Energy consumption per capita (3d) Fishing licenses (6th)	Miles per gallon of gas consumed (50th) State environmental policy initiatives (50th) Toxics released to surface water per capita (47th) Local funds for parks and recreation (50th)
California	State environmental policy initiatives (1st) Renewable energy (1st)	Municipal solid waste generated (49th) Shellfishing waters limited (49th) Population with air violating CO standards (48th) Sustainable farming practices (49th)
Colorado	Municipal solid waste generated (2d) Cancer deaths (3d)	Cropland erosion (47th) Air violating carbon monoxide standards (45th) Military hazardous sites (42nd) Fresh water withdrawals (46th)
Connecticut	Workplace deaths (1st) Fertilizer use per capita (2d)	Toxics released to air per square mile (50th) Air violating carbon monoxide standards (50th) Electricity from nuclear power (50th) Loss of fish landings (49th)
Delaware	Municipal waste recycled or composted (3d) Public health spending (6th)	Workers in most toxic industries (50th) Herbicide use per cropland acre (49th) Cancer death rate (48th) Non-Superfund hazardous waste sites (49th)
Florida	Households without adequate plumbing (2d) Solar collection systems (2d)	Total toxics released to land (50th) Low-income homes weatherized (50th) Herbicide use per cropland acre (50th) Pesticide-contaminated groundwater (49th)
Georgia	Acres in conservation reserves (2d) Impaired rivers and streams (3d)	Hazardous waste remaining in state (50th) State spending to manage waste (50th) Nerve-damaging toxins released (46th) Disability benefits for injured workers (50th)
Hawaii	Miles per gallon of gas consumed (1st)	Military hazardous sites (48th)

State	BEST INDICATORS (RANKING AMONG 50 STATES)	WORST INDICATORS (RANKING AMONG 50 STATES)
Hawaii (*cont.*)	Metro life quality (1st)	Emissions without end-of-stack controls (48th) Curbside recycling (48th) Use of conservation tillage (50th)
Idaho	Renewables as percent of all energy (3d) Low-income homes weatherized (4th)	Doctors delivering patient care (50th) Fresh water withdrawals (50th) Workers in high-injury industries (48th) LCV Congressional voting score (47th)
Illinois	Maximum disability benefits (4th) Growth of carbon emissions (5th)	Citations of nuclear plants (50th) Share of U.S. radioactive waste (50th) Impaired lakes and reservoirs (49th) Toxics released to surface water (48th)
Indiana	Impaired lakes and reservoirs (2d) Population with SDWA violations (4th)	Toxics released to land per square mile (50th) Release of toxins causing birth defects (50th) Sulfur dioxide emissions (49th) Acid rain (47th)
Iowa	Population without insurance (3d) Premature deaths (5th)	Pesticide-contaminated groundwater (50th) Pesticide use (50th) Impaired rivers and streams (50th) Release of toxins causing birth defects (43d)
Kansas	Municipal solid waste generated (3d) Households without adequate plumbing (3d)	Toxics sent off site per capita (50th) Nitrates in well water (49th) Total toxics injected underground (48th) Oil and gas injection wells (48th)
Kentucky	Cropland irrigated (3d) State funds for parks (5th)	Gasoline use per capita (50th) Sulfur dioxide emissions (47th) Households without adequate plumbing (49th) Workers in high-risk jobs (42d)
Louisiana	Commercial fish landings (2d) Inland recreational waters (5th)	Total toxics released per capita (50th) Facilities posing high cancer risk (50th) Cancer death rate (46th) Oil spills in state waters (50th)
Maine	State spending to manage waste (1st) Population with SDWA violations (1st)	Acid rain (50th) Facilities posing high cancer risk (49th) Paper, cardboard, and pulp mills (50th) Hazardous waste workers (50th)
Maryland	Mass transit spending (3d) Public health spending (3d)	Cancer death rate (50th) Municipal solid waste generated (50th) Population with air violating CO standards (49th) Toxics to surface water per square mile (47th)
Massachusetts	Doctors in patient care (1st) LCV Congressional voting score (1st)	Air violating ozone standards (50th) Investment required for adequate sewers (50th) Toxics sent to public sewers per square mile (49th) Use of municipal waste incineration (48th)
Michigan	Military hazardous sites (1st) Population with health insurance (2d)	Total toxics sent off site (49th) Workers in most toxic industries (49th) Public sewers in noncompliance (49th) Pesticide-contaminated surface and groundwater (47th)
Minnesota	Water systems violating SDWA (1st) Curbside recycling (2d)	Pesticide use per capita (46th) Impaired rivers and streams (45th) Pesticide-contaminated groundwater (44th) Release of toxins causing birth defects (44th)
Mississippi	Unsafe nitrates in wells (3d)	Laws for worker safety (50th)

FINAL RANKINGS   13

State	BEST INDICATORS (RANKING AMONG 50 STATES)	WORST INDICATORS (RANKING AMONG 50 STATES)
Mississippi (cont.)	Impaired rivers and streams (6th)	LCV Congressional voting score (50th) Premature deaths (49th) Toxics released to air per capita (45th)
Missouri	Non-hazardous waste impoundments (1st) Impaired lakes and reservoirs (4th)	Toxics sent to public sewers per capita (50th) Total toxics released to land (47th) Infant mortality (47th) Percent of wetlands lost (47th)
Montana	Ozone-depleting emissions per capita (1st) Low-income homes weatherized (1st)	Toxics released to land per capita (50th) Workplace death rate (48th) Superfund NPL sites per capita (46th) Water violating Safe Drinking Water Act (45th)
Nebraska	Hazardous waste management facilities (3d) Households without adequate plumbing (3d)	Fertilizer use per capita (50th) Pesticide-contaminated groundwater (48th) Gasoline use per capita (49th) State funds for public health (49th)
Nevada	Ozone-depleting emissions per capita (1st) Herbicide use per cropland acre (1st)	Cropland erosion (49th) Growth of carbon emissions (49th) Gasoline use per capita (48th) Cancer death rate (44th)
New Hampshire	Pesticide-contaminated groundwater (1st) Workers in high-risk jobs (2d)	Release of cancer-causing toxins (44th) Investment for sewer needs (49th) Ozone-depleting emissions facilities (49th) Investment required for adequate sewers (49th)
New Jersey	Curbside recycling (1st) LCV Congressional voting score (5th)	Total toxics released per square mile (50th) Toxics sent to sewers per square mile (50th) Population with SDWA violations (50th) Density of vehicle traffic (50th)
New Mexico	Cancer-causing toxics released per capita (1st) Cancer deaths (4th)	Population without insurance (50th) Military hazardous sites (49th) Toxics released to land per capita (47th) Mass transit versus highway spending (50th)
New York	Per-capita energy consumption (1st) Mass transit versus highway spending (1st)	Municipal incineration (50th) Percent of state budget for environment (50th) Investment required for adequate sewers (48th) Deaths from nine diseases (48th)
North Carolina	Acres in conservation reserve (5th) Unsafe nitrate levels in wells (8th)	Low-level radioactive waste sent off site (50th) Hazardous materials transportation accidents (48th) Low-income homes weatherized (47th) Release of cancer-causing toxins (42d)
North Dakota	Premature deaths (1st) Total toxics released per capita (1st)	Growth in energy consumption (49th) Carbon dioxide and nitrogen oxide emissions (49th) Pesticide use per capita (49th) Loss of farms (50th)
Ohio	Maximum unemployment benefits (4th) Cropland irrigated (5th)	Total toxics sent off site (50th) Total toxics released to air (49th) State funds for public health (48th) Sulfur dioxide emissions (46th)
Oklahoma	Reliance on nuclear power (1st) State funds for parks (2d)	Oil and gas injection wells (49th) Spending on water quality (49th) Unemployed with unemployment insurance (49th) Nitrates in well water (47th)
Oregon	Municipal waste recycled (2d) Acid rain (2d)	State funds for public health (50th) Oil spills in state waters (48th)

State	BEST INDICATORS (RANKING AMONG 50 STATES)	WORST INDICATORS (RANKING AMONG 50 STATES)
Oregon (cont.)		Forest acres lost (48th)
		Toxics sent to public sewers per capita (42d)
Pennsylvania	Gasoline use per capita (3d)	Hazardous waste generators (48th)
	Curbside recycling (4th)	Tons of carbon dioxide emissions (48th)
		Total toxics sent off site (47th)
		Local funds for parks, recreation (46th)
Rhode Island	Open municipal landfills (1st)	Nitrates in well water (50th)
	Pesticide use per capita (1st)	Public sewers in significant noncompliance (50th)
		Toxics released to air per capita (49th)
		Density of vehicle traffic (49th)
South Carolina	Miles per gallon of gas consumed (2d)	Share of nation's radioactive waste (49th)
	Impaired lakes and reservoirs (3d)	Premature deaths (50th)
		Infant mortality (50th)
		Nerve-damaging toxics released (47th)
South Dakota	Hazardous waste generated (1st)	State environmental policy initiatives (49th)
	Total toxics released to land (1st)	Fertilizer and pesticide use (47th)
		Energy vs. population growth (48th)
		Impaired rivers and streams (43d)
Tennessee	Price of electricity (1st)	Hazardous waste generated (50th)
	Cropland irrigated (7th)	Nerve-damaging toxics released (49th)
		Birth defect toxics released (49th)
		Toxics released to water or underground (50th)
Texas	Emissions without end-of-stack controls (5th)	Total toxics released (50th)
	Number of private tree farms (5th)	Total toxics injected underground (50th)
		Electricity from renewable sources (49th)
		State spending for environmental protection (50th)
Utah	Cancer death rate (1st)	Toxics released to air per capita (50th)
	Acid rain (1st)	LCV Congressional voting score (49th)
		Total toxics released per capita (48th)
		Workplace death rate (45th)
Vermont	Infant mortality (1st)	Cleanup of Superfund sites (50th)
	LCV Congressional voting score (2d)	Nuclear plant decommissioning costs (50th)
		Urban mass transit use (50th)
		Hazardous waste transport accidents (40th)
Virginia	Use of conservation tillage (4th)	Nerve-damaging toxics released (50th)
	Highway deaths (7th)	State funds for parks (50th)
		Total toxics released to surface water (49th)
		Impaired rivers and streams (46th)
Washington	Municipal waste recycled (1st)	Workers in high-injury industries (49th)
	Renewables as percent of all energy (1st)	Total toxics released to surface water (47th)
		Water violating Safe Drinking Water Act (48th)
		Investment required for adequate sewers (47th)
West Virginia	State funds for parks (1st)	Cancer-causing toxics released (50th)
	Farms gained (2d)	Impaired lakes and reservoirs (50th)
		Sulfur dioxide emissions (50th)
		Acid rain (48th)
Wisconsin	Hazardous materials transport accidents (2d)	Paper, cardboard, and pulp mills (49th)
	Miles per gallon of gas consumed (3d)	Impaired lakes and reservoirs (48th)
		Toxics sent to public sewers per capita (45th)
		Open municipal landfills (47th)
Wyoming	Spending on water quality (1st)	Workers in high risk jobs (50th)
	Investment for sewer needs (1st)	Oil and gas injection wells (50th)
	Population density (2d)	Carbon dioxide emissions per capita (50th)
		Workplace death rate (49th)

CHAPTER 2

Air Sickness

INDICATORS

Population with air violating ground-level ozone standard
Population with air violating carbon monoxide standard
State spending to control air pollution
Density of motor vehicles
Density of motor vehicle traffic
Volume of toxic chemicals released into the air
Toxics per capita released into the air
Toxics per square mile released into the air
End-of-pipe emission controls
High-risk cancer-causing factories
Volume of ozone-depleting chemicals released into the air
Factories emitting ozone-depleting chemicals
Acid rain levels
Emissions of sulfur dioxide
Emissions of nitrogen oxides
Emissions of carbon dioxide

Half the people in the United States are routinely exposed to polluted air, and more than half the pollutants come from their own cars and trucks. Much of the rest comes from power plants that burn fossil fuels and from industrial facilities that poured 2.5 billion pounds of toxic chemicals into the air in 1988 alone.

The Clean Air Act of 1970 and its 1977 amendments targeted emissions from motor vehicles, especially lead and carbon monoxide. But since more Americans now drive more miles — four times as many as in 1950 — the air is still badly polluted. "All the progress we are making through [fuel efficient] technology is being eaten up by growth," says James Bond, executive officer of the California Air Resources Board. The introduction of lead-free gasoline has cut that pollutant's presence by 95 percent since 1970, but the rate of decline for carbon monoxide and smog is far less dramatic, especially in the last decade.

Worse, 20 years after the first Earth Day and Clean Air Act, the federal government has yet to set standards for thousands of the chemicals that industries pump into the air we breathe. Passage of the 1990 Clean Air Act means a full-scale crackdown is still years away, with standards geared to the limits of current technology rather than to eliminating threats to human health. Of the 300-odd toxic chemicals EPA now requires companies to monitor, 123 are carcinogens, yet the agency has set emission standards for only seven.* According to EPA, "The implementation of [federal standard-setting authority] has become increasingly difficult with frequent litigation and consequently few regulatory actions have been completed in recent years."

While corporate lawyers hold up action, Americans continue to pay an extremely high cost for air pollution. The American Lung Association estimates that 120,000 people die unnecessarily or prematurely each year from motor vehicle exhaust, more than twice the number killed in traffic accidents. Many more have their lives cut short by carcinogens and other factory emissions. Lakes, forests, and buildings are destroyed by acid rain created by fossil-fuel combustion. Even indoor air can be contaminated with radon, asbestos, and formaldehyde.

* The seven are arsenic, asbestos, benzene, beryllium, mercury, radon-222, and vinyl chloride.

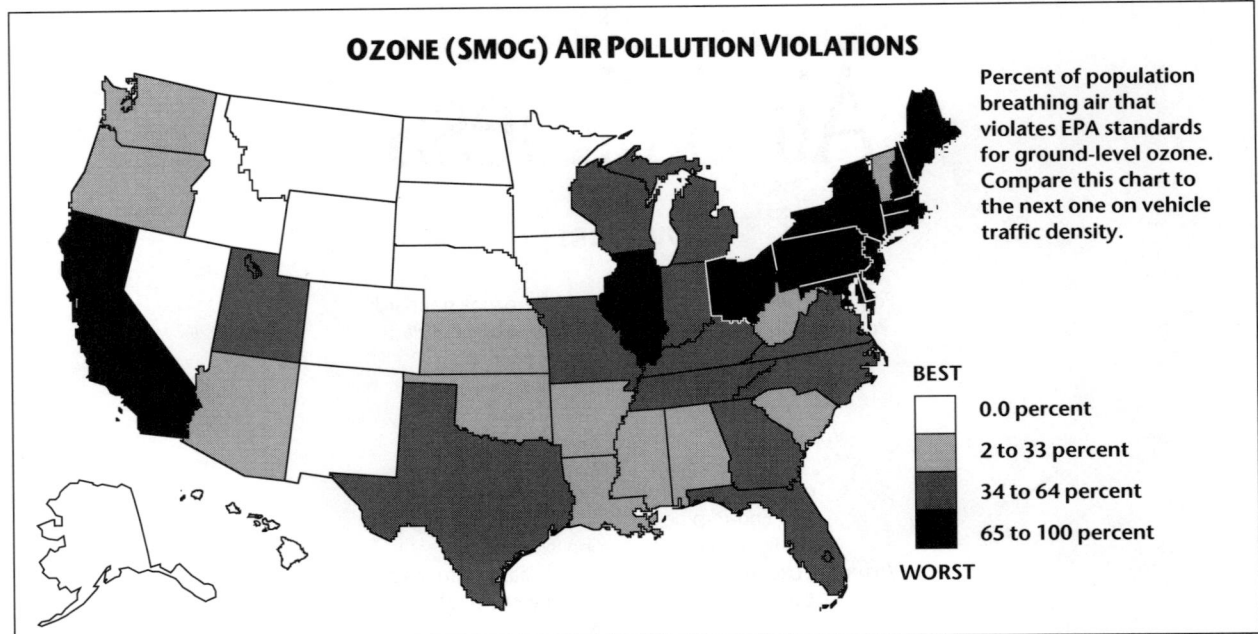

THE SMOKING GUN

There is little doubt that the automobile is the most lethal weapon in America. In addition to highway deaths, the car is the biggest single source of greenhouse gases that threaten to raise temperatures worldwide; even "clean fuels" produce 20 pounds of carbon dioxide for each gallon of gas consumed. Leaky air conditioners in vehicles account for one-fourth of the chlorofluorocarbons (CFCs) that are eating a hole in the upper atmosphere's protective ozone layer. And billions of pounds of nitrogen oxides from our tailpipes return to Earth as acid rain. The car is also the driving force behind the petrochemical industry, the biggest source of environmental poisons not on wheels. More than four million gallons of used motor oil are dumped into sewers each week, billions of tires crowd landfills, and exhaust fumes — brimming with carcinogens like butadiene — are choking us to death.

During one hot August week in 1988, New Jersey residents with respiratory problems were warned to stay indoors; hospitals reported a sharp increase in admissions of patients with lung problems. That year, New Jersey had one of the worst records for ground-level ozone (commonly called smog) in the country, violating federal standards for 45 days. Although the violations declined in 1989 — in large part because cool, moist air prevailed instead of the dry, hot air conducive to ozone formation — the problem of controlling groundlevel ozone remains.

The prime component of smog, ozone is created when fuel vapors (hydrocarbons) from vehicles and power plants break down in the presence of heat and sunlight. In the upper atmosphere, ozone protects the earth from ultraviolet rays, but at ground-level it causes respiratory ailments in humans and ruins forests and crops. Carbon monoxide, another byproduct of fossil-fuel combustion, can increase the chance of heart failure. Vehicle exhaust, particularly from diesel combustion, also increases the risk of cancer.

New Jersey, highly industrialized and heavily traveled, ranks at the bottom of the ground-level ozone (or smog) indicator, with 100 percent of the population breathing air violating ozone standards in 1989. The state also ranked poorly in carbon monoxide emissions, with over 80 percent of the people breathing air that violated federal air pollution standards at least one day during the year.

Connecticut, Massachusetts, and Rhode Island score just as poorly as New Jersey on air pollution indicators, partly due to the prevailing winds, but also because of their own cars and industry. In fact, on a per-capita basis, the five states with the most factories spewing out ozone-depleting chemicals are all in New England. To their credit, several New England states have taken steps to curb air pollution by toughening tailpipe emissions standards, requiring pollution control devices on gas pumps, promoting use of cleaner fuels, and requiring industries to reduce their toxic chemical emissions.

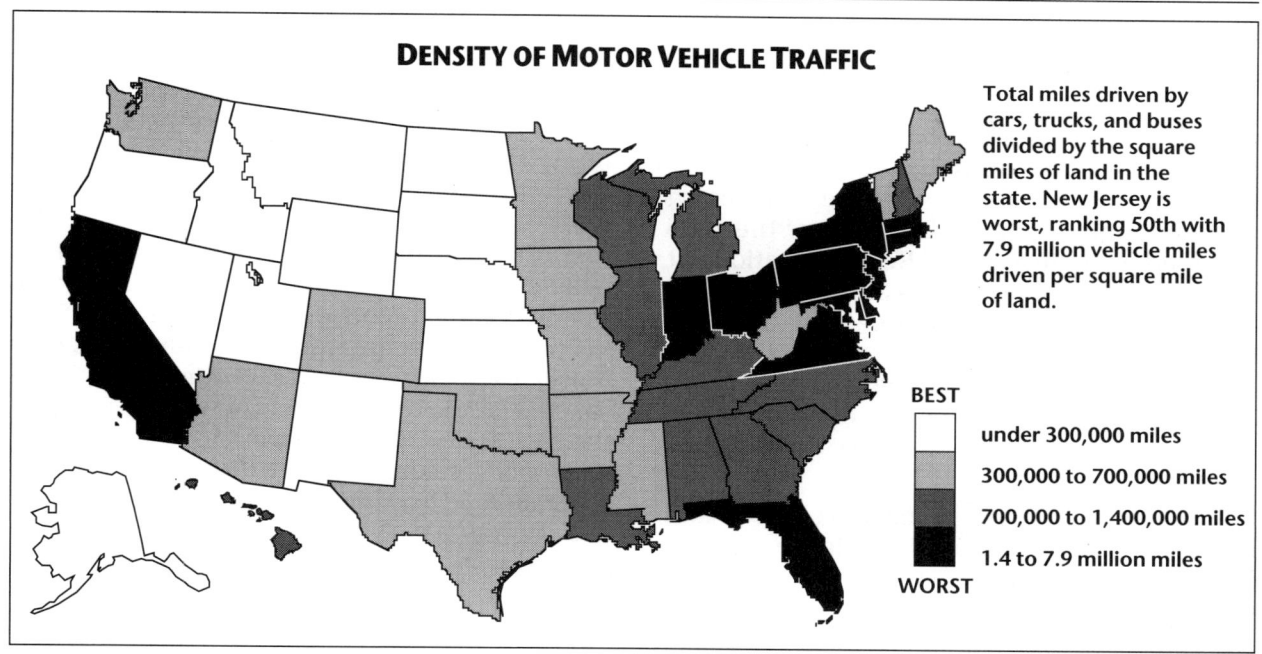

In states along the densely populated, heavily traveled Washington–New York corridor, large numbers of people are also at risk. Maryland, Delaware, and Pennsylvania rank with New Jersey and New York among the worst 10 states for smog and/or carbon monoxide pollution. In the West, Colorado, Washington, Nevada, and Arizona join California in the bottom 10 for carbon monoxide violations because of the foul air in their largest metropolitan areas. Other Sunbelt states (Florida, Georgia, Tennessee, Virginia, North Carolina, and Texas) still promote their pristine environment to new arrivals, but 40 percent or more of their citizens live in cities with repeated smog violations.

California, where smog was first diagnosed, faces enormous problems. Years of severe auto-generated pollution in the heavily populated valleys has affected not only people, but also fruit crops in the San Joaquin Valley and trees in the San Bernardino National Forest. A 1989 study concluded that the Los Angeles basin could save $9.4 billion in health and lost-time costs if it met federal clean air standards. The state already spends more than twice as much as any other state per person on air pollution programs. Innovative programs proliferate. San Francisco, for example, formulated a plan in the winter of 1990 to reduce vehicle emissions by increasing tolls, calling for employer-funded carpools, and improving the rail system.

Although California is ahead of most states in air pollution legislation, the results have been disappointing. In 1989 Los Angeles called for the production of cars powered by methanol and other clean fuels that would reduce tailpipe emissions, but a year later the cars and new fuels were still in the experimental stages. Between 1987 and 1988, smog levels increased for most counties, and in 1990 about 90 percent of the state's residents breathed air violating ozone and carbon monoxide standards.

INDUSTRIAL TOXICS

Control of industrial emissions in California and elsewhere have been even more disappointing. Residents of Port Neches, in southeast Texas, live in the shadow of the U.S. factory that poses the highest risk of cancer from a single chemical. According to EPA, Texaco's Neches West Chemical Plant puts its neighbors at a 1-in-10 risk of getting cancer from exposure to the one million pounds of butadiene it emits each year. Townspeople have seen friends and relatives in their thirties and forties die of the disease. For years, their complaints fell on deaf ears. Finally, in March 1990, Texaco and another plant, Ameripol-Synpol, were sent notices of violations for emissions of cancer-causing styrene and butadiene.

The notices came from state, not federal, officials. Despite passage of the 1970 Clean Air Act, EPA has dragged its feet in issuing regulations for toxic air emissions. In fact, many industries under pressure to reduce their discharge of water pollutants have simply switched technologies to burn them, sending even more poisons up the stack.

While EPA does not regulate, much less stop, most chemical air emissions, it does add up the pounds released by major industrial producers. The numbers come from the companies' own measurements, as required by the Emergency Planning and Community Right-to-Know Act of the 1986 Superfund Amendments and Reauthorization Act (Title III of SARA). Even with its limitations, the act gives citizens access to information about 300 chemicals released into their communities. For two years, EPA has published the totals in its Toxic Release Inventory (TRI), a survey of chemical discharges to water, air, the land, public sewers, or injection wells.

TRI data for industrial emissions in 1987 and 1988, the only two years available, is the basis for several of our air pollution indicators. Some highlights:

- *Total Air Toxics.* The six states with the most toxic releases into the air are Texas, Ohio, Tennessee, Louisiana, Utah, and Virginia. The top polluters are the chemical producers, steel and other metal manufacturers, paper makers, and the auto industry. Nearly 110 million of Utah's total release of 119 million pounds came from the AMAX Magnesium complex in Tooele the nation's single largest industrial source of air toxics. The second largest, Kodak's Tennessee Eastman in Kingsport, puts out 40 million pounds, mainly the eye, nose, throat, liver, and kidney irritants acetone and methyl isobutyl ketone. Studies confirm that children in the area have more respiratory problems than normal.

- *Toxics Per Capita.* When ranked by pounds-per-person, 10 of the 15 states with the largest releases are in the South. One third of West Virginia's air emissions are in Kanawha County (Charleston), and half of that amount, or 5 million pounds, comes from Union Carbide's plant in Institute — a sister plant to the one that killed at least 3,500 people in Bhopal, India. In February 1990, a small amount of methyl isocyanate, the Bhopal killer, leaked out and injured seven workers in Institute. Among the toxics the county's dozen chemical facilities dumped into the environment in 1988 were 1.6 million pounds of known carcinogens.

- *Toxics Per Mile.* Based on pounds of toxics released per square miles, the New England states of Connecticut, Rhode Island, and Massachusetts sink to the bottom, joined by New Jersey and Ohio. In Cranston, Rhode Island, the Davol Company sterilizes medical equipment with ethylene oxide, but its rooftop release of the same chemical poses a 1-in-1,000 cancer risk to the plant's neighbors. When Rhode Island set a standard for ethylene oxide in 1987, Davol avoided regulation for two years by contending it used the chemical as a pesticide to kill micro-organisms.

- *End-of-Pipeline Controls.* Four out of five of the facilities reporting TRI data in 1988 had no end-of-pipe air pollution control devices (bag house, flare, electrostatic precipitator, carbon absorber, condenser, etc.) The worst rates were in Alaska, South Dakota, Hawaii, Wyoming, and New Hampshire. Big chemical states, like Delaware, West Virginia, Louisiana, and Texas, at least took this step to cut gross pollutants and had among the best rates.

- *High-Risk Factories.* Using the 1987 data, EPA prepared a study of the facilities posing the greatest cancer risk from exposure to a single chemical. Texas had the most plants — 33 out of 179 on the list. Next came Louisiana with 17, California and Georgia with 11 each, and Washington with 10. The order changes when the states are ranked on the basis of their plants per person. Maine, with four plants (all paper-pulp) posing up to a 1-in-1,001 cancer risk from their chloroform emissions, ranks 49th just ahead of Louisiana (rank 50). "Our operations are safe," protested International Paper's Keith Morgan in Jay, Maine. "I don't think these figures have any meaning whatsoever," echoed Eric Baxter of Boise Cascade in nearby Rumford.

- *Cancer Sources.* The Natural Resources Defense Council (NRDC) took the data a step further by identifying the 1,500 largest sources of 11 cancer-causing chemicals spewed into the air. The biggest for each substance include Monsanto's Soda Springs, Idaho factory, which released 100,250 pounds of cadmium into the air; Eastman Kodak's sprawling complex in Rochester, New York, which released 8.9 million pounds of methylene chloride; and ALCOA of Riverdale, Iowa, with 2.3 million pounds of perchloroethylene.

- *Ozone Hole.* NRDC also published a "Who's Who of American Ozone Depleters" identifying the leading sources of chlorofluorocarbon-113, methyl chloroform, and carbon tetrachloride. These chemicals are used in cleaning agents, aerosols, coolants, and other products. In addition to speeding global warming, they release chlorine which destroys the stratospheric ozone layer protecting life below from deadly ultraviolet radiation. Other CFCs and halogens not included in EPA's Toxic Release Inventory expand the hole, but these three are responsible for 37 percent of the ozone-depleting chlorine traced to human activity. Unless the ozone hole is plugged, increased ultraviolet radiation exposure will cause between 163 million and 308 million additional cases of skin cancer among Americans alive today or born by the year 2075. While California has twice the number of ozone-depleting factories (led by IBM) and twice the emissions of any other state, on a per-capita basis five New England states rank much worse, with Connecticut ranking 50th on both indicators.

WHAT WE DON'T KNOW

Right-to-Know legislation has given residents of polluted areas an important tool in their fight for cleaner air. In Lima, Ohio, for example, citizens received federal funding to monitor a British Petroleum plant that released 8.6 million pounds of toxins in 1987, including probable carcinogens. Groups in at least 10 other states have filed petitions to have sources of dangerous toxins declared "hot spots" by EPA, a designation that requires polluters to revise their discharge permits.

On the other hand, the Toxic Release Inventory only monitors manufacturing processes; it exempts utilities, government-owned plants, mining operations, and, ironically, waste management firms. If all these sources were included in our indicators of toxic poisons, the relative ranking of the states may not significantly change. Generally, the states that host factories producing loads of toxins are also the ones with other hazardous facilities. Louisiana is a perfect example.

Louisiana ranks 50th in high-risk factories, 47th in total pounds of air toxins, and 48th on a per-capita basis. Its "Chemical Corridor" from Baton Rouge to New Orleans produces a fifth of the nation's chemicals, and is also nicknamed "Cancer Alley" for its above-normal rates of cancer. The state also attracts poisons from all over the country to its waste facilities, but none of their emissions are counted in the TRI.

For example, Marine Shale Processors in Morgan City burns 100,000 tons of hazardous waste each year, making it the largest commercial incinerator in the United States. The company first burned oil field waste, then began incinerating other wastes illegally, without updating its permits. The substances burned included mercury, DDT, cyanide, and dioxin-tainted wastes. At the same time, the number of respiratory problems, birth defects, miscarriages, and cancers in the area shot up. Neuroblastoma, a fatal nervous system cancer, struck five children in 18 months among 64,000 residents near Marine Shale; the normal rate is one in 100,000.

But since Marine Shale is a waste handler rather than a manufacturer, none of its emissions are tracked by the TRI. EPA's inventory also omits thousands of chemicals that pose serious harm to human health and the environment. For example, the chemical industry is a major producer of sulfur dioxide, which is not on the TRI list even though it is the chief precursor for acid rain. In September 1990, a huge cloud of sulfur dioxide left the Tennessee Chemical Company and floated over nearby McCaysville, Georgia. State air pollution monitors shut down from overload, but the damage was obvious and immediate. At least six people went to hospitals with respiratory distress, and within two days hundreds of acres of trees and other vegetation were scorched brown — the result of instant acid rain.

ACID RAIN

When the sulfur dioxide and nitrogen oxides produced from burning fossil fuels react with water in the atmosphere, the product is acid rain. And when the rain, snow, or mist falls to Earth, the chemical reaction continues. Hundreds of lakes and streams from New Jersey's Pine Barrens through New York's Adirondacks to the forests of Maine have become acidic solutions. Fish and trees die, marble or limestone buildings corrode, and people with breathing or heart problems face increased health risks. Acid rain can also ruin drinking water supplies and food because it causes traces of aluminum, mercury, and other metals naturally present in the soil to bond together.

Acid raid is not simply a problem for the Northeast. More than half the streams and lakes in northern Florida have acidic pH levels; so do a fifth of the lakes in the Appalachians as far south as Tennessee and North Carolina; and so do a sixth of the lakes and streams in northern Wisconsin and the Michigan peninsula.

John Mahoney, director of the federally funded National Acid Precipitation Assessment Program, is actually encouraged by these figures. "Acid rain does cause damage," he told a conference of scientists in early 1990, "but the amount of damage is less than we once thought, and it's much less than some of the characterizations we sometimes hear."

Studies by Mahoney's organization show both

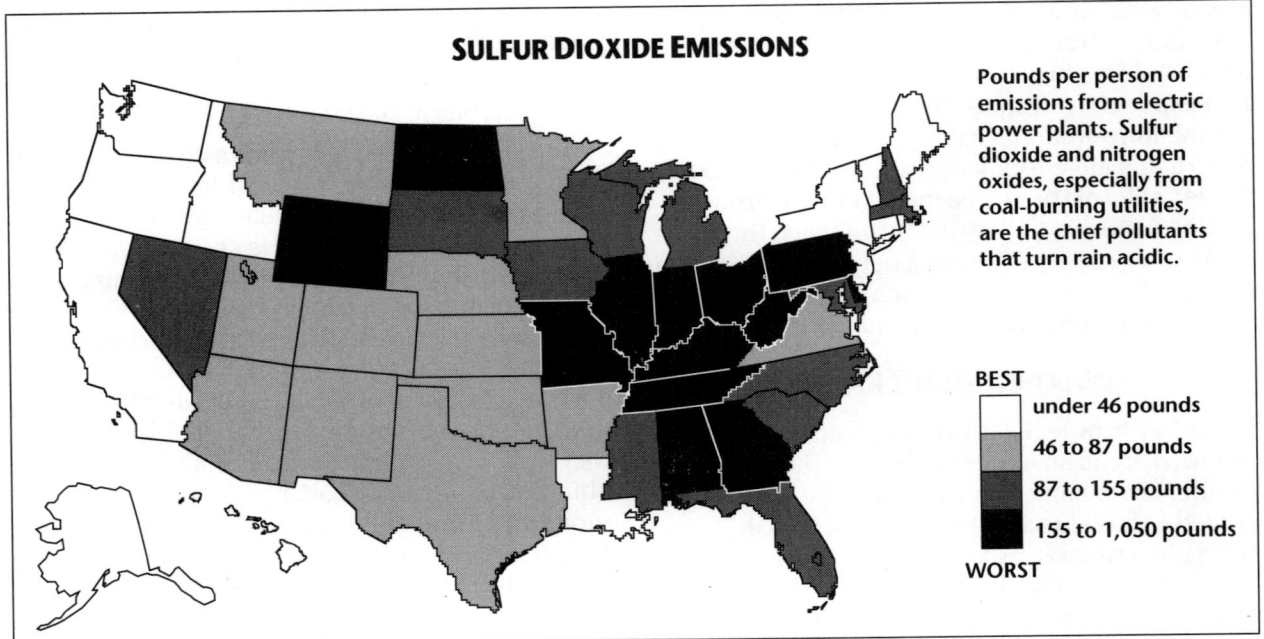

SULFUR DIOXIDE EMISSIONS

Pounds per person of emissions from electric power plants. Sulfur dioxide and nitrogen oxides, especially from coal-burning utilities, are the chief pollutants that turn rain acidic.

BEST
- under 46 pounds
- 46 to 87 pounds
- 87 to 155 pounds
- 155 to 1,050 pounds

WORST

good and bad news. First the good news: Between 1973 and 1988, sulfur dioxide emissions dropped by nearly a fourth, even though electric utilities burned a steadily growing volume of coal. The decrease followed the phase-out of some of the dirtiest power plants, installation of scrubbers to capture sulfur leaving the stacks, and a shift to burning more low-sulfur coal. Emissions of nitrogen oxides have also dropped, from 4.6 billion pounds in 1978 to 4 billion pounds in 1988.

Now for the bad news: The improvements peaked in 1982 and emissions have remained fairly constant since then. While acidic conditions may have stabilized in parts of the Northeast, the oxides coming from power plants in the Rocky Mountain energy states are producing more acidic rain in that region. Wyoming, Montana, New Mexico, Nevada, and North Dakota now rank among the 10 states with the largest per-capita releases of nitrogen oxides or sulfur dioxide, and in several Western states the rain tests below pH 5.6, the threshold for normal rain.

Understandably, the coal-rich Ohio Valley has the greatest concentration of coal-fired power plants in the country, and their emissions have been linked to increased rates of childhood bronchitis in places like Steubenville, Ohio and Monroeville, Pennsylvania. Ohio ranks 46th in sulfur dioxide and 40th in acidic rain. West Virginia ranks 50th on the sulfur dioxide indicator, generating twice the pounds of the next worst state, Indiana; the two states reap the consequences with acid rain pH levels below 4.5, ranking them 48th and 47th respectively. Kentucky is 47th in emissions, but thanks to the prevailing winds, most of its acid drifts hundreds of miles eastward.

To stop acid rain and revive the damaged ecosystem will require substantial new initiatives, beginning with the control of coal-burning power plants (source of 70 percent of the sulfur dioxide, 35 percent of nitrogen oxides) and vehicle emissions (the second greatest source). But while the U.S. Capitol is itself a victim of acid rain corrosion, legislators inside from the big coal and auto states have opposed acid rain regulation proposed by New Englanders.

Maine and Connecticut, the two states with the worst acid rain measurements, catch the fallout from the Midwest. Like Vermont and Rhode Island, the two states don't rely much on coal-fired turbines but they suffer from the emissions of Midwestern plants. Frustrated by federal inaction, Massachusetts and New Hampshire started their own programs to promote acid rain reduction. The University of Massachusetts coordinated a project to document acid levels in that state's waters. The results led to increased public awareness and the passage of state legislation requiring a cap on sulfur dioxide emissions from utilities and industry.

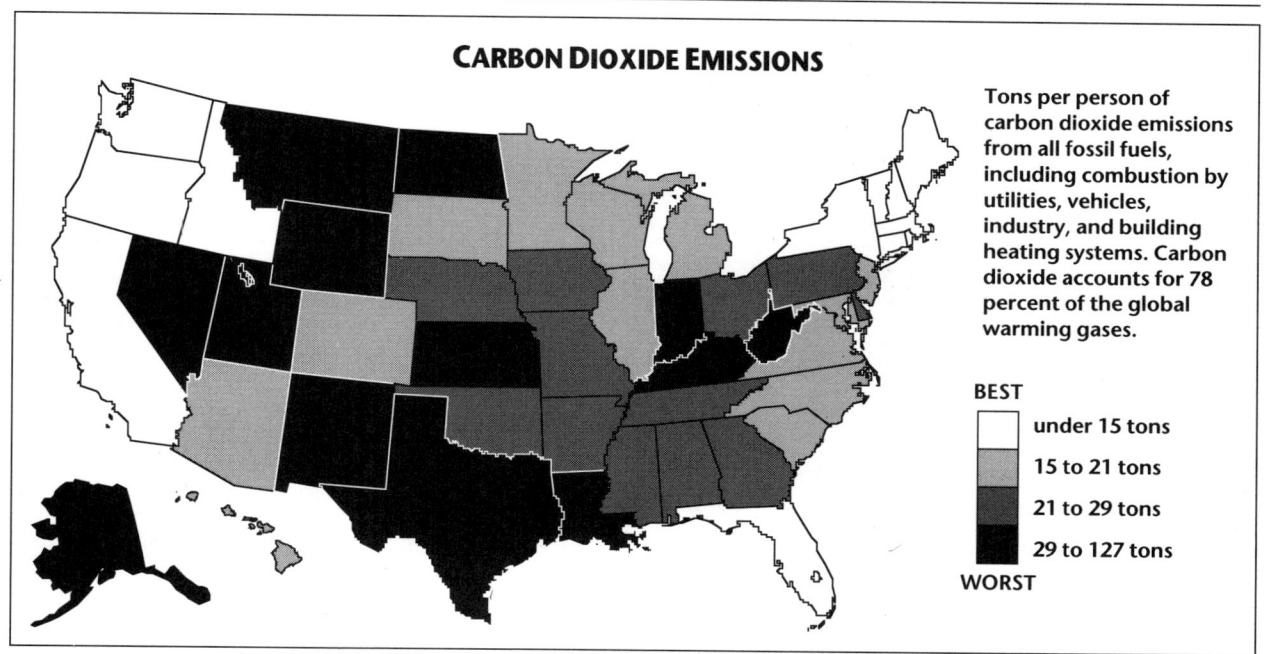

BURNING CARBON

The New England states are also well ahead of the federal government in controlling carbon dioxide, the leading cause of global warming. The byproduct of burning hydrocarbons, carbon dioxide acts as a shield in the upper atmosphere, allowing sunlight through and trapping the heat below, much like a greenhouse canopy. Other gases, including CFCs, methane, and nitrous oxide, perform the same role. Instead of keeping the Earth from becoming another frigid planet, the escalating volume of these greenhouse gases now threatens to melt the polar ice caps, hasten the rise in sea levels, distort rainfall patterns, kill plants, and eventually destroy human life.

With 5 percent of the world's people, the United States produces 25 percent of carbon dioxide released from burning fossil fuels. About a third of that share comes from our vehicles, and another third comes from electric utilities. Understandably, the nations of the world expect the United States to tackle the problem aggressively. But the Bush administration has chosen to stall, claiming more data is needed, despite the consensus among the international scientific community that immediate action is required.

Bush's adopted home state, Texas, generates more carbon dioxide than all of Canada or the United Kingdom. California tops France's output, and Pennsylvania, Ohio, Indiana, and Illinois together match the reunited Germany. On a per-capita basis, the worst states are all big energy producers, from Wyoming (rank 50) and North Dakota to Kentucky and New Mexico (rank 41). The ranking shifts significantly in only a few cases when the focus is on carbon dioxide emissions solely from electric utilities. For example, Louisiana, Alaska, and Oklahoma score better on this indicator because their utilities rely less on coal, the most carbon-intensive fuel, while the rankings for such coal-dependent states as Georgia, Colorado, Missouri, and Nevada get worse. Overall, most states show considerable consistency in their per-capita rankings for emissions of carbon, nitrogen, and sulfur dioxides.

In the vacuum left by the federal government, several states in the Northeast have taken concrete steps to curb these emissions. In 1989, the governors of New Jersey and Vermont issued executive orders to reduce greenhouses gases and energy consumption from nonrenewable sources. New York is studying ways to cut its 200 million tons of annual carbon dioxide emissions, now the eighth worst volume in the nation. And in 1990, Connecticut became the first state with a global warming law that penalizes new buildings that fail energy conservation standards and requires new state-owned vehicles to average 45 miles per gallon by the year 2000. Meanwhile the state's native son, George Bush, embraces Big Oil and rejects the connection between gas guzzling cars, wasteful energy consumption, and deadly air pollution.

AIR POLLUTION

State	POP. WITH AIR VIOLATING STANDARDS FOR OZONE %	Rank	CARBON MONO. %	Rank	STATE SPENDING ON AIR POLLUTION 1,000 $	Per Capita $	Rank	# Motor Vehicles in 1,000s	Per Sq. Mile	Rank	# Vehicle Miles Driven in Millions	1,000s Per Sq.Mile	Rank
Alabama	32.7	25	3.7	24	1,855	0.45	28	4,075	80.3	29	39,684	781.7	28
Alaska	0.0	1	28.3	34	751	1.43	2	367	0.6	1	3,841	6.7	1
Arizona	28.7	23	57.7	41	3,162	0.91	10	2,785	24.5	11	34,247	301.7	14
Arkansas	2.1	14	2.1	19	647	0.27	43	1,436	27.6	14	19,219	369.0	16
California	91.8	45	84.9	48	92,380	3.26	1	21,657	138.6	39	241,575	1,545.6	40
Colorado	0.0	1	75.6	45	4,562	1.38	3	2,932	28.3	15	27,665	267.0	13
Connecticut	100.0	50	97.0	50	3,451	1.07	7	2,695	553.2	48	26,062	5,349.3	47
Delaware	100.0	50	33.0	36	552	0.84	12	529	273.8	45	6,404	3,314.7	45
Florida	51.5	32	0.0	1	6,241	0.51	25	11,378	210.1	42	105,319	1,944.8	42
Georgia	41.9	27	0.0	1	2,415	0.38	36	5,385	92.8	31	62,262	1,072.4	32
Hawaii	0.0	1	0.0	1	1,215	1.11	6	719	111.9	35	7,419	1,154.7	34
Idaho	0.0	1	0.0	1	302	0.30	40	953	11.6	8	8,127	98.6	7
Illinois	69.0	39	2.6	21	5,362	0.46	27	8,091	145.4	40	78,483	1,410.4	37
Indiana	46.2	29	0.0	1	2,468	0.44	30	4,265	118.7	36	51,124	1,422.8	38
Iowa	0.0	1	0.0	1	401	0.14	50	2,613	46.7	20	21,907	391.4	17
Kansas	23.4	21	0.0	1	416	0.17	48	2,237	27.4	13	21,161	258.8	11
Kentucky	48.5	30	0.0	1	3,222	0.86	11	2,841	71.6	27	31,614	796.9	29
Louisiana	17.8	19	0.0	1	1,865	0.42	32	2,984	67.0	26	34,682	779.0	26
Maine	65.6	38	0.0	1	1,221	1.01	8	988	31.9	16	11,401	367.8	15
Maryland	88.7	44	87.9	49	2,532	0.55	23	3,539	359.8	46	37,498	3,811.9	46
Massachusetts	100.0	50	75.1	44	1,340	0.23	45	3,791	484.5	47	43,334	5,538.6	48
Michigan	59.2	35	0.0	1	4,685	0.51	24	7,293	128.1	38	77,899	1,367.8	36
Minnesota	0.0	1	55.8	39	1,720	0.40	35	3,267	41.1	19	36,447	458.2	18
Mississippi	2.4	16	2.4	20	518	0.20	47	1,811	38.3	18	22,043	466.7	19
Missouri	55.0	34	18.2	30	1,814	0.35	38	3,873	56.2	24	45,570	661.0	25
Montana	0.0	1	14.3	26	451	0.56	22	733	5.0	2	8,138	56.0	2
Nebraska	0.0	1	0.0	1	235	0.15	49	1,340	17.5	10	13,407	174.9	10
Nevada	0.0	1	82.5	46	1,237	1.17	4	835	7.6	4	8,989	81.8	4
New Hampshire	72.0	40	57.5	40	302	0.28	42	976	108.5	34	9,507	1,057.2	31
New Jersey	100.0	50	84.4	47	5,062	0.66	16	5,894	789.2	50	58,671	7,856.3	50
New Mexico	0.0	1	32.1	35	900	0.60	20	1,247	10.3	7	15,283	126.0	8
New York	77.6	42	65.9	42	7,372	0.41	33	10,184	215.0	43	103,692	2,188.7	44
North Carolina	44.1	28	24.5	32	3,242	0.50	26	5,201	106.5	33	57,943	1,186.3	35
North Dakota	0.0	1	0.0	1	195	0.29	41	662	9.6	6	5,765	83.2	5
Ohio	76.5	41	26.5	33	7,566	0.70	15	8,820	215.1	44	81,990	1,999.6	43
Oklahoma	11.1	18	14.9	27	740	0.23	44	2,581	37.6	17	32,388	471.8	20
Oregon	21.4	20	52.6	38	2,509	0.91	9	2,367	24.6	12	25,204	262.0	12
Pennsylvania	84.6	43	15.7	28	7,537	0.63	18	7,922	176.5	41	81,238	1,809.8	41
Rhode Island	100.0	49	0.0	1	300	0.30	39	687	651.2	49	5,853	5,547.9	49
South Carolina	32.3	24	0.0	1	1,544	0.44	29	2,474	81.9	30	31,759	1,051.5	30
South Dakota	0.0	1	0.0	1	157	0.22	46	707	9.3	5	6,634	87.3	6
Tennessee	53.0	33	17.6	29	2,853	0.58	21	4,382	106.5	32	44,193	1,073.8	33
Texas	49.4	31	3.4	22	13,939	0.83	13	12,565	48.0	21	156,458	597.1	22
Utah	62.5	37	45.7	37	609	0.36	37	1,188	14.5	9	13,263	161.6	9
Vermont	3.3	17	0.0	1	242	0.43	31	473	51.0	22	5,553	598.8	23
Virginia	60.6	36	22.9	31	3,847	0.64	17	4,729	119.1	37	57,453	1,447.0	39
Washington	2.4	15	66.0	43	3,379	0.73	14	4,075	61.3	25	41,813	628.7	24
West Virginia	28.5	22	3.6	23	754	0.40	34	1,321	54.8	23	13,884	575.6	21
Wisconsin	40.7	26	4.3	25	2,944	0.61	19	4,043	74.3	28	42,458	780.1	27
Wyoming	0.0	1	0.0	1	560	1.17	5	491	5.1	3	5,658	58.3	3
U.S. Total	**56.6**		**32.4**		**213,573**	**0.87**		**188,401**	**53.2**		**2,022,181**	**571.4**	

AIR POLLUTION

State	Total Pounds	Rank	Pounds Per Capita	Rank	Pounds Per Sq. Mile	Rank	TOXIC EMISSIONS WITHOUT END-OF-STACK CONTROLS %	Rank	HIGH-RISK CANCER FACILITIES #	Rank	Output in 100 Tons	Per Capita Rank	# Big Facilities	Per Capita Rank
Alabama	97,124,680	42	23.5	46	1,879.0	38	78.9	23	5	41	17.2	28	37	20
Alaska	21,996,215	19	42.9	49	37.2	7	97.1	50	1	45	0.1	3	1	4
Arizona	14,780,075	14	4.3	12	129.6	10	75.3	13	3	34	24.7	46	56	39
Arkansas	46,801,874	30	19.3	42	879.9	25	84.4	37	1	22	14.1	41	38	37
California	81,594,258	37	2.9	6	514.1	19	79.4	25	11	21	121.8	29	353	31
Colorado	11,129,196	12	3.4	8	106.9	9	79.7	26	2	27	14.7	30	38	27
Connecticut	23,950,336	20	7.4	23	4,772.9	50	78.3	20	2	28	60.7	50	128	50
Delaware	4,873,438	10	7.4	22	2,384.3	41	64.0	2	1	43	1.5	16	4	12
Florida	53,107,471	33	4.3	13	905.3	26	81.9	31	7	26	22.2	9	65	10
Georgia	82,538,859	38	12.9	36	1,401.1	31	82.5	34	11	44	11.8	11	55	19
Hawaii	874,145	2	0.8	2	135.1	11	92.3	48	0	1	0.2	4	1	3
Idaho	3,982,578	9	4.0	11	47.7	8	78.4	21	1	35	1.3	7	2	5
Illinois	104,592,707	43	9.1	24	1,856.3	37	80.4	27	2	16	55.9	33	166	33
Indiana	110,075,627	44	19.7	43	3,042.0	44	81.9	31	2	19	53.2	49	92	40
Iowa	43,135,115	27	15.2	39	766.5	23	88.3	43	0	1	15.7	37	52	43
Kansas	24,631,652	21	9.9	28	299.4	15	82.6	36	2	32	5.7	15	21	18
Kentucky	43,739,655	28	11.8	34	1,082.4	27	73.0	9	3	31	15.6	27	39	24
Louisiana	133,070,512	47	30.1	48	2,786.8	42	70.7	6	17	50	7.8	8	26	11
Maine	16,553,882	15	13.7	38	497.6	18	77.1	17	4	49	7.6	44	19	38
Maryland	17,383,926	16	3.7	10	1,661.9	34	74.3	10	2	24	8.5	10	29	13
Massachusetts	26,494,040	22	4.5	14	3,198.2	46	81.6	30	0	1	33.3	39	147	46
Michigan	95,641,067	41	10.3	30	1,634.1	33	76.1	15	4	23	32.4	24	108	28
Minnesota	49,388,024	32	11.5	33	585.2	20	82.3	33	1	17	26.1	43	66	36
Mississippi	53,968,917	34	20.5	45	1,131.7	28	85.1	39	2	30	8.0	21	28	25
Missouri	48,634,108	31	9.5	26	697.8	22	81.2	28	0	1	23.2	31	64	30
Montana	2,384,167	6	3.0	7	16.2	3	68.0	4	1	40	0.0	1	0	1
Nebraska	17,499,077	17	10.9	32	226.2	14	88.9	45	0	1	9.0	38	24	35
Nevada	724,620	1	0.7	1	6.6	1	71.7	7	0	1	0.0	1	0	1
New Hampshire	11,654,930	13	10.6	31	1,256.1	29	91.6	47	0	1	9.7	48	39	49
New Jersey	36,522,739	26	4.7	15	4,690.2	48	74.4	11	5	29	16.4	12	85	26
New Mexico	1,883,293	5	1.2	3	15.5	2	76.3	16	0	1	4.4	19	8	9
New York	92,806,469	40	5.2	16	1,889.8	39	78.8	22	2	15	54.2	20	137	14
North Carolina	88,335,109	39	13.5	37	1,677.2	35	82.5	34	7	39	29.5	32	124	44
North Dakota	1,236,260	3	1.9	4	17.5	4	84.6	38	0	1	0.3	6	3	8
Ohio	136,453,929	49	12.6	35	3,301.6	47	77.6	19	4	20	52.9	34	188	42
Oklahoma	31,100,849	24	9.5	27	444.6	17	88.5	44	0	1	7.1	13	33	22
Oregon	19,887,098	18	7.3	21	204.9	13	78.9	23	3	38	6.0	14	28	23
Pennsylvania	80,987,641	36	6.7	20	1,787.5	36	75.3	13	7	25	59.4	35	141	29
Rhode Island	5,774,024	11	5.8	17	4,764.0	49	87.5	40	1	36	4.9	36	31	48
South Carolina	62,613,127	35	17.9	41	2,012.4	40	71.8	8	3	33	25.3	47	57	41
South Dakota	2,478,960	7	3.5	9	32.1	6	94.5	49	0	1	2.5	23	6	17
Tennessee	133,697,458	48	27.2	47	3,172.4	45	81.2	28	7	42	28.4	40	67	32
Texas	169,936,759	50	10.1	29	636.9	21	70.3	5	33	46	44.5	17	132	15
Utah	119,410,265	45	70.6	50	1,406.5	32	63.9	1	0	1	12.1	45	25	34
Vermont	1,519,293	4	2.7	5	158.0	12	75.0	12	0	1	2.3	26	15	47
Virginia	119,593,757	46	19.9	44	2,933.6	43	87.8	41	2	18	19.3	22	58	21
Washington	27,604,148	23	6.0	18	405.1	16	77.1	17	10	47	12.3	18	38	16
West Virginia	31,885,186	25	16.9	40	1,315.9	30	64.9	3	5	48	7.3	25	8	7
Wisconsin	44,412,636	29	9.1	25	790.9	24	88.0	42	5	37	29.3	42	99	45
Wyoming	2,923,126	8	6.2	19	29.9	5	91.4	46	0	1	0.2	5	1	6
U.S. Total	2,453,387,277		10.0		678.0		78.6		179		1,020.0		2,981	

AIR POLLUTION

State	ACID RAIN		AIR EMISSIONS FROM U.S. ELECTRIC UTILITIES						CARBON DIOXIDE EMISSIONS FROM ALL FUELS				COMPOSITE FOR AIR POLLUTION INDICATORS	
			Sulfur Dioxide Per Capita		Nitrogen Oxides Per Capita		Carbon Dioxide Per Capita		Million		Tons Per			
	pH	Rank	Pounds	Rank	Pounds	Rank	Tons	Rank	Tons	Rank	Capita	Rank	Score	Rank
Alabama	4.4	41	244.8	40	87.3	37	12.4	40	120.2	37	29.3	37	604	47
Alaska	5.5	7	3.8	5	0.0	1	0.9	6	30.8	11	58.6	47	293	7
Arizona	5.1	23	67.1	20	60.2	29	9.0	30	63.1	22	18.1	21	412	16
Arkansas	4.8	28	60.1	17	63.5	31	9.5	33	55.6	18	23.1	30	497	32
California	5.2	21	1.0	4	10.7	7	0.2	4	341.7	49	12.0	6	432	19
Colorado	5.5	8	67.9	21	61.8	30	9.5	32	67.2	24	20.4	24	355	12
Connecticut	4.1	49	38.4	10	14.2	8	4.0	11	40.7	14	12.6	7	542	40
Delaware	4.4	37	266.7	41	100.0	40	13.7	41	18.6	7	28.2	36	536	38
Florida	5.5	11	118.2	32	49.5	20	6.7	21	186.3	41	15.1	11	426	18
Georgia	4.8	30	282.2	42	69.1	34	10.5	36	146.6	40	23.1	29	551	42
Hawaii	5.7	5	45.5	13	14.6	9	6.0	20	18.7	8	17.1	17	220	2
Idaho	5.7	6	0.0	1	0.0	1	0.0	1	11.0	3	10.9	4	169	1
Illinois	5.0	25	155.8	38	56.5	24	5.3	17	208.3	45	18.0	19	545	41
Indiana	4.1	47	538.9	49	159.5	46	17.1	42	213.8	46	38.5	45	679	50
Iowa	5.4	14	139.0	36	64.9	33	9.8	34	66.9	23	23.6	33	475	23
Kansas	5.4	13	86.6	25	57.7	25	8.9	29	73.9	26	29.5	38	415	17
Kentucky	4.9	27	434.1	47	184.6	47	21.5	46	132.3	39	35.4	42	526	35
Louisiana	5.5	10	40.8	11	54.0	23	4.9	14	203.9	44	46.3	46	464	22
Maine	4.0	50	24.9	8	3.3	5	2.3	9	18.3	6	15.2	12	387	14
Maryland	4.3	43	119.9	33	39.4	15	5.9	19	75.0	27	16.2	14	476	24
Massachusetts	4.4	42	89.3	27	29.5	14	4.9	15	83.2	29	14.1	9	568	43
Michigan	4.7	32	91.3	28	59.3	27	8.0	27	191.8	42	20.7	25	509	33
Minnesota	5.2	19	69.7	22	46.4	18	7.3	24	80.1	28	18.6	22	459	21
Mississippi	4.5	35	107.6	31	39.7	16	5.1	16	55.1	17	21.1	26	483	27
Missouri	4.6	33	354.8	44	113.6	43	11.7	39	113.5	33	22.0	27	539	39
Montana	5.3	18	72.0	23	154.0	45	23.9	47	30.6	10	38.1	44	302	8
Nebraska	5.1	22	62.4	18	88.6	38	9.1	31	35.6	13	22.3	28	403	15
Nevada	5.8	4	127.1	35	123.3	44	19.9	45	33.4	12	31.7	39	251	3
New Hampshire	4.8	29	151.2	37	49.8	21	5.6	18	15.1	5	14.0	8	523	34
New Jersey	4.4	38	22.3	7	16.1	11	1.7	7	117.9	36	15.3	13	492	28
New Mexico	5.0	26	86.3	24	110.2	42	19.3	44	52.2	16	34.6	41	319	9
New York	4.2	45	43.1	12	15.9	10	3.3	10	203.9	43	11.4	5	495	30
North Carolina	4.5	36	98.6	29	48.7	19	7.2	23	114.6	35	17.6	18	574	44
North Dakota	5.8	3	491.8	48	362.8	49	45.5	49	48.3	15	72.4	49	331	11
Ohio	4.4	40	421.0	46	93.8	39	11.2	38	275.6	47	25.4	34	666	49
Oklahoma	5.4	15	59.8	16	78.3	35	8.6	28	88.5	30	27.3	35	433	20
Oregon	5.8	2	0.0	1	0.0	1	0.0	1	28.7	9	10.4	3	258	5
Pennsylvania	4.4	39	215.5	39	64.3	32	9.8	35	282.2	48	23.5	32	590	46
Rhode Island	4.6	34	10.1	6	4.0	6	0.8	5	9.8	2	9.8	2	479	26
South Carolina	5.0	24	99.7	30	46.1	17	7.0	22	62.6	21	18.1	20	493	29
South Dakota	5.5	9	87.0	26	53.3	22	4.7	13	11.8	4	16.4	15	260	6
Tennessee	4.7	31	348.1	43	80.5	36	10.8	37	114.6	34	23.4	31	642	48
Texas	5.2	20	66.9	19	59.3	26	7.8	26	609.6	50	36.2	43	476	24
Utah	5.8	1	46.2	14	101.8	41	18.0	43	55.9	19	33.1	40	495	30
Vermont	4.2	44	0.0	1	0.0	1	>.1	3	5.2	1	9.4	1	252	4
Virginia	4.2	46	54.2	15	24.9	13	4.1	12	99.1	32	16.5	16	529	37
Washington	5.4	16	26.7	9	18.1	12	2.1	8	67.6	25	14.6	10	356	13
West Virginia	4.1	48	1,041.6	50	338.0	48	43.9	48	122.4	38	65.0	48	581	45
Wisconsin	5.3	17	124.8	34	59.3	28	7.7	25	91.1	31	18.8	23	527	36
Wyoming	5.5	12	375.8	45	605.4	50	93.9	50	60.7	20	126.4	50	330	10
U.S. Total			135.3		56.4		7.4		5,256.9		21.6			

SOURCES FOR AIR POLLUTION INDICATORS

Air violating ground-level ozone standard
Percent of state's population living in counties with air that failed to meet Clean Air standard for ground-level ozone more than one day a year, on average, during 1987, 1988, and 1989.
Source: "Ozone and Carbon Monoxide Areas Violating the National Ambient Air Quality Standards," September 12, 1990. Published by Office of Air Quality Planning and Standards, U.S. Environmental Protection Agency, Research Triangle Park, North Carolina.

Air violating carbon monoxide standard
Percent of state's population living in counties with air that failed to meet Clean Air standard for carbon monoxide more than one day a year, on average, during 1988 and 1989.
Source: "Ozone and Carbon Monoxide Areas Violating the National Ambient Air Quality Standards," September 12, 1990. Published by Office of Air Quality Planning and Standards, U.S. Environmental Protection Agency, Research Triangle Park, North Carolina.

Spending on air pollution control
State and local funds spent for air quality management, fiscal 1988. Total dollars in thousands, per-capita spending, and ranking for per-capita spending.
Source: Office of Air Quality Planning and Standards, U.S. Environmental Protection Agency, Research Triangle Park, North Carolina, October 1988.

Density of motor vehicle traffic and pollution
Motor vehicle travel, the single greatest source of air pollutants, is measured by number of motor vehicles per square mile and by number of motor vehicle miles driven per square mile. Motor vehicle miles equals the total miles driven by cars, trucks, and buses in 1989. Additional vehicle indicators are included in Energy Use and Auto Abuse chapter.
Source: "MVMA Motor Vehicle Facts & Figures, 1990." Published by Motor Vehicle Manufacturers Association of the United States, 7430 Second Avenue, Detroit, MI 48202; telephone (313) 872-4311.

Toxic chemicals released into the air
Total pounds, pounds per capita, and pounds per square mile reported by manufacturing facilities using 50,000 pounds or more of any of 322 chemicals, including 123 carcinogens. Includes fugitive and point-source releases.
Source: "Toxics in the Community: The 1988 Toxic Release Inventory National Report," September 1990. Published by Office of Toxic Substances, U.S. Environmental Protection Agency, Washington.

Toxic air emissions without end-of-stack controls
Percent of point-source air releases that lack "end-of-pipe" control devices such as flares or electrostatic precipitators, based on data from EPA's Toxic Release Inventory.
Source: "Working Notes on Community Right-to-Know," May 1990. Published by Working Group on Community Right-to-Know, 215 Pennsylvania Avenue, SE, Washington, DC 20003; telephone (202) 546-9707.

Facilities posing a high risk of cancer
Number of facilities, ranked per capita, from which one chemical released into air poses a cancer risk of greater than 1 in 100,000 for someone living 200 meters from the factory's "fenceline" for 70 years. The effect of multiple chemical releases is not considered. Data based on an EPA analysis of 1988 releases conducted at request of Congressman Henry Waxman.
Source: Press packet dated January 12, 1990, released by Honorable Henry A. Waxman, Chairman, Subcommittee of Health and the Environment, U.S. House of Representatives.

Ozone-depleting emissions
Pounds per capita of chlorofluorocarbon-113 (CFC-113), methyl chloroform, and carbon tetrachloride released by industrial facilities. These three chemicals account for 37 percent of the ozone-depleting chlorine created by human activity and now found in the stratosphere. They are the only major ozone-depleting chemicals monitored by EPA's 1987 Toxic Release Inventory, the database for this indicator.
Source: "A Who's Who of American Ozone Depleters," January 1990. Published by Natural Resources Defense Council, 40 West 20th Street, New York, NY 10011; telephone (212) 727-2700.

Ozone-depleting factories
Number of major industrial facilities, ranked per capita, which released one or more of the three ozone-destroying chemicals monitored by EPA's 1987 Toxic Release Inventory.
Source: "A Who's Who of American Ozone Depleters," January 1990. Published by Natural Resources Defense Council.

Acid rain
Acid rain measured on pH scale. The lower the pH reading, the more acidic the rain. Because the pH scale is logarithmic, rain with a pH of 4.6 is 10 times more acidic than normal rain (pH 5.6). Numbers are average of readings taken in February, July, and September 1990 by the Citizens Acid Rain Network.
Source: Press releases dated March 19 and October 11, 1990, from National Audubon Society, 950 Third Avenue, New York, NY 10022; telephone (212) 832-3200.

Sulfur dioxide emissions from electric power plants
Pounds per capita of sulfur dioxide released in 1988 by fossil-fuel steam-electric generating plants.
Source: "Electric Power Annual, 1988." Published by Energy Information Administration, U.S. Department of Energy, December 1989.

Nitrogen oxides from electric power plants
Pounds per capita of nitrogen oxides released in 1988 by fossil-fuel steam-electric generating plants.
Source: "Electric Power Annual, 1988." Published by Energy Information Administration, U.S. Department of Energy, December 1989.

Carbon dioxide emissions from electric power plants
Pounds per capita of carbon dioxide released in 1988 by fossil-fuel steam-electric generating plants. Carbon dioxide is major greenhouse gas, contributing to global warming.
Source: "Electric Power Annual, 1988." Published by Energy Information Administration, U.S. Department of Energy, December 1989.

Carbon dioxide emissions from fossil-fuel combustion
Millions of tons and pounds per capita of carbon dioxide released in 1988 from combustion of all fossil fuels, including combustion by utilities, vehicles, industry, and building heating systems. These emissions account for 78 percent of global warming gases.
Source: "The Statehouse Effect: State Policies to Cool the Greenhouse," July 26, 1990. Published by Natural Resources Defense Council, 40 West 20th Street, New York, NY 10011; telephone (212) 727-2700.

Composite air quality score
Rankings on 15 indicators are totaled to produce a composite score. Lowest score receives lowest (best) composite rank for air quality.

CHAPTER 3

Water Pollution

INDICATORS

Per-capita water consumption
Toxic chemicals released to surface water
Toxic chemicals sent to public sewage systems
Toxic chemicals pumped into the ground
Sewage systems in noncompliance with EPA standards
Investment needed for adequate sewage systems
Miles of river and streams not meeting designated use
Acres of lakes not meeting designated use
Spending on water quality protection
Population dependent on groundwater
Households with their own wells
Households relying on septic tanks
Groundwater potentially contaminated with pesticides
Surface and groundwater potentially contaminated
Water systems violating Safe Drinking Water Act (SWDA)
Community water systems in significant noncompliance
Water used for drinking

Few substances affect our health and well-being as profoundly as water. The essential ingredient of life, it flows in vast underground aquifers and covers three-quarters of the Earth's surface in oceans, lakes, rivers, and streams. But this bountiful supply is now polluted enough to cause 10 million deaths a year worldwide.

About half the drinking water consumed in the United States comes from surface water — rivers, lakes, streams, and reservoirs. Although their pollution has been regulated since the 1950s, one-fourth of these waters now fail to meet their designated uses for drinking and recreation. Poorly treated factory effluent, run-off from farms, acid rain, as well as the chemicals, bacteria, oil, and dirt washed into aging sewers, all pollute our surface waters.

Wetlands act as nature's filter for water and a haven for wildlife, but they are fast disappearing. Fishing has been prohibited in many areas because the fish contain chemicals or metals (see chapter 7). Laws that should stop such destruction are enforced poorly, and the problems could get worse because lawmakers are preparing poorly for future sewage, land management, and water-use needs.

Surface water feeds and is fed in part by underground aquifers, or groundwater. Many urban residents and 97 percent of rural residents (about half of the population) depend on groundwater for drinking. Like surface water, groundwater is susceptible to contamination from agricultural and industrial chemicals. It is also vulnerable to leaking landfills, waste lagoons, and underground tanks. Groundwater moves slowly, often along an unpredictable path, and contaminants may concentrate in plumes for years, making cleanup difficult or impossible. Too often, water from our taps or wells contains some of these dangerous pollutants.

TOXIC TOILET

A third of industry's most toxic point-source water pollution (end-of-pipe effluent) comes from *direct factory discharges*. The remaining two-thirds pass through *public sewage treatment facilities* and then into our waterways. Because these facilities cannot neutralize most toxic pollutants, EPA requires generators to cleanse, or "pretreat," their waste before it reaches the public sewage system. However, an extensive survey by the U.S. General Accounting Office reveals that 41 percent of the pretreating companies exceeded one or more discharge limits during the study year.

Companies get rid of even more toxic chemicals through *underground injection,* which jeopardizes the purity of groundwater. Altogether, industry flushed away 2.2 billion pounds of toxic waste in 1988 through direct discharge into surface water, transfers to sewage systems, or underground injection. The Toxic Release Inventory (TRI) monitors all three mediums for wastewater disposal.

• *Direct Discharges to Water.* The 150-mile section of the Mississippi River between Baton Rouge and New Orleans, the toilet for at least 136 major industrial facilities, receives more toxins than any other stretch of water in the country. In fact, Louisiana has one-half of all chemical waste directly discharged into surface waters by TRI-monitored companies. Many local residents rely on the Mississippi for their drinking water and suffer a higher than normal incidence of cancer and miscarriages. By volume, most of the chemicals (71 percent of Louisiana's total and 36 percent of the national total) come from two plants belonging to one company in Saint James Parish — Freeport McMoran's Agrico Division. The company's wastewater includes phosphoric acid, ammonia, and sulfuric acid.

• *Direct Discharges Per Capita.* On a per-capita basis, Louisiana again ranks last in toxins piped to surface water. Alaska, Virginia, Arkansas, and Washington round out the bottom five. In Alaska (rank 49), Unocal Chemicals in Kenai discharges over 150,000 pounds of ammonia, which can cause lung damage, 8,000 pounds of ethylene glycol, which can cause birth defects and kidney damage, and 250 pounds of the carcinogen formaldehyde. The best five states of this and many other water indicators — Nevada, New Mexico, Arizona, North Dakota, and South Dakota — are relatively dry and less industrialized. Washington state more than doubled its TRI discharges to water between 1987 and 1988, putting it among the worst 10. Arkansas also experienced a substantial jump and joined the bottom 10 for the first time.

• *Direct Discharges Per Mile.* Louisiana is at the bottom, followed by the Eastern Seaboard states of Connecticut, Virginia, Maryland, Rhode Island, and Delaware. The waste from Maryland's two biggest water polluters, W.R. Grace and Bethlehem Steel, continues to forestall restoring the once fertile Chesapeake Bay. Even though thousands of fishers have lost jobs, Bethlehem Steel has used its workforce of 8,000 as leverage to negotiate reduced fines and repeated delays in meeting emission limits for various chemicals.

• *Toxic Transfers to Sewers.* Missouri sends the most chemicals to public sewage systems — 77.6 million pounds or 14 percent of the U.S. total, with 74 percent coming from St. Louis County alone. A single St. Louis company, Columbian Chemicals, accounts for 9 percent of the national total. According to the TRI, the company increased its ammonium sulfate transfer by more than 3.5 million pounds between 1987 and 1988. Monsanto Company, also in St. Louis, increased its discharge of the same chemical by 5.2 million pounds in the same period. Across the river in Cahokie, Illinois, another Monsanto plant decreased its transfer by 11.7 million pounds — but Illinois still ranks 49th on this indicator. Sewage systems in New Jersey, California, Texas, and Virginia also receive large volumes of industrial toxins, each accounting for 7 percent or more of the U.S. total.

• *Per-Capita Transfers to Sewers.* Missouri again ranks 50th in pounds per person of toxics sent to sewers. New Jersey, Virginia, Illinois, and Tennessee follow, each handling twice the national per-capita average. The Dakotas and several Rocky Mountain states (Montana, Nevada, Wyoming, New Mexico) rank best; like Alaska (rank 2), they lack the infrastructure or inclination to manage industrial waste through public sewage systems. By contrast, almost a third of New Jersey's total TRI emissions to air, water, or land pass through its public sewage treatment plants. The sheer volume of this waste helps explain why the state ranks 45th in sewage systems out of compliance with EPA standards, 44th in investment needed for adequate treatment facilities, and 2d in per-capita spending to protect water resources.

• *Per-Mile Transfers to Sewers.* New Jersey, Massachusetts, Rhode Island, Missouri, and Delaware send the most chemicals to sewage systems for their land area. Monsanto's Indian Orchard Plant in Springfield, Massachusetts discharged almost 7 million pounds of methanol, sodium hydroxide, sulfuric acid, and other chemicals to sewers in 1987. The Bay state ranks 40th in total transfers to sewage systems, 43d in per-capita transfers, and 49th per square mile; it also ranks 50th in the in-

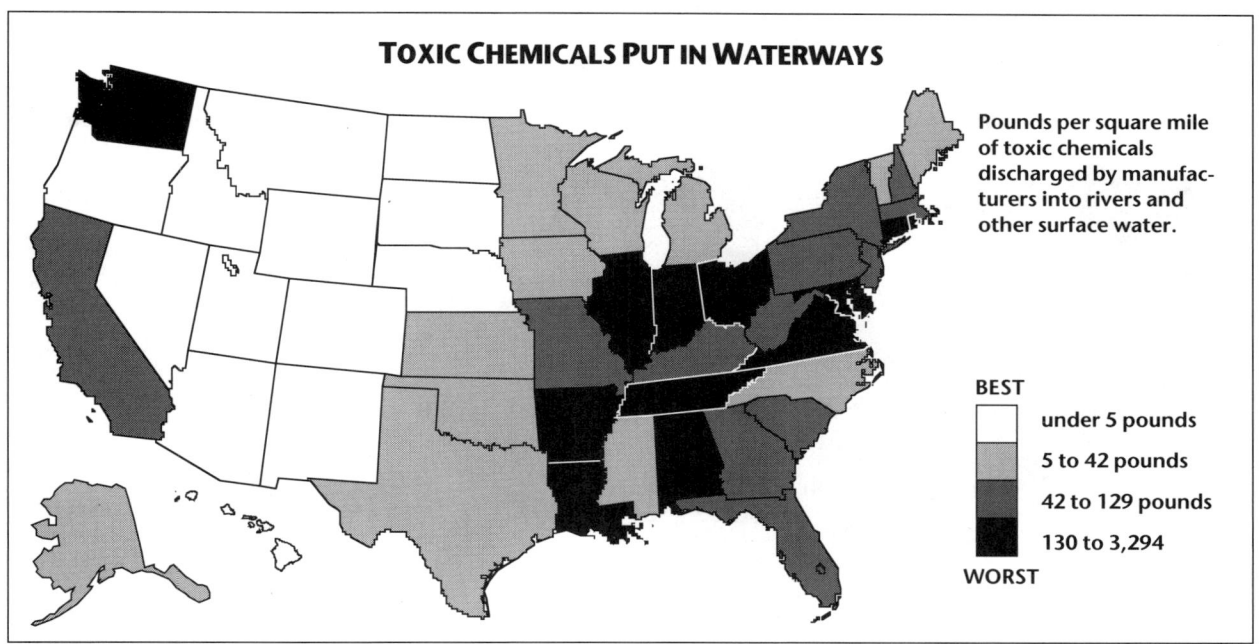

TOXIC CHEMICALS PUT IN WATERWAYS

Pounds per square mile of toxic chemicals discharged by manufacturers into rivers and other surface water.

BEST
- under 5 pounds
- 5 to 42 pounds
- 42 to 129 pounds
- 130 to 3,294
WORST

vestment required for its sewage facilities to meet the state's needs by the year 2008.

• *Toxics Injected Underground.* Texas and Louisiana create 69 percent of the toxins pumped underground, with Louisiana ranking last in injections per capita and per square mile, while Texas is 50th in total volume. In Alvin, Texas, Monsanto increased by 50 percent the amount of acrylonitrile, a probable carcinogen, it sent underground between 1987 and 1988. American Cyanamid in Westwego, Louisiana injected almost 27 million pounds of volatile organic chemicals into the ground in 1988, including over half a million pounds of acrylonitrile. Shell Oil, another major Louisiana polluter, put an astonishing 152 million pounds of hydrochloric acid into the ground in 1988.

• *Injections Per Capita.* Wyoming, ranked 49th in underground injections per capita, hosts Wycon Chemical in Cheyenne. The company's waste includes ammonium nitrate, ammonia, hydrochloric acid, chlorine, ethylene glycol, and phosphoric acid. Like Wyoming, the other states with the most injections — Louisiana, Kansas, Texas, Mississippi, Tennessee, Kentucky, and Indiana — have major chemical plants that feed off fossil fuels and then pump their wastes back underground.

• *Injections Per Mile.* Texas, Ohio, Tennessee, and Kansas rank at the bottom (along with Louisiana) for pounds of toxic injections per square mile. Vulcan Chemicals of Wichita, Kansas sent over 90 million pounds of hydrochloric acid, sulfuric acid, and 22 other chemicals into the ground in 1988. Toxic injections in the state jumped an amazing 38 percent from 1987 to 1988. Because of Vulcan and another Wichita chemical company, Racon Inc., Sedgwick County is the third largest producer of TRI wastes in the nation (Louisiana's Jefferson and St. Charles parishes are first and second).

When the rankings for all nine of these toxic wastewater indicators are added and re-ranked, Tennessee emerges as the worst state overall. The biggest generators are the chemical companies, led by DuPont's two facilities in Memphis and New Johnsonville and Kodak's huge Tennessee Eastman plant in Kingsport. But a dozen other firms that span business lines, from food processing to textiles to papermaking, also send a million or more pounds of toxins to sewage systems, rivers, or underground caverns each year.

Too often, getting state and company officials to control, much less reduce, these wastes remains difficult, even when drinking water quality is at stake. Consider the example of Avtex Fiber in Virginia, another Southern state that ranks in the bottom five in overall water-borne toxins. In 1978, and for the next decade, Avtex Fibers consistently disregarded requests from Virginia's Water Control Board and EPA to clean up the toxic waste it dumped into the Shenandoah River. Located in the Blue Ridge Mountains, the plant was the sole producer of carbonized rayon for the Defense Depart-

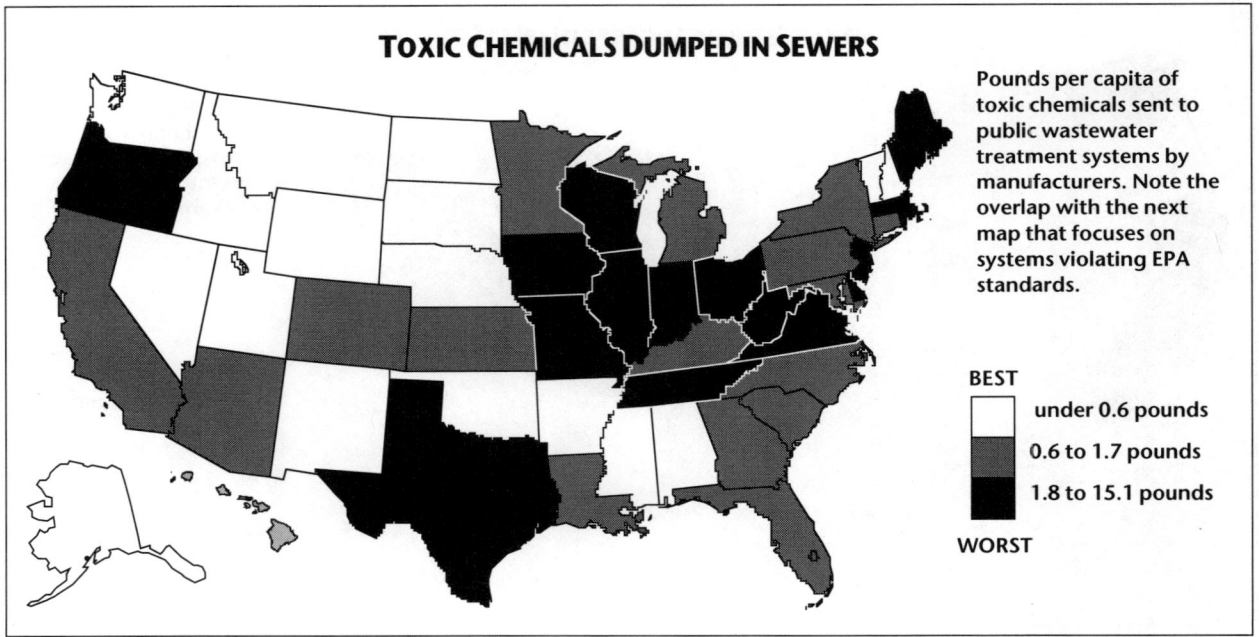

TOXIC CHEMICALS DUMPED IN SEWERS

Pounds per capita of toxic chemicals sent to public wastewater treatment systems by manufacturers. Note the overlap with the next map that focuses on systems violating EPA standards.

BEST
- under 0.6 pounds
- 0.6 to 1.7 pounds
- 1.8 to 15.1 pounds

WORST

ment and space program. Its discharge included zinc, chlorine, sulfuric acid, and PCBs. Despite evidence of chemical pollution in wells across from the plant in 1981, high toxin levels in fish in 1985, and a PCB spill in 1986, the Water Control Board and EPA issued only weak warnings.

Finally, in late 1988, after the Natural Resources Defense Council threatened to sue the company, the state decided to sue Avtex itself. In November 1989, following new PCB emissions from the company, Avtex was shut down and fined $6 million. The cleanup is expected to cost at least $100 million. "So far, the state has failed to understand the basic problem with environmental pollution, that the price for environmental damage will be extracted," says David S. Bailey, former head of enforcement for Water Control Board and current director of the Environmental Defense Fund's Virginia office. "If you don't make the company pay for it, the environment will pay for it, and the citizens bear the cost."

TOXIC DRAINS

In addition to the danger posed by TRI chemicals created by industry, detergents, motor oil, fertilizer, construction waste, and pesticides wash off lawns and city streets into storm drains or sewers. If poorly treated, or not treated at all, these pollutants can threaten the health of our lakes, rivers, and harbors.

Throughout the country, aging sewage plants are failing to handle the waste load from new industry and more people. In 1988, some 6,250 of the nation's 15,600 treatment facilities reported water quality or public health problems. In Boston, 12 billion tons of raw or partially treated sewage reach Boston Harbor each year — about 500 million gallons per day. Construction of a secondary treatment facility to clean the water more thoroughly is underway but won't be completed until after the year 2000. Massachusetts' shortsightedness shows up on the indicator measuring funds required to manage each state's sewage. It ranks last, with $991 per capita needed to provide adequate sewage treatment through the year 2008. Other states that face large bills include Oregon, Washington, and Alaska in the West, and New Hampshire, New York, Connecticut, New Jersey, and Florida in the East.

Massachusetts, Florida, New Jersey, and Washington also rank poorly for public sewage plants violating EPA standards. Another New England state, Rhode Island, ranks even worse. With 40 percent of its sewers in noncompliance, the state falls to the bottom on this indicator. Century-old sewer overflow pipes in Pawtucket, Central Falls, Providence, Fall River, and Newport spew raw sewage into Narragansett Bay during heavy rainfalls, forcing the closing of local shellfishing beds.

Environmentalists have pressured Rhode Island cities to clean up. Most towns have made an effort to stop the pollution, but the expense is sometimes overwhelming. "They say it will cost

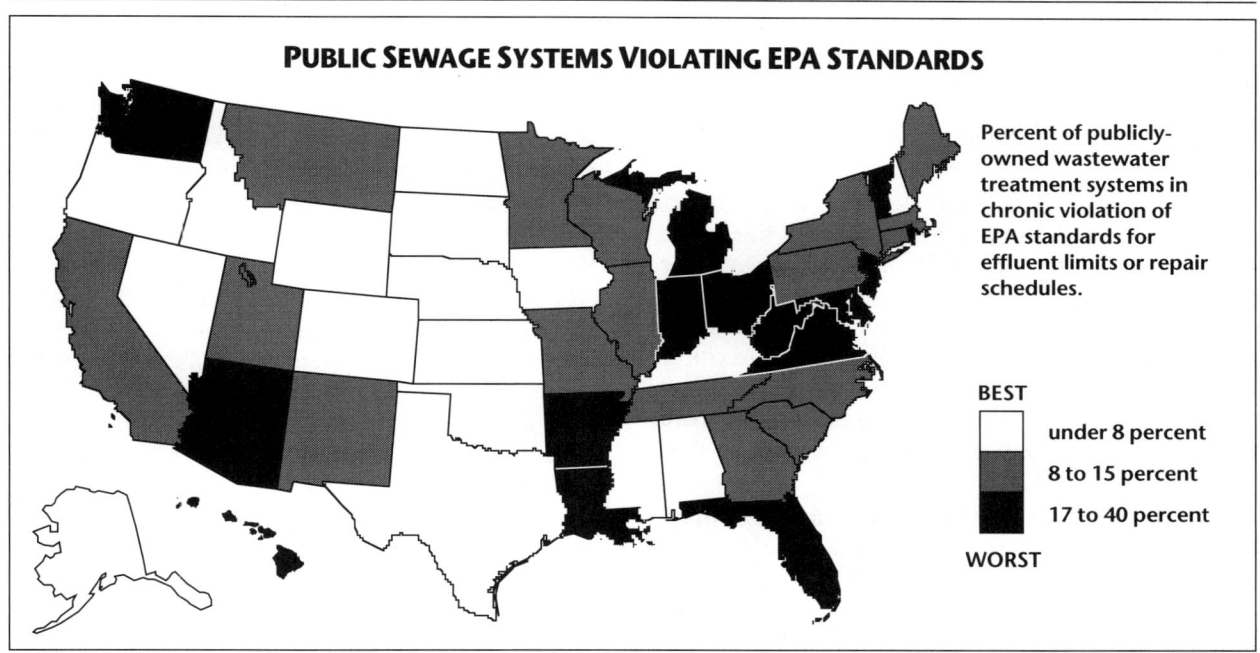

$50 million to correct this in Pawtucket alone," says Mayor Brian J. Sarault. "The people in Pawtucket just can't afford it." Rhode Island ranks 40th in the investment needed for proper sewage systems. Since it ranks 42d in toxics piped to public sewers per square mile, it's a safe bet that the overflow and poorly treated sewage reaching the Narragansett Bay is laced with chemical toxins.

RIVERS AND LAKES

The toll such waste is taking on the nation's inland waters is difficult to gauge, but it's clear the impact is widespread. Ten percent of the river and stream miles assessed by the states are already ruined; they can no longer support their designated uses for fishing, recreation, and/or drinking. Another 20 percent only partially support their designated use, and a seventh of the remaining 70 percent face imminent danger of becoming impaired. The breakdown is about the same for acres of lakes and reservoirs. Most contaminants come from industry, development and urban sewers, agriculture and forestry, mining, landfills, and dredging.

The states ranking worst on fresh water quality are in the Great Lakes and Farmbelt (Ohio, Illinois, Wisconsin, Minnesota, and Iowa) or are mining states (West Virginia, Montana, New Mexico, Oklahoma, and Alaska). Among the best are Alabama, Mississippi, and Georgia, even though Alabama and Mississippi ranked among the worst 10 states for drinking water violations, and Alabama and Georgia ranked 42d and 41st in toxic discharges to surface water. The impairment rankings can be deceptive because each state decides how much to test and how to define fully, partially, or non-supporting waters.

In Minnesota, which is second only to Alaska in total surface water miles, monitoring includes an analysis of fish tissues. Nearly two-thirds of the state's rivers and streams fail to meet designated uses, ranking Minnesota 45th. Its lakes had a better standing (rank 24), but scientists identified serious problems with mercury and PCB contamination. Rain-borne mercury from coal-burning electric plants and incineration is accumulating in fish in the state's northeastern lakes, harming or killing fish-eating animals. The scientists also found high levels of toxic chemicals in fish down river from major municipalities. In June 1990, two Minneapolis-based environmental groups warned 28 companies that they were violating the Clean Water Act for excessive discharges of chromium, nickel, cyanide, and fecal coliform.

Dioxin, a deadly poison that can cause birth defects, miscarriages, and nerve damage, is another significant threat to surface water quality (see page 102). In 1908, when Champion International built the South's first paper mill on the banks of North Carolina's Pigeon River, the river was clear and full of trout. Today, the Pigeon is discolored, practically dead, and contaminated with dioxin from Champion's wastewater. Four major rivers in

Arkansas, recipients of waste from paper companies like Nekoosa Papers in Ashdown, also have dangerous levels of dioxin. Arkansas ranks 42d, with 58 percent of its assessed rivers and streams impaired.

Maine is one of the chief targets of dioxin reduction measures promoted by EPA. Two of the seven companies targeted, Scott Paper and James River Company, have filed suit, arguing that the standards are too stringent. Acid rain is another serious problem for surface water in Maine and other New England states. The region's lakes and rivers catch the brunt of sulfur dioxide emissions from more heavily industrial states to the south and west (see pages 19-20).

The greatest single threat to aquatic life in inland surface waters is agricultural run-off. Pesticides, herbicides, fertilizers, other nutrients, and sediment wash, dribble, or blow into the water, impairing 55 percent of the nation's river miles. A study by the U.S. Geological Survey released in January 1990 reveals that 98 percent of the streams tested in 10 Midwest states contain the pesticides atrazine and alachlor, both likely carcinogens. Of the 127 streams examined, 71 had atrazine levels above EPA safety limits and 44 exceeded the limit for alachlor.

Agriculture is also a major consumer of the nation's freshwater supply, especially in the Midwest and Rocky Mountains. Seven of the dozen states with the nation's highest per-capita consumption of water (Idaho, Wyoming, Nebraska, Colorado, Nevada, Kansas, New Mexico) are among the dozen that rely most heavily on artificial irrigation for their crops (see page 109). While Kansas and New Mexico have helped deplete the aquifers of the High Plains by more than half, several of the other states continue draining the Colorado River as their chief source of surface water.

THE NOT-SO GREAT LAKES

The Great Lakes hold one-fifth of the world's fresh water, furnishing 3 billion gallons a day for domestic use, yet they have become a toxic soup. Their wide expanse, strategic location, and neighboring natural resources turned the region into America's industrial heartland. People and pollution blossomed in Buffalo, Cleveland, Detroit, Chicago, Milwaukee, and all points between. Today, 73 percent of the five Great Lakes' shoreline miles fail to support designated uses for fishing, drinking, or recreation. While deeper waters in the Lakes' centers may be cleaner, only 372 of 4,479 shoreline miles assessed still fully support their intended uses.

Violations of metal pollution are the primary reason that much of Lake Erie's shoreline only partially supports intended uses. Right next to the lake, in Ecorse, Michigan, National Steel dumps thousands of pounds of zinc, manganese and lead compounds, aluminum oxide, ammonia, and ethylene glycol into surface water.

Fish in Lake Michigan contain dioxin, PCBs, DDT, dieldrin, and chlordane flushed through sewage plants or directly released by lakeshore industries. Studies show that babies born to mothers who eat Lake Michigan fish are more likely to be premature, underweight, and slow learners. The U.S. General Accounting Office (GAO) estimates it will cost $1.8 billion just to bring Michigan's Rouge River, one of the region's 42 major areas of concern, up to the state's public health standards by the year 2005.

Toxic reduction is as important as cleanup, says the GAO, and too little is being done. For example, Eastman Kodak in Rochester, New York, on Lake Ontario increased its wastewater discharge of cancer-causing dichloromethane by 16,200 pounds between 1987 and 1988. Levels of dioxin and PCBs found in Lake Ontario's fish still exceed safe-food limits.

States bordering the Great Lakes, including Wisconsin, Illinois, Michigan, Ohio, and New York, score poorly on lakes and reservoirs supporting designated uses. All of the states monitor toxins in fish, and programs to reduce phosphorus levels in the Lakes have been successful; however, nitrogen levels are on the rise and sediment contamination continues to threaten the entire Lakes system.

DEEP THROAT

Underground aquifers in the United States contain up to 16 times as much water as the Great Lakes. They feed public water systems and private wells, and supply billions of gallons of free water daily to mining, industrial, and agribusiness concerns. In North Carolina, for example, Texasgulf's phosphate operation sucks out more water than is consumed by the entire city of Charlotte.

Groundwater pollution comes from many sources. Poisons leach from Superfund or other dump sites, and agricultural chemicals seep through the soil. Saltwater invades when coastal wetlands lose their recharging capacity. Underground storage tanks leak benzene and other dangerous substances. A 1986 EPA report estimated that 300,000 underground gasoline storage tanks

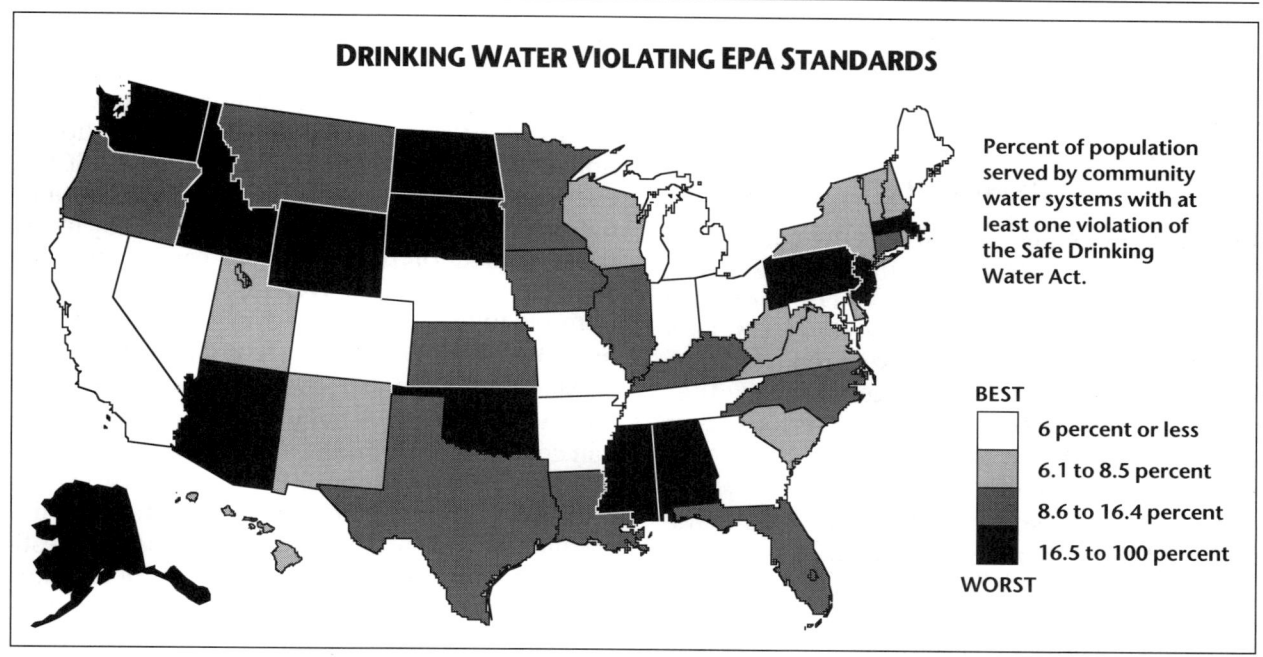

DRINKING WATER VIOLATING EPA STANDARDS

Percent of population served by community water systems with at least one violation of the Safe Drinking Water Act.

BEST
- 6 percent or less
- 6.1 to 8.5 percent
- 8.6 to 16.4 percent
- 16.5 to 100 percent

WORST

were leaking; one gallon of gasoline can contaminate a million gallons of water.

In 1980, at the behest of Senator Bennett Johnston of Louisiana, Congress exempted companies drilling for oil and gas from hazardous waste disposal laws. That decision has had a profoundly negative impact on the environment, especially the nation's groundwater. Under the exemption, oil producers can dump "non-hazardous" waste mud from their drilling into open pits, even though the sludge and brine contaminate groundwater. In addition, oil and gas producing states — such as Louisiana, Texas, Wyoming, Indiana, Kansas, Oklahoma, and Ohio — are dotted with injection wells holding wastes that make their way into shallow aquifers.

All seven of the states listed are also among the worst dozen for toxic chemicals pumped underground by manufacturers. In Ohio (rank 47), the 160-square-mile Great Miami Aquifer was contaminated by the Chem-Dyne Corporation in the 1970s and cleanup is still underway. Rat poisons, acids, cyanide sludges, and other hazardous chemicals were dropped in gravel pits over the aquifer, which supplies one-third of Ohio's groundwater. Over a million fish died in the Great Miami River as a result, and residents near the Chem-Dyne site have suffered a high rate of respiratory illness.

Pesticides, another potential groundwater pollutant, do their worse damage in the big agricultural states. Seven of these states — Iowa, Florida, Nebraska, Mississippi, Minnesota, Wisconsin, Idaho — are also among the 10 most dependent on groundwater for their drinking water. In Iowa and Kansas more than 20 percent of wells tested had unsafe levels of nitrates, the result of seepage from fertilizers, animal waste, and septic tanks. The problems are not limited to the big farm states. For example, nitrates and other organic pollutants have closed 20 public water supplies in upstate New York; on Long Island, 33 water systems closed and the pesticide aldicarb (used on potato fields) exceeds safe limits in a fourth of the wells tested.

Groundwater protection is largely left to the states. Out of necessity, Wisconsin, Iowa, California, Florida, and New York are among the states with the toughest legislation. Florida's Ground-Water Protection Strategy not only requires data collection, but implements federal underground injection and storage tank control programs, a groundwater discharge permitting program, septic tank regulations, and aquifer protection. Per capita spending of federal and state funds to protect and improve water quality in the Sunshine state ranks 9th nationally.

Florida needs all the help it can get. It ranks 49th in pesticide contaminated groundwater, 47th in reliance on groundwater for drinking, 46th in public water systems and 39th in sewage systems in non-compliance, 46th in impaired lakes, and 43rd on the composite toxic wastewater score. Overall, Florida takes last place on our clean water indicators. The dying Everglades, symbolic of the state's problems, feed the aquifer that feeds south

Florida's ballooning population, but state officials have stood by (or even helped) as the sugar and oil interests pollute, siphon, and otherwise destroy these unique wetlands.

DRINK WELL

Drinking water sources all across the nation face similar threats. Twenty-one hundred different chemicals turned up in a survey of public water systems between 1971 and 1985, and 111,228 cases of disease from drinking water were reported. The pollutants included 97 carcinogens and 93 other contaminants suspected of causing serious harm to humans. Currently, only 83 of these 190 health-threatening pollutants are regulated by federal law.

In 1974, Congress passed the Safe Drinking Water Act (SDWA), requiring states to monitor and enforce standards set by EPA. A 1986 amendment expanded the number of substances covered by the SDWA, but out of over 36,000 violations of EPA standards the following year, states took enforcement action on only 2.5 percent. In June 1990, the U.S. General Accounting Office reported that (a) "the number of violations is considerably understated," (b) water system operators are "inadequately trained or inexperienced" and occasionally engage in "intentional falsification of data," (c) state enforcement against systems with SWDA violations is "often neither timely nor appropriate," including in three-fourths of the cases involving significant noncompliance, (d) and "some [violators] posing health risks have persisted for years."

The worst five states for water systems with one or more SDWA violation in a year are Alaska (rank 50), New Jersey, Washington, Wyoming, and Arizona. Nevada, the Dakotas, Florida, Illinois, and Vermont are also among the worst 10 when it comes to states failing to act against systems with significant noncompliance. A study in Massachusetts, which ranks 44th for population served by violators, shows that residents who rely on public drinking water tainted with industrial chemicals have a significantly higher chance of developing leukemia.

Maine has one of the best drinking water programs in the country with only 2 percent of its water systems experiencing SWDA violations. A small population, relatively little industry, strict monitoring, and follow-up enforcement all enhance compliance with EPA standards. Only Minnesota ranks better; it has instituted a Local Water Planning Project to organize, fund, and provide technical assistance to local groups monitoring groundwater and surface water.

EPA regulations only apply to public water systems that serve 25 people or more for at least 60 days a year. Private wells, which serve one household in seven, are not monitored under the SDWA, even though evidence suggests many are contaminated. For example, a 1986 California study found that a quarter of the 8,000 wells tested contained pesticides. In Florida, over 1,000 wells were condemned following the discovery of groundwater laced with the pesticide ethylene dibromide.

Many rural states that depend the most on private wells also rely heavily on septic tanks, which can contaminate groundwater. Maine, New Hampshire, and Vermont score in the bottom five on both indicators. The problems are even worse for rural communities in Farmbelt states that also face pesticide contamination, or for those in Southern states like Tennessee, Mississippi, and Kentucky which allow huge injections of toxic chemicals beneath the ground.

The state with the largest percentage of its population served by wells is North Carolina. The Tarheel state also ranks 30th in surface and groundwater that may be contaminated and 49th in households using septic tanks. Some areas don't even enjoy the luxury of septic tanks. A small community of black families in Camden County, North Carolina lives in a swampy area where sewage from outhouses runs through open drainage ditches less than 10 feet from their wells.

Similar problems plague parts of Appalachia. "The vital connection between poverty and sickness is bad water," observes a West Virginia health official. "So much of the disease comes from the wells. It starts with the baby. You're basically mixing a formula with sewer water."

West Virginia officials say kidney disease, worms, and parasites are common. Many families have no running water at all, and no money to install pipes or septic systems. Some still haul water from creeks which may be contaminated by mining, industrial, or household waste. In fact, 80 percent of West Virginia's streams and 100 percent of its lakes are impaired, putting it dead last for surface water quality. The state also ranks 39th in households served by wells, 47th in households dependent on septic tanks, 47th in water used for nondrinking purposes, 43d in spending for water quality, and 46th in investment needed for adequate sewage facilities. For too many West Virginians, a drink of cool, clean mountain water goes with the myth of country living, not the reality.

WATER POLLUTION

State	FRESH WATER WITHDRAWALS Gal. Per Capita	Rank	TOXIC CHEMICAL RELEASE TO SURFACE WATER Total Pounds	Rank	Pounds Per Capita	Rank	Pounds Per Sq. Mile	Rank	TOXIC CHEMICAL TRANSFERS TO PUBLIC SEWERS Total Pounds	Rank	Pounds Per Capita.	Rank	Pounds Per Sq. Mile	Rank
Alabama	2,736	42	6,908,442	42	1.7	44	133.6	38	1,223,368	17	0.3	11	23.7	16
Alaska	421	7	4,274,455	35	8.3	49	7.2	15	1,000	1	0.0	2	0.0	1
Arizona	2,309	35	9,850	5	0.0	3	0.1	5	4,524,493	30	1.3	27	39.7	18
Arkansas	2,925	44	7,446,055	45	3.1	47	140.0	40	1,108,236	16	0.5	12	20.8	15
California	1,518	30	11,017,789	46	0.4	27	69.4	31	48,609,149	47	1.7	34	306.3	35
Colorado	4,949	46	87,843	8	0.0	7	0.8	7	1,879,125	19	0.6	18	18.1	14
Connecticut	409	6	7,305,148	44	2.3	45	1,455.8	49	2,795,903	25	0.9	24	557.2	42
Delaware	225	2	574,167	20	0.9	38	280.9	45	2,271,089	21	3.4	44	1,111.1	46
Florida	642	12	7,198,454	43	0.6	33	122.7	35	16,678,069	40	1.3	28	284.3	34
Georgia	1,122	20	6,509,879	41	1.0	40	110.5	34	8,658,999	35	1.4	29	147.0	31
Hawaii	1,237	23	10,000	6	0.0	6	1.5	9	835,250	12	0.8	20	129.1	28
Idaho	17,928	50	296,220	12	0.3	22	3.5	12	515,514	11	0.5	14	6.2	9
Illinois	1,473	29	14,304,086	48	1.2	41	253.9	44	59,151,864	49	5.1	47	1,049.8	45
Indiana	2,545	38	4,873,432	38	0.9	39	134.7	39	12,067,445	36	2.2	38	333.5	36
Iowa	1,111	19	1,563,824	26	0.6	32	27.8	23	6,262,070	31	2.2	39	111.3	27
Kansas	2,695	41	801,192	23	0.3	23	9.7	17	3,387,911	27	1.4	30	41.2	19
Kentucky	1,234	22	1,697,760	28	0.5	29	42.0	26	2,358,242	22	0.6	19	58.4	21
Louisiana	2,676	39	157,333,611	50	35.6	50	3,294.9	50	3,565,551	28	0.8	22	74.7	23
Maine	730	13	439,516	17	0.4	24	13.2	20	2,733,459	24	2.3	40	82.2	25
Maryland	319	3	3,756,283	33	0.8	37	359.1	47	3,959,217	29	0.9	23	378.5	38
Massachusetts	429	8	699,295	22	0.1	14	84.4	32	16,649,263	39	2.8	43	2,009.8	49
Michigan	1,651	31	1,147,387	25	0.1	15	19.6	22	15,833,193	38	1.7	33	270.5	33
Minnesota	740	14	2,758,505	31	0.6	34	32.7	24	6,557,312	32	1.5	32	77.7	24
Mississippi	1,110	18	1,984,907	29	0.8	35	41.6	25	1,366,669	18	0.5	15	28.7	17
Missouri	1,379	27	4,091,507	34	0.8	36	58.7	30	77,606,284	50	15.1	50	1,113.5	47
Montana	13,333	49	124,874	10	0.2	18	0.8	8	1,312	2	0.0	1	0.0	2
Nebraska	7,481	47	309,468	14	0.2	19	4.0	13	875,885	13	0.5	17	11.3	12
Nevada	3,830	45	250	1	0.0	1	0.0	1	19,505	4	0.0	3	0.2	4
New Hampshire	381	4	484,711	18	0.4	28	52.2	29	504,434	10	0.5	13	54.4	20
New Jersey	383	5	1,003,447	24	0.1	16	128.9	37	53,823,264	48	7.0	49	6,911.9	50
New Mexico	2,690	40	750	2	0.0	2	0.0	2	36,116	5	0.0	5	0.3	5
New York	450	9	2,084,783	30	0.1	13	42.5	27	25,643,490	44	1.4	31	522.2	40
North Carolina	1,294	24	695,661	21	0.1	9	13.2	19	7,493,240	34	1.1	25	142.3	30
North Dakota	1,460	28	3,600	4	0.0	5	0.1	4	52,681	6	0.1	6	0.7	6
Ohio	1,303	25	5,897,407	39	0.5	31	142.7	41	22,193,113	41	2.0	37	537.0	41
Oklahoma	513	10	363,208	15	0.1	12	5.2	14	424,512	9	0.1	7	6.1	8
Oregon	2,529	37	303,696	13	0.1	11	3.1	11	7,067,786	33	2.6	42	72.8	22
Pennsylvania	1,349	26	4,453,168	37	0.4	25	98.3	33	15,437,749	37	1.3	26	340.7	37
Rhode Island	176	1	385,645	16	0.4	26	318.2	46	1,930,025	20	1.9	36	1,592.4	48
South Carolina	1,740	32	1,599,365	27	0.5	30	51.4	28	2,688,403	23	0.8	21	86.4	26
South Dakota	975	15	2,400	3	0.0	4	0.0	3	156,884	8	0.2	10	2.0	7
Tennessee	2,098	34	6,398,920	40	1.3	42	151.8	42	24,623,468	43	5.0	46	584.3	43
Texas	976	16	4,306,731	36	0.3	21	16.1	21	40,459,590	46	2.4	41	151.6	32
Utah	2,494	36	255,653	11	0.2	17	3.0	10	900,304	14	0.5	16	10.6	11
Vermont	636	11	113,058	9	0.2	20	11.8	18	72,765	7	0.1	8	7.6	10
Virginia	982	17	19,780,454	49	3.3	48	485.2	48	38,704,548	45	6.5	48	949.4	44
Washington	1,861	33	13,511,390	47	2.9	46	198.3	43	977,544	15	0.2	9	14.3	13
West Virginia	2,893	43	3,122,244	32	1.7	43	128.9	36	3,338,844	26	1.8	35	137.8	29
Wisconsin	1,215	21	535,849	19	0.1	10	9.5	16	22,406,583	42	4.6	45	399.0	39
Wyoming	10,392	48	42,050	7	0.1	8	0.4	6	10,350	3	0.0	4	0.1	3
U.S. Total	1,529		312,868,389		1.3		86.5		570,441,070		2.3		157.6	

WATER POLLUTION

State	TOXIC CHEMICAL UNDERGROUND INJECTIONS						SUMMARY FOR 9 TOXIC INDICATORS		PUBLIC SEWERS IN NON-COMPLIANCE		INVESTMENT FOR SEWER NEEDS TO YEAR 2008		
	Total Pounds	Rank	Pounds Per Capita	Rank	Pounds Per Sq. Mile.	Rank	Score	Rank	%	Rank	Mill. $	$ Per Capita	Rank
Alabama	1,634,717	36	0.40	35	31.62	35	274	31	4	7	781	190	15
Alaska	1,018	26	0.00	30	0.00	21	180	18	5	10	221	422	41
Arizona	0	1	0.00	1	0.00	1	91	9	19	39	979	281	27
Arkansas	7,036,201	39	2.91	41	132.29	39	294	37	20	42	370	154	11
California	946,853	34	0.03	32	5.97	34	320	41	8	18	6,539	231	21
Colorado	0	1	0.00	1	0.00	1	76	7	4	7	196	59	3
Connecticut	0	1	0.00	1	0.00	1	232	26	10	23	1,392	431	42
Delaware	0	1	0.00	1	0.00	1	217	25	29	46	127	192	16
Florida	34,651,596	43	2.80	40	590.68	42	338	43	19	39	6,186	501	45
Georgia	52,800	31	0.01	31	0.90	32	304	39	10	23	1,007	159	13
Hawaii	1,051,509	35	0.96	38	162.50	40	194	22	18	37	413	376	38
Idaho	1,400	28	0.00	29	0.02	27	164	15	4	7	124	124	8
Illinois	7,340,184	40	0.64	37	130.27	38	389	49	14	31	2,958	255	23
Indiana	34,820,650	44	6.25	43	962.30	44	357	45	32	47	1,721	310	33
Iowa	0	1	0.00	1	0.00	1	181	20	6	14	646	228	20
Kansas	90,766,710	48	36.50	48	1,103.18	46	281	35	2	6	720	289	30
Kentucky	30,000,250	42	8.06	44	742.42	43	274	31	7	17	1,457	391	39
Louisiana	423,320,002	49	95.77	50	8,865.15	50	372	48	23	44	1,189	270	25
Maine	0	1	0.00	1	0.00	1	153	11	8	18	341	283	28
Maryland	2	20	0.00	1	0.00	20	248	28	19	39	919	199	18
Massachusetts	4,000	30	0.00	28	0.48	30	287	36	15	32	5,836	991	50
Michigan	5,617,060	37	0.60	36	95.97	37	276	34	39	49	3,321	359	36
Minnesota	0	1	0.00	1	0.00	1	180	18	12	27	1,106	257	24
Mississippi	46,806,563	45	17.82	46	981.50	45	275	32	5	10	548	209	19
Missouri	500	24	0.00	25	0.01	25	321	42	9	22	1,222	238	22
Montana	0	1	0.00	1	0.00	1	44	5	8	18	69	86	5
Nebraska	68,208	32	0.04	33	0.88	31	184	21	5	10	114	71	4
Nevada	0	1	0.00	1	0.00	1	17	1	0	1	165	157	12
New Hampshire	0	1	0.00	1	0.00	1	121	10	0	1	854	787	49
New Jersey	2,750	29	0.00	27	0.35	29	309	40	25	45	3,754	486	44
New Mexico	0	1	0.00	1	0.00	1	24	2	10	23	130	86	6
New York	251	23	0.00	21	0.01	24	253	29	12	27	12,721	710	48
North Carolina	250	21	0.00	22	0.00	23	204	24	8	18	1,799	277	26
North Dakota	0	1	0.00	1	0.00	1	34	3	6	14	34	51	2
Ohio	56,920,293	47	5.24	42	1,377.21	48	367	47	32	47	3,579	330	34
Oklahoma	6,353,464	38	1.95	39	90.82	36	178	17	5	10	476	147	10
Oregon	1	19	0.00	1	0.00	1	153	11	0	1	1,273	460	43
Pennsylvania	750	25	0.00	24	0.02	26	270	30	15	32	1,644	137	9
Rhode Island	0	1	0.00	1	0.00	1	195	23	40	50	408	411	40
South Carolina	0	1	0.00	1	0.00	1	158	13	13	30	684	197	17
South Dakota	0	1	0.00	1	0.00	1	38	4	0	1	87	122	7
Tennessee	49,906,110	46	10.15	45	1,184.18	47	394	50	11	26	1,467	300	32
Texas	490,826,922	50	29.25	47	1,839.63	49	343	44	6	14	4,975	295	31
Utah	0	1	0.00	1	0.00	1	82	8	15	32	583	345	35
Vermont	0	1	0.00	1	0.00	1	75	6	17	35	209	375	37
Virginia	1,373	27	0.00	26	0.03	28	363	46	17	35	957	159	14
Washington	0	1	0.00	1	0.00	1	176	16	21	43	2,685	578	47
West Virginia	97,712	33	0.05	34	4.03	33	301	38	18	37	976	520	46
Wisconsin	250	22	0.00	23	0.00	22	238	27	12	27	1,399	288	29
Wyoming	27,113,559	41	57.57	49	277.21	41	162	14	0	1	18	38	1
U.S. Total	**1,315,343,908**		**5.36**		**363.48**				**11**		**81,379**	**332**	

WATER POLLUTION

State	RIVERS & STREAMS			LAKES & RESERVOIRS			SPENDING ON WATER QUALITY & DEVEL.		PEOPLE SERVED BY GROUNDWATER		HOUSEHOLDS SERVED BY OWN WELLS		HOUSEHOLDS WITH SEPTIC TANK ONLY	
	Miles	% Impaired	Rank	1,000 Acres	% Impaired	Rank	$ per Capita	Rank	%	Rank	%	Rank	%	Rank
Alabama	40,600	9.5	5	504	17.5	25	3.24	42	54	28	18.4	29	46.8	44
Alaska	365,000	47.0	34	12,787	46.9	39	14.33	18	69	39	21.0	32	32.0	33
Arizona	6,671	30.5	20	111	14.2	19	4.97	35	65	38	4.0	4	18.8	9
Arkansas	11,508	58.3	42	na			3.78	38	50	23	24.0	38	42.1	40
California	26,970	33.5	26	1,418	47.2	40	25.49	5	46	16	3.9	3	10.5	1
Colorado	14,655	14.0	9	266	1.3	6	5.01	34	15	1	7.2	7	12.8	4
Connecticut	8,400	33.9	27	83	57.1	43	5.02	33	32	4	21.1	33	31.7	32
Delaware	500	40.0	30	na			14.45	17	60	31	22.9	37	25.2	17
Florida	12,659	33.4	25	2,085	67.3	46	20.28	9	90	47	13.4	17	28.1	25
Georgia	20,000	2.8	3	418	1.3	5	1.61	48	48	17	20.1	30	39.7	39
Hawaii	349	24.1	15	na			8.05	24	95	50	0.2	1	18.5	7
Idaho	7,310	17.3	12	363	0.0	1	22.10	6	88	46	24.7	40	36.3	38
Illinois	14,080	55.4	40	247	87.5	49	21.08	8	49	19	10.3	12	15.1	6
Indiana	90,000	32.1	22	105	0.2	2	3.32	41	61	33	26.5	43	34.1	35
Iowa	18,300	99.2	50	81	66.6	45	16.38	14	82	44	21.1	34	25.9	19
Kansas	19,791	42.0	31	175	32.9	34	9.44	20	62	35	12.3	14	20.9	12
Kentucky	18,465	28.6	19	228	16.4	23	6.73	26	41	9	18.3	28	45.7	43
Louisiana	14,180	32.5	23	714	27.3	30	21.89	7	69	40	13.0	15	28.3	27
Maine	31,672	1.2	1	995	3.7	8	3.78	39	57	30	34.9	49	50.0	48
Maryland	9,300	7.2	4	17	15.0	21	8.57	22	28	3	16.3	21	20.4	11
Massachusetts	10,704	56.7	41	na			28.70	3	33	5	6.2	5	26.1	21
Michigan	36,350	2.2	2	841	28.3	32	11.01	19	43	13	27.1	45	28.6	28
Minnesota	91,944	65.0	45	3,411	16.5	24	4.56	36	75	42	25.0	41	25.2	16
Mississippi	15,623	11.3	6	500	3.7	7	1.96	46	93	49	16.7	23	43.5	41
Missouri	19,630	48.3	35	288	0.8	4	8.34	23	34	6	15.6	20	27.7	23
Montana	20,532	37.1	29	756	47.9	41	26.72	4	54	25	25.6	42	36.2	37
Nebraska	10,212	43.0	32	145	3.8	9	4.29	37	82	44	18.2	27	20.3	10
Nevada	na			na			18.68	11	50	22	7.2	6	12.7	3
New Hampshire	14,544	28.6	18	151	12.8	17	15.86	15	60	31	31.7	48	47.7	46
New Jersey	6,450	71.2	48	19	28.0	31	58.29	2	45	15	8.4	8	13.5	5
New Mexico	3,500	50.0	36	127	39.5	37	6.92	25	92	48	14.2	18	26.7	22
New York	70,000	23.7	14	750	39.4	36	5.11	32	35	7	9.8	11	21.3	13
North Carolina	37,378	32.8	24	305	3.9	10	1.91	47	55	29	37.0	50	53.2	49
North Dakota	11,284	30.6	21	626	7.8	13	17.90	13	62	34	21.4	35	27.8	24
Ohio	43,917	68.0	47	117	65.9	44	2.49	45	42	12	17.0	25	23.8	15
Oklahoma	19,791	64.3	44	na			1.58	49	41	10	13.4	16	26.1	20
Oregon	90,000	54.8	39	611	25.9	29	6.30	28	63	37	16.6	22	31.4	30
Pennsylvania	50,000	27.2	17	na			5.54	30	44	14	17.7	26	25.5	18
Rhode Island	724	15.8	10	17	8.7	15	18.04	12	24	2	9.4	10	31.6	31
South Carolina	9,900	25.6	16	525	0.3	3	2.52	44	42	11	26.5	44	46.9	45
South Dakota	9,937	63.0	43	1,598	14.3	20	6.35	27	77	43	21.0	31	29.5	29
Tennessee	19,124	36.6	28	539	16.1	22	5.61	29	49	18	14.9	19	43.6	42
Texas	80,000	13.1	8	1,410	13.1	18	1.05	50	49	20	8.9	9	18.7	8
Utah	na			na			9.01	21	63	36	3.0	2	12.3	2
Vermont	5,162	12.2	7	229	21.7	28	3.72	40	54	25	29.7	47	53.3	50
Virginia	27,240	65.7	46	162	8.5	14	5.30	31	41	8	22.8	36	34.2	36
Washington	40,492	50.3	38	614	21.5	27	14.73	16	50	21	11.8	13	32.3	34
West Virginia	28,361	80.0	49	19	100.0	50	3.11	43	53	24	24.6	39	48.3	47
Wisconsin	na			971	74.4	48	19.78	10	70	41	29.7	46	28.1	26
Wyoming	19,437	17.3	11	427	7.1	12	145.11	1	54	25	16.9	24	21.9	14
U.S. Total	1,522,792	30.4		35,754	25.7		12.47		51		15.1		26.0	

WATER POLLUTION

State	PESTICIDE CONTAMINATED GROUNDWATER %	Rank	SURF.& GROUND WATER POSSIBLY CONTAMINATED %	Rank	WATER SYSTEMS VIOLATING SDWA %	Rank	WATER SYSTEMS SIGNIFICANT NONCOMPLIANCE %	Rank	POPULATION WITH SDWA VIOLATIONS %	Rank	WATER USE FOR DRINKING & COOKING %	Rank	COMPOSITE WATER POLLUTION Score	Rank
Alabama	16.0	35	39.0	34	20.9	27	0.15	4	17.5	41	0.023	37	689	38
Alaska	na		na		78.8	50	78.29	50	48.0	48	0.070	12	647	30
Arizona	28.8	42	47.2	38	62.0	46	24.14	48	59.9	49	0.025	35	575	19
Arkansas	8.5	27	16.3	20	4.0	8	0.00	1	5.8	11	0.020	42	711	41
California	6.6	21	15.2	19	9.4	19	2.25	34	4.6	9	0.035	30	612	27
Colorado	3.4	13	25.8	24	26.2	32	0.93	19	2.3	5	0.012	46	332	2
Connecticut	0.3	5	1.4	6	1.8	4	1.22	24	14.5	34	0.142	6	554	17
Delaware	35.9	45	70.5	48	9.4	20	0.91	17	6.2	15	0.245	2	584	22
Florida	56.5	49	65.0	45	43.1	41	4.18	46	16.2	36	0.091	10	830	50
Georgia	8.3	26	26.0	26	36.5	40	0.64	12	3.7	6	0.056	16	628	29
Hawaii	na		na		23.6	28	1.53	29	6.3	17	0.046	21	553	16
Idaho	22.5	39	27.0	27	35.7	39	1.79	31	17.0	40	0.002	50	598	25
Illinois	24.2	41	63.8	44	6.7	14	3.32	43	8.9	27	0.041	25	800	46
Indiana	38.1	47	66.9	46	4.3	9	1.40	27	2.2	4	0.034	31	815	49
Iowa	56.6	50	75.5	50	25.8	30	3.26	42	16.2	37	0.052	17	666	34
Kansas	36.8	46	70.8	49	26.1	31	1.60	30	12.7	32	0.022	39	731	43
Kentucky	6.7	22	44.9	37	27.1	35	1.06	22	12.5	31	0.048	19	666	34
Louisiana	15.3	33	25.9	25	13.5	22	0.34	7	9.1	28	0.023	37	774	44
Maine	4.0	16	19.0	21	1.7	3	0.00	1	1.2	1	0.112	8	437	8
Maryland	6.9	23	57.3	42	1.8	5	0.84	15	4.3	8	0.196	4	487	12
Massachusetts	0.5	7	1.7	8	4.8	10	0.74	14	20.8	44	0.047	20	579	20
Michigan	14.0	31	69.8	47	3.7	7	0.26	6	1.3	2	0.039	28	652	31
Minnesota	33.1	44	50.9	39	1.0	1	0.00	1	13.1	33	0.069	13	580	21
Mississippi	22.7	40	24.9	23	26.9	34	0.21	5	23.8	46	0.058	15	657	32
Missouri	1.9	11	5.8	11	10.2	21	0.92	18	6.0	13	0.042	24	601	26
Montana	3.7	14	10.4	14	53.2	45	1.40	28	16.0	35	0.005	48	478	11
Nebraska	47.8	48	61.3	43	19.6	25	1.32	25	1.5	3	0.008	47	595	24
Nevada	0.0	1	0.0	1	33.8	38	28.35	49	5.9	12	0.013	45	287	1
New Hampshire	0.0	1	0.0	1	7.6	15	0.88	16	8.0	24	0.073	11	418	5
New Jersey	16.3	36	35.4	32	75.4	49	0.63	11	100.0	50	0.175	5	695	40
New Mexico	0.5	6	0.5	5	29.0	36	2.97	40	7.5	22	0.021	40	428	6
New York	6.9	24	31.4	29	8.8	17	0.48	9	6.1	14	0.099	9	552	15
North Carolina	4.7	18	31.7	30	9.4	18	1.03	21	8.7	26	0.040	27	621	28
North Dakota	6.2	20	12.1	17	26.2	33	3.39	44	20.8	45	0.030	33	410	4
Ohio	18.7	37	56.7	40	8.0	16	0.37	8	4.1	7	0.043	22	791	45
Oklahoma	4.2	17	15.2	18	15.7	24	2.18	33	16.5	38	0.140	7	505	14
Oregon	0.6	8	2.0	9	52.9	44	2.50	36	9.7	29	0.021	40	585	23
Pennsylvania	10.7	29	42.8	36	46.5	43	2.74	38	16.6	39	0.043	22	677	37
Rhode Island	1.0	10	6.5	12	1.6	2	1.16	23	7.7	23	0.390	1	437	8
South Carolina	9.2	28	40.0	35	6.2	13	1.33	26	6.8	18	0.025	36	556	18
South Dakota	15.7	34	22.0	22	25.4	29	3.70	45	20.2	43	0.052	18	445	10
Tennessee	14.9	32	38.3	33	43.2	42	0.55	10	4.6	10	0.028	34	805	47
Texas	5.2	19	11.9	16	20.7	26	2.69	37	11.5	30	0.041	25	670	36
Utah	0.0	1	0.0	1	33.5	37	0.73	13	7.2	19	0.020	42	392	3
Vermont	0.0	1	0.0	1	6.0	12	3.22	41	7.3	21	0.212	3	434	7
Virginia	3.7	15	31.3	28	14.8	23	1.01	20	7.3	20	0.060	14	720	42
Washington	6.9	25	10.8	15	66.6	48	18.68	47	44.5	47	0.031	32	662	33
West Virginia	2.2	12	5.5	10	5.3	11	2.47	35	6.3	16	0.018	44	807	48
Wisconsin	30.1	43	56.8	41	2.4	6	1.85	32	8.5	25	0.036	29	691	39
Wyoming	0.6	9	1.4	7	64.6	47	2.85	39	18.7	42	0.004	49	492	13
U.S. Total	**14.9**		**34.1**				**3.37**		**14.5**					

SOURCES FOR WATER POLLUTION INDICATORS

Fresh water withdrawals
   Total per-capita consumption in gallons of fresh water from all surface and groundwater sources, including agriculture and industry use but excluding hydroelectric instream pass-through.
   Source: "National Water Summary, 1985," Table 23. Published by U.S. Geological Survey, U.S. Department of Interior, 1988.

Toxic chemicals released into surface water
   Total pounds, pounds per capita, and pounds per square mile of direct surface water discharges reported by manufacturing facilities using or releasing at least 50,000 pounds of any of 322 chemicals, including 123 carcinogens.
   Source: "Toxics in the Community: The 1988 Toxic Release Inventory National Report," September 1990. Published by Office of Toxic Substances, U.S. Environmental Protection Agency, Washington.

Toxic chemicals sent into public sewage systems
   Total pounds, pounds per capita, and pounds per square mile of public sewer transfers reported by manufacturing facilities using or releasing at least 50,000 pounds of any of 322 chemicals, including 123 carcinogens.
   Source: "Toxics in the Community: The 1988 Toxic Release Inventory National Report," September 1990. Published by Office of Toxic Substances, U.S. Environmental Protection Agency, Washington.

Toxic chemicals injected underground
   Total pounds, pounds per capita, and pounds per square mile of underground injections reported by manufacturing facilities using or releasing at least 50,000 pounds of any of 322 chemicals, including 123 carcinogens.
   Source: "Toxics in the Community: The 1988 Toxic Release Inventory National Report," September 1990. Published by Office of Toxic Substances, U.S. Environmental Protection Agency, Washington.

Composite toxic water score
   Each state's rank for the nine indicators above was totaled to produce a composite score. Lowest score receives best composite rank for toxic chemical releases threatening water quality.

Sewage systems in noncompliance
   Percent of publicly-owned wastewater treatment works (POTWs) in significant noncompliance with final effluent limits for secondary treatment or better, and/or with interim effluent limits, and/or with construction schedules.
   Source: Office of Water Enforcement and Permits, U.S. Environmental Protection Agency, Washington, for quarter ending June 30, 1988.

Sewage system investment needs
   Funds needed for publicly-owned wastewater treatment facilities to meet anticipated demand by 2008, including cost of new, expanded, upgraded, or better managed systems. Total dollars in millions, per-capita dollars, and per-capita ranking.
   Source: "1988 Needs Survey Report to Congress: Assessment of Needed Publicly Owned Wastewater Treatment Facilities." Published by Office of Municipal Pollution Control, U.S. Environmental Protection Agency, Washington, February 1989.

Impaired rivers and streams
>Total miles of rivers and streams, and percent of total miles that partially or completely fail to meet their designated use for drinking, recreation, or fishing.
>*Source:* "National Water Quality Inventory: 1988 Report to Congress." Published by Office of Water Regulations and Standards, U.S. Environmental Protection Agency, March 1990.

Impaired lakes and reservoirs
>Total acres of lakes and reservoirs, and percent of total acres that partially or completely fail to meet their designated use for drinking, recreation, or fishing.
>*Source:* "National Water Quality Inventory: 1988 Report to Congress." Published by Office of Water Regulations and Standards, U.S. Environmental Protection Agency, March 1990.

Funds for water quality and development
>Per-capita spending in fiscal 1988 for SWDA and public drinking water programs, water quality protection, and water resource conservation and development. Includes state, federal, and other funds (fines, licences, etc.) that pass through state budgetary process. Excludes funds for coastal water and marine protection.
>*Source:* "Resource Guide to State Environmental Management," second edition, 1991. Published by Council of State Governments, P.O. Box 11910, Lexington, KY 40578; telephone (606) 231-1939.

Population served by groundwater
>Percent of population dependent on groundwater for public or self-supplied water systems.
>*Source:* "National Water Summary, 1985," Table 23. Published by U.S. Geological Survey, U.S. Department of Interior, 1988.

Households with wells
>Percent of households with their own wells.
>*Source:* "General Housing Characteristics, U.S. Summary, 1980, U.S. Census of Population." Published by Bureau of Census, U.S. Department of Commerce, Washington.

Households with septic tanks only
>Percent of households with their own septic tanks or no public sewer service.
>*Source:* "General Housing Characteristics, U.S. Summary, 1980, U.S. Census of Population." Published by Bureau of Census, U.S. Department of Commerce, Washington.

Groundwater potentially contaminated by pesticides
>Percent of state's population served by public water supplies in counties potentially contaminated with pesticides or agricultural chemicals.
>*Source:* Elizabeth G. Nielsen and Linda K. Lee, "The Magnitude and Costs of Groundwater Contamination from Agricultural Chemicals." Agricultural Economic Report No. 576, October 1987. Published by the Economic Research Service, U.S. Department of Agriculture, Washington.

Surface and groundwater potentially contaminated
>Percent of state's population served by public water supplies in counties potentially contaminated by pesticides or agricultural chemicals.
>*Source:* Elizabeth G. Nielsen and Linda K. Lee, "The Magnitude and Costs of Groundwater Contamination from Agricultural Chemicals." Agricultural Economic Report No. 576, October 1987. Published by the Economic Research Service, U.S. Department of Agriculture, Washington.

Water systems with SDWA violations
   Percent of public water systems with one or more violations of the Safe Drinking Water Act during fiscal 1987.
   Source: Norman L. Dean, "Danger On Tap: The Government's Failure to Enforce the Federal Safe Drinking Water Act," October 1988. Published by the National Wildlife Federation, 1400 16th Street, NW, Washington, DC 20036; telephone (202) 797-6820.

Water systems in significant noncompliance
   Percent of community water systems in significant, chronic violation of the Safe Drinking Water Act during fiscal 1987.
   Source: "Danger On Tap: The Government's Failure to Enforce the Federal Safe Drinking Water Act," October 1988. Published by the National Wildlife Federation.

Population with SDWA violations
   Percent of population in 1987 served by community water systems with at least one violation of the Safe Drinking Water Act. Each of the nation's 60,000 community water systems serves at least 15 connections or 25 people year-round.
   Source: "Danger On Tap: The Government's Failure to Enforce the Federal Safe Drinking Water Act," October 1988. Published by the National Wildlife Federation.

Water use for drinking purposes
   Percent of total public and self-supplied withdrawals of water consumed for domestic drinking and cooking purposes. The vast majority of water is consumed by industry, utilities, and agriculture.
   Source: "Estimated Use of Water in the United States in 1985," U.S. Geological Survey Circular 1004. Published by U.S. Department of Interior, 1988. Percentages calculated by Chris Nichols in "Drinking Water," Renew America, Washington, 1989.

Composite water quality score
   Rankings on 25 indicators were totaled to produce a composite score. Lowest scores receives lowest (best) composite rank for water quality.

CHAPTER 4

Energy Use and Auto Abuse

INDICATORS

Coal production	Share of nation's radioactive waste
Oil production	Cost of electricity to residential versus industrial customers
Natural gas production	Electricity from coal
Gross state product from energy industry	Electricity from oil or gas
Pipeline violations	Electricity from hydro or other sources
Oil and related spills in state waters	Gas use per capita
Oil and gas injection wells	Miles per gallon of gas
Growth of carbon emissions per capita	Highway deaths per billion miles driven
Carbon emissions per $1,000 of gross state product	Persons per registered vehicles
Energy consumption per capita	Cars per transit bus
Growth in energy consumption, 1960-1975	Employment in vehicle-related jobs
Growth in energy consumption, 1975-1987	Vehicle-related taxes as percent of state revenues
Growth in energy consumption versus population growth	Highway spending as percent of vehicle-related taxes
Low-income homes weatherized	Highway spending as percent of spending for public transportation
Electricity from nuclear power	Urban mass transit
Cost of decommissioning nuclear power plants	Energy from renewable sources
Funds set aside to pay for decommissioning	Electricity from renewable sources
Safety citations at nuclear power plants	Electricity from non-hydro renewable sources
Low-level radioactive waste shipped	Energy from burning municipal solid waste
Accumulated radioactive waste generated	Solar collection systems

Americans are accustomed to seemingly unlimited, cheap supplies of fuel and electric power. With the help of federal and state subsidies, we've become fossil-fuel junkies, demanding more and more power for our cars, timesaving gadgets, air conditioners, and computer games. We now consume a third of the world's energy and emit one-fifth of its global warming gases.

As demand increases, more land is stripped for coal, more holes are drilled for oil and natural gas, and more power plants are built by the electric utilities. For decades, fuel and electricity sold at radical discounts to the largest customers, encouraging expansion, waste, and pollution. But after the oil embargo of the early 1970s, the annual rate of growth in energy consumption plummeted, proving that conservation and market pricing can work. In the late 1980s, consumption began climbing again, proof that the nation still lacks a comprehensive energy policy aimed at weaning us from fossil fuels, whether produced here or abroad. In fact, between 1985 and 1989, oil imports jumped from 27 percent to 41 percent of U.S. supply, while the federal government pared down its already meager support for the development of renewable energy sources and mass transit.

"We have a growing dependency on foreign oil and a growing dependence on the automobile," says Nancy Hirsh, policy analyst for the Energy Conservation Coalition. "We have tax incentives that encourage employers to subsidize parking costs for their employees but not to subsidize their use of mass transit."

Soon the world will have no choice about find-

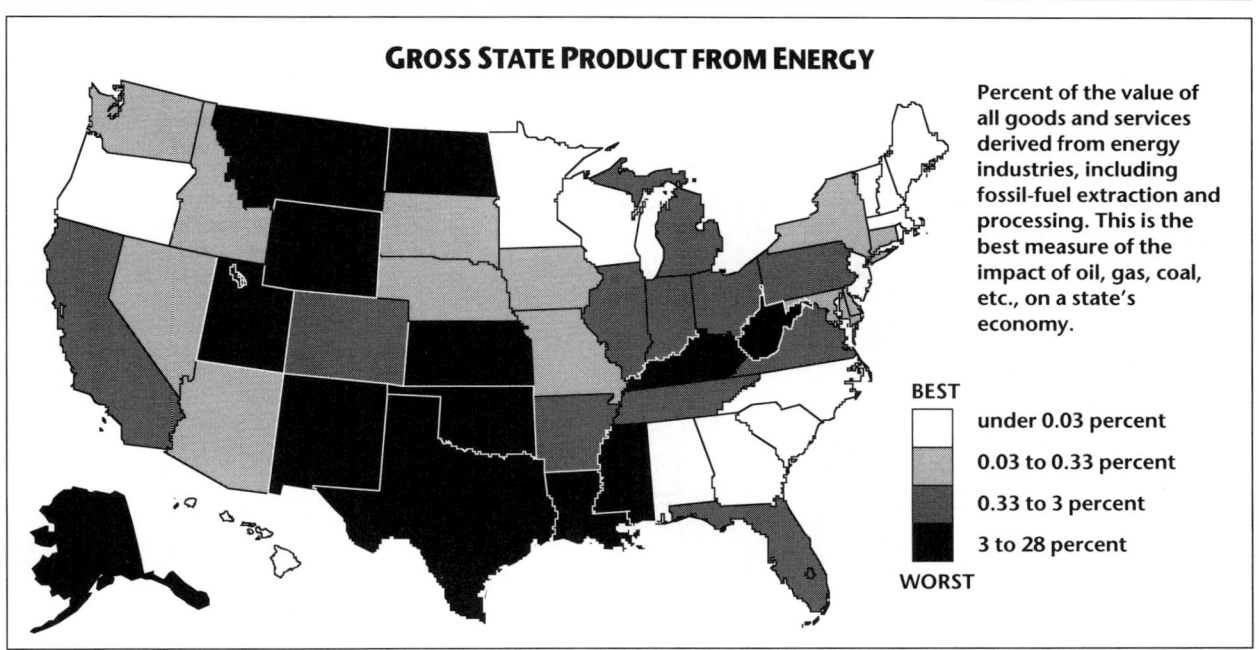

GROSS STATE PRODUCT FROM ENERGY

Percent of the value of all goods and services derived from energy industries, including fossil-fuel extraction and processing. This is the best measure of the impact of oil, gas, coal, etc., on a state's economy.

BEST
- under 0.03 percent
- 0.03 to 0.33 percent
- 0.33 to 3 percent
- 3 to 28 percent

WORST

ing alternatives. Global reserves of oil are expected to last only 30 more years and natural gas supplies may last only 60 years.

THE ENERGY BUSINESS

Energy is big business in the United States — 33 of the 50 states produce oil and/or gas. Alaska, Wyoming, and Louisiana are the most heavily dependent on fossil-fuel production to drive their economies, with each deriving over 20 percent of their gross state product from energy industries. Alaska nudges out Texas as the nation's top domestic source of crude oil, while every one of Louisiana's 64 parishes (counties) yields oil or, more commonly, natural gas. Texas, dependent on energy production for almost 13 percent of its gross state product, sells a larger combined volume of oil and gas than any other state.

These big fossil-fuel producing states — Alaska, Louisiana, Texas, Wyoming — are also the four biggest per-capita consumers of energy. Oklahoma, Montana, North Dakota, West Virginia, and Kansas are five more states that rank among the dozen biggest energy consumers and producers, reflecting the fact that the energy business feeds on itself and attracts big users of its products, such as chemical manufacturers. Pollution also comes with the business. For example, with the exception of Alaska, all nine of these major energy producer/consumer states rank among the dozen biggest producers of global-warming carbon emissions per dollar of gross economic output.

Oil spills are the most visible polluting byproduct of oil production. The Wilderness Society documented 10,000 spills in the United States during the year following the *Exxon Valdez* disaster. Most of the petroleum in our coastal waters comes from normal drilling operations at a rate of about 1 ton for every 1,000 tons produced. For the years 1984 through 1986, the Coast Guard says Louisiana led the nation in oil and other hazardous spills into navigable waters. In May 1990, another 38,000 gallons of oil leaked into the state's coastal waters, this time from an off-shore Texaco rig.

Citizens are working hard to guard their coastlines from spills. California officials have stopped transport of oil from wells near Santa Barbara; an Alabama district attorney has sued Shell for dumping drilling waste into the Gulf of Mexico; and North Carolinians have insisted on extensive studies before allowing Mobil Oil to begin exploratory drilling 35 miles off the Outer Banks. Congress has also begun to respond by declaring temporary drilling moratoriums for some states, including Florida, California, and Alaska.

Besides causing spills, oil and natural gas drilling disturbs delicate ecosystems and produces toxin-contaminated wastes. The toxic sludge is left in unlined pits where it can leach into water supplies. Kansas, a significant oil producer despite its Farmbelt stereotype, is the only state to require lined pits for such waste. Oil and gas injection wells can also pollute groundwater, and pipelines carrying gaseous or liquid fuel often fail to meet

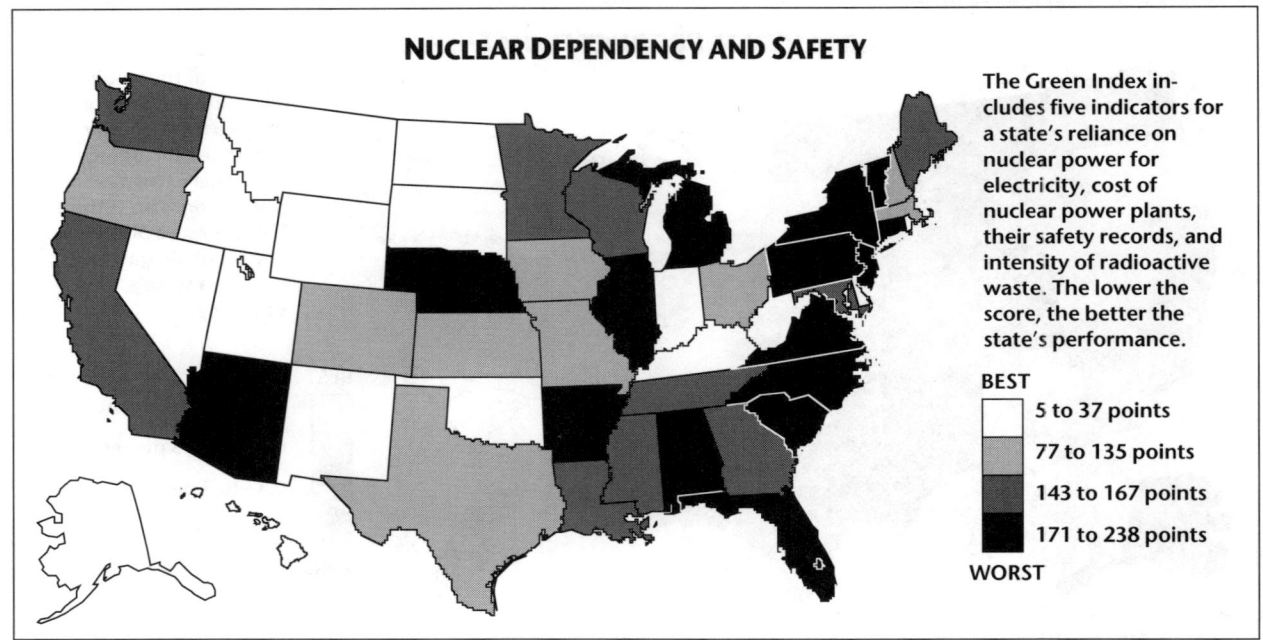

federal safety standards. On a per-capita basis, Arizona leads the nation in pipeline violations and Wyoming leads in injection wells. But in absolute numbers, Texas has more pipelines in noncompliance (nearly 5,000) and more oil and gas injection wells (almost 50,000) than any other state. The Lone Star state also leads the nation in total carbon dioxide emissions, the global-warming gas that results from burning fossil fuels.

Coal, the dirtiest and most abundant of the fossil fuels, fires the boilers producing 60 percent of the nation's electricity. The fuel is extracted either by underground mining, which puts workers at high risk for lung disease and accidents, or by strip mining, which leaves land barren and leads to erosion as well as sediment-filled rivers and streams. When coal is burned, it yields sulfur dioxide and nitrogen oxides that cause acid rain, along with carbon dioxide that warms the Earth.

Wyoming now leads in coal output, reflecting the rapid expansion of mining in the Rocky Mountains and Southwest following the oil embargo. The next two producers — Kentucky and West Virginia — are Appalachia's traditional leaders, although their increasing shift to machine-intensive stripmining has left tens of thousands of miners jobless. All three states rank among the worst 10 for carbon emissions, occupational deaths, and high-risk jobs. They also host some of the nation's dirtiest, most coal-dependent utilities, which put the states in the worst 10 for emissions of sulfur dioxide and carbon dioxide. Other big coal states, such as Pennsylvania, Illinois, North Dakota, Ohio, and Alabama, show similarly poor rankings for dangerous jobs, dangerous emissions, or both.

NUCLEAR COSTS

Nuclear energy, which accounts for 14 percent of the nation's electric capacity, has been lauded by industry representatives as a cheap, clean alternative to fossil-fuel powered plants. But as people learn more about the life-threatening nature of its radioactive byproducts, they have pressured legislators to block siting of nuclear plants or require expensive safety features that make their construction less attractive to utilities.

One of the least discussed issues is the cost of safely securing or disposing of the tons of material in a power plant once its useful life ends. Electric utilities put the price tag for "decommissioning" their 124 nuclear plants at over $25 billion, but they have collected less than one-seventh of that amount. As a consequence, states that depend heavily on nuclear power, including Nebraska, Arizona, Illinois, and several others in New England and the Southeast, face a mothballing charge of $200 or more per resident. Since a fail-safe method for disposing high-level radioactive waste still eludes us, the cost will likely be much greater.

While the plants operate, accidents are a daily occurrence. In 1987, nuclear plants in the U.S. re-

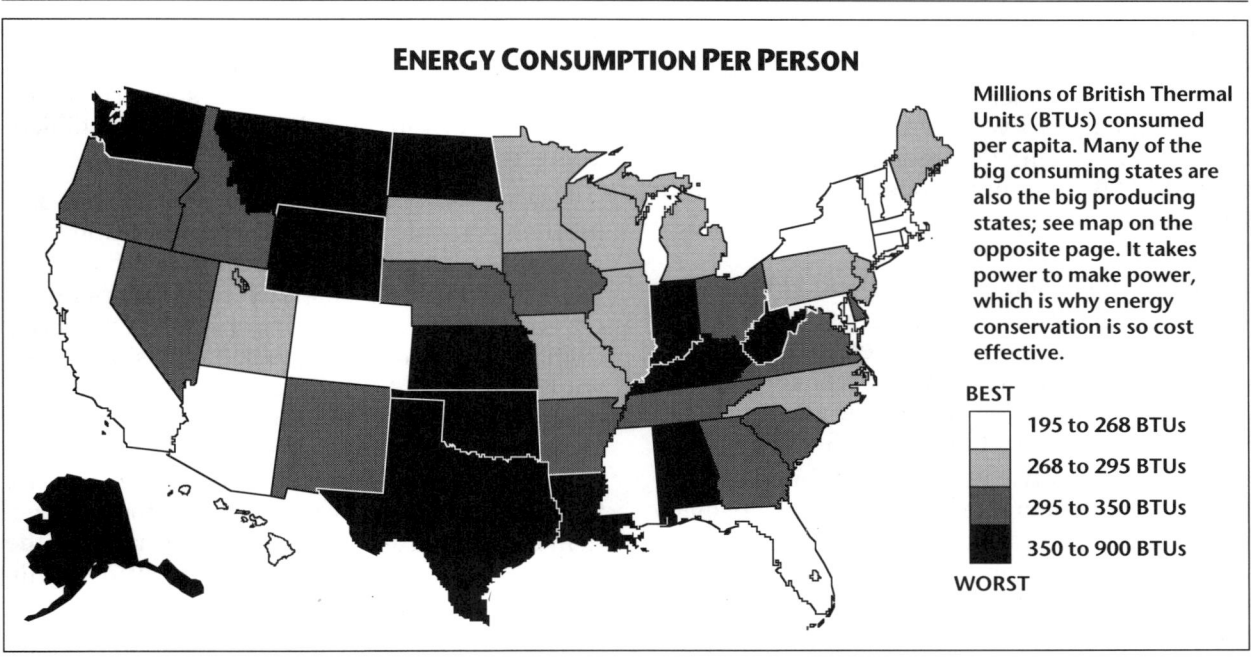

ported 3,000 mishaps, over 400 emergency shutdowns, and 104,000 incidents where workers were exposed to radiation. One two-millionth of a curie (a measure of radioactivity) of plutonium can cause lung cancer, yet the United States produces waste which radiates 11.2 billion curies each year. Ninety-three percent of the radwaste comes from nuclear power plants. Even at low levels, radiation can cause cancer, sterility, cataracts, premature aging, and genetic mutations. Studies have linked above-normal rates of leukemia and other cancers to radiation leaks from upwind nuclear power plants in Pennsylvania, Massachusetts, and Oregon (sites of the Three Mile Island, Pilgrim, and Trojan reactors), as well as in Illinois and South Carolina, the two states with the most Nuclear Regulatory Commission violations.

Radioactive waste is shipped to a few central repositories, and more storage or treatment sites are planned as part of various multi-state compacts. South Carolina, home of seven nuclear power plants and the Savannah River complex that makes components for nuclear weapons, ranks 49th in curies of radioactivity generated. The federal government wants to convert the 34 million gallons of radioactive waste stored at Savannah River into glass logs that can later be shipped to the planned high-level waste repository in the West. Cross-country transport is just part of the problem. Leaks have already contaminated parts of the Savannah River site, and workers continually report unsafe conditions. Nevertheless, the government has decided to expand operations to replace contaminated sites at the Hanford Reservation in Washington and the Rocky Flats Plant in Colorado.

South Carolina is also home to the Barnwell repository, the nation's largest low-level radioactive waste disposal site. Three similar sites — in West Valley, New York; Maxey Flats, Kentucky; and Sheffield, Illinois — have closed because radioactive elements were discovered in soil where the waste was buried.

Illinois is a perfect example of the mounting problems and price of nuclear power. It leads the nation in the potency of its accumulated radioactive waste and in the number of safety violations at its nuclear power plants. It also has the worst mix of making electricity from nuclear and fossil fuels, rather than renewable sources. The bottom line: Residential customers in Illinois pay 30 percent more per kilowatt hour than the national average (only New Jersey utilities charge more) and 88 percent more than what industrial customers pay (the gap is larger in only New York and Ohio).

POWER PEAKS

Nuclear power is also amazingly unreliable. In 1989, two out of every five nuclear plants produced less than 60 percent of their boilerplate capacity. Customers wind up paying for power plants that don't work. For some people, the increasing price of electricity means they must survive without it. In nuclear-rich Illinois, for example, 73,000 Chicagoans went without electricity in a typical year during the mid-1980s. At the same time, 40,000 people in Houston and 80,000 in Florida lost their power because they couldn't afford the bill.

Interestingly, Illinois, Texas, and Florida rank near or at the bottom in the percent of their low-income homes that are weatherized to conserve energy bills. By contrast, utility shareholders earned almost twice as much as the average industrial stockholder between 1980 and 1985.

Although electric utilities must build generators to meet their customers' peak demand, many build power plants that far exceed need. Since 1975, the United States has had over 40 percent excess electric-generating capacity, at a cost of more than $9 billion to ratepayers. Iowa, which scores poorly on per-capita energy consumption and utility emissions, is homebase for the utility with the highest reserve margin (generating capacity beyond what is needed for peak use). Iowa Public Service capacity exceeds peak demand by 112 percent and creates excess costs of $198 per customer annually, according to Environmental Action's 1986 study "Gambling for Gigabucks."

Many excess generators have avoided state regulation through multi-state contracts that place them under the jurisdiction of the Federal Regulatory Commission, which is more friendly to new plant construction. Some states, however, are forcing the utilities to slow down. State regulators rejected substantial portions of rate hikes designed to pay for the Wolf Creek nuclear plant in Kansas, the Susquehanna 2 nuclear plant in Pennsylvania, and the Valmy 2 plant in Idaho.

In Alaska, the federal government is making it easy for utilities to install excess capacity, even though the state's per-capita consumption of energy is the highest in the country and its use of renewables is among the lowest (rank 40). With federal aid, a group of politicians, utilities, unions, and Alaska's only commercial coal company plan to build a controversial coal-powered utility. The plant will cost $161 million to build, will not be needed for 5 to 10 years, and will raise the overall price of electricity by replacing cheaper natural gas power. Proponents see the plant as a way to diversify the energy base and give inland areas their own power source; but when opponents say the plant is "economically absurd," supporters almost agree. "If the feds hadn't come in with $93 million like Santa Claus," says Bob LeResche, director of the Alaska Energy Authority and a supporter of the plant, "nobody in their right mind would think of doing this."

Large utilities also use their political ties and lobbying muscle to minimize competition from suppliers who sell electricity at lower cost. One such battle in New Jersey pits independent cogenerators against Public Service Electric & Gas Company. Cogeneration, which yields both electricity and heat from burning a single fuel, is a cheaper, more efficient means of producing energy. Although PSE&G has supplemented its own power generation in the past with cogenerators, the utility is now losing customers to the independent companies and is attempting to undercut the competition by lobbying against existing tax incentives for cogenerators.

Some states, recognizing the need to regulate utility costs, have developed least-cost planning strategies. These programs require utilities to submit plans outlining ways to meet demand at the lowest feasible cost, through increased efficiency, load management, conservation measures, cogeneration, and/or renewable sources. To date, the New England states have the best existing least-cost energy programs. Massachusetts, for example, mandates open hearings for evaluating a utility's plan and authorizes an Energy Facilities Siting Council to review options before certifying new plant construction.

ENERGY GUZZLERS

The price of oil is lower in the United States than elsewhere because of government subsidies. If we paid the full price of extracting, importing, refining, and cleaning up after oil, the bill would probably exceed $4 a gallon. For example, the United States spent $47 billion in 1987 to provide military protection to petroleum interests in the Persian Gulf. And that figure pales in comparison to the investment made following Iraq's invasion of Kuwait in August 1990.

Forcing consumers to pay the full price for gasoline and electricity may be the last, best hope for the environment — that is, if such an approach leads to conservation rather than simply fueling America's sense that the world's resources should be under its control. The energy consumption indicators reveal how conservation took hold after the 1973 oil embargo. Nationally, per-capita consump-

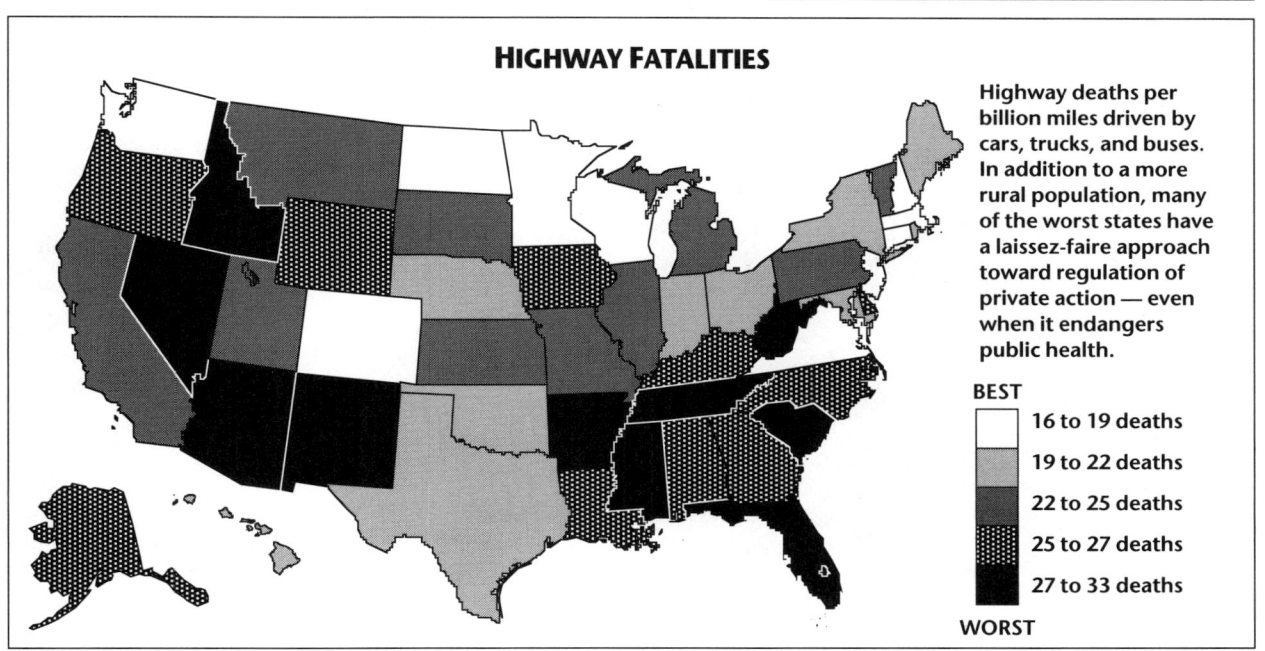

HIGHWAY FATALITIES

Highway deaths per billion miles driven by cars, trucks, and buses. In addition to a more rural population, many of the worst states have a laissez-faire approach toward regulation of private action — even when it endangers public health.

BEST
- 16 to 19 deaths
- 19 to 22 deaths
- 22 to 25 deaths
- 25 to 27 deaths
- 27 to 33 deaths

WORST

tion jumped 37 percent between 1960 and 1975, but actually declined by 5 percent between 1975 and 1987.

The reversal in energy consumption growth rates is most dramatic in several low population states (Mississippi, Arkansas, Utah, Idaho, Nebraska, Hawaii) where conservation measures by industrial and other big energy users showed quick results. Many of the high-density, economically diversified states had relatively slow growth rates in per-capita consumption before the embargo and tightened even further to achieve negative growth between 1975 and 1987. These states include New York, California, Pennsylvania, Massachusetts, Rhode Island, Ohio, and Connecticut. The notable exceptions among this group are chemical-intensive New Jersey, Maryland, and Delaware; each ranked among the best 10 before the embargo but among the worst 10 afterwards. Energy producing states and several in the fast-growing South (Georgia, Virginia, North and South Carolina) posted the biggest jumps in per-capita consumption during both periods.

Almost half of the energy consumed comes from petroleum (42 percent), and half of that is pumped into cars, buses, and trucks. Our addiction to the automobile is as strong as ever. Americans now own a third of the world's cars and drive as many miles as the rest of world combined. In fact, American cars and trucks cover more than two trillion miles a year, the equivalent of a trip to Pluto and back every day. And while French and Italian drivers get 34 miles per gallon of gas, we manage barely 18. Wyoming, Nevada, North Dakota, Iowa, Kansas, Nebraska, and Kentucky, all sizable states with dispersed populations, rank in the bottom dozen in both per-capita gasoline consumption and miles-per-gallon efficiency.

Kentucky has the same people-to-vehicles ratio as Maryland and California (4 to 3), but its cars and trucks burn about 50 percent more gas per unit per year, ranking the Bluegrass State last in per-capita gas use. Wyoming depends on trucking and vehicle manufacturing for more of its jobs than any other state, even Michigan; it also ranks last in people per vehicles (1 to 1), last in support for public transportation, and 49th on the miles-per-gallon efficiency indicator.

Detroit's automakers improved fuel efficiency in cars following the gas crunch of the 1970s, but they have balked at implementing the radical changes needed. While Renault and Volvo have developed cars that get over 60 miles per gallon, most U.S. manufacturers aggressively market their low-efficiency vehicles, arguing that consumers want and need size, horsepower, and luxury more than high gas mileage.

"Cars rated at 40 mpg or better are now available but attract less than 3 percent of the U.S. sales," argues Thomas Hannan, president of the Motor Vehicle Manufacturers Association. "The only way for a manufacturer to reach a 40-plus cor-

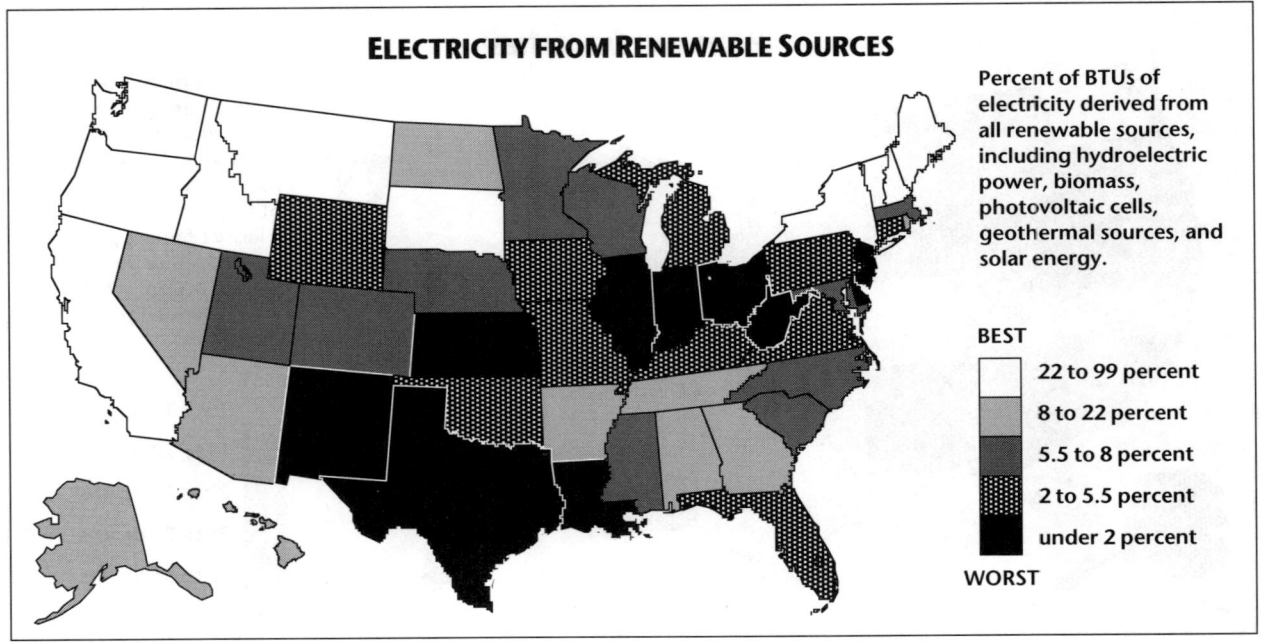

ELECTRICITY FROM RENEWABLE SOURCES

Percent of BTUs of electricity derived from all renewable sources, including hydroelectric power, biomass, photovoltaic cells, geothermal sources, and solar energy.

BEST
- 22 to 99 percent
- 8 to 22 percent
- 5.5 to 8 percent
- 2 to 5.5 percent
- under 2 percent

WORST

porate average is to slash the size and selection of its vehicles. The availability of full- and mid-size vans and pick-up trucks — the backbone of small businesses and farms because of their cargo capacity — would be seriously reduced, while the family vehicle would be limited chiefly to compact and subcompact cars."

AUTO GLUT

The poorer, rural states tend to have fewer cars per people, but more highway fatalities per miles driven. For example, Arkansas follows New York with the fewest registered cars per capita (rank 2), but its highway death rate is 32 percent above the U.S. average (rank 45). Interestingly, the dozen states with highest highway death rates are all in the Rocky Mountains or the South, the two regions known for lax regulations in general. When applied to highway safety, their laissez-faire philosophy leads directly to more fatalities.

Reflecting their low regard for public standards, 11 states from the same two regions, plus Kansas, contribute no state funds at all for public transportation. Several of the same rural states, along with others like Oklahoma and Maine, also have a low ratio of buses to cars; Arkansas ranks 50th on this indicator of mass transit use. By contrast, many of the states making the strongest commitments to public transit also enjoy the best records for fuel efficiency and highway deaths. These states include New York, Massachusetts, Maryland, Connecticut, Hawaii, Washington, Wisconsin, Michigan, Minnesota, and California.

California has earned the reputation as the nation's worst auto polluter for good reason. Los Angeles alone violated EPA ozone standards an average of 137.5 days per year between 1987 and 1989. That record compares with 17.4 days in violation for New York, 13 for Chicago, and 10 for Boston. Several booming metropolitan areas in the South are also emerging as pollution zones. Houston, Raleigh, and Atlanta have repeatedly exceeded national air quality standards. Florida's per-capita carbon emissions doubled between 1966 and 1986, and Georgia's increased even more, ranking the two states 44th and 45th on this indicator of fossil-fuel pollutants.

Halting the rising use of transportation fuels and their emissions requires tough policy initiatives, yet auto dependency remains highly subsidized by federal and state governments. Subsidies for the nation's 3,000,000 miles of paved roads, 40,000 miles of the interstate highway system, military escorts to the Persian Gulf, and work-related auto use amount to $300 billion, while public transit receives only $1.9 billion each year. Fuel taxes are one way to bring down gas use. Connecticut, one of the best states for fuel efficiency and one of the few to reduce carbon emissions in recent years, adds 20 cents to the federal tax for each gallon of gasoline.

Along with taxes, states are beginning to regulate fumes at the gas pump. Programs have been enacted in New Jersey and New England states requiring gas stations to install vapor-catching nozzles on pumps. Michael J. Bradley, executive director of the Northeast States for Coordinated Air Use Management, says the nozzles can reduce hydrocarbon emissions — "one of the few sizable uncontrolled sources out there" — by 3 to 5 percent. Station owners, oil industry representatives, and some legislators are campaigning against the nozzles, saying the fixtures are expensive and unnecessary. Even Vermont's Senator James Jeffords, usually a friend of environmental legislation, proposed an amendment to the 1990 Clean Air Act that would exempt Vermont from having to install the new equipment on the grounds that the state's low level of ozone pollution didn't justify its expense.

More radical options include new automobile technology and mass transit. New engine and transmissions designs, weight reduction, aerodynamic changes, and energy storage devices have already been developed by major auto manufacturers and have the potential for dramatically reducing emissions and improving mileage. Improved public transportation is an even better alternative. Rural states from Wyoming to Vermont rank lowest on mass transit, while highly urbanized New York ranks first. After a major cleanup and investment in new trains, ridership on Manhattan's subways leaped 61 percent between 1982 and 1989.

"The greatest potential for reducing smog lies in providing people with first-class options for getting around," says Sierra Club Transportation Chair Ken Ryan. San Francisco, Boston, Pittsburgh, Atlanta, Washington, Buffalo, Portland, Sacramento, and San Diego have all recently begun or expanded their commuter train systems, but big spending for highways remains the norm. Thirty-seven state governments even spend more on roads than they bring in from gasoline and vehicle-related taxes. Thirty-one put less than $3 into public transit for every $100 spent on highways.

SUSTAINABLE ENERGY

Alternatives to fossil-fuel use are often seen as esoteric, expensive, and impractical. But hydroelectric and geothermal power already account for 21 percent of the world's electricity. Other renewable energy sources, including biomass, solar, wind, and ocean power, are also on the rise. According to Public Citizen's report, "The Power of the States," renewables now provide 13 percent of the nation's electricity and 10 percent of all energy needs. If the price of power included each energy source's full social and environmental impact (its life-cycle cost), then renewables would easily win the price battle over fossil or nuclear fuels and supply more of our energy needs.

Falling water, or hydropower, has long established itself as an inexpensive, reliable source for baseload and peak capacity, and it still accounts for four-fifths of the electricity generated by renewables. The biggest concentration of hydropower projects is in the Pacific Northwest, led by Washington. The state's Grand Coulee Dam can provide massive amounts of electricity — 6,180 megawatts — cheaply, with no carbon or sulfur dioxide emissions. Construction of huge dams like the Grand Coulee can have a harmful effect on aquatic life, but smaller dams offer a clean, low-impact supplement or alternative to fossil-fuel driven plants. In New England, for example, over 1,700 aging or unused dams could be renovated to provide energy. Hydropower projects are currently being slowed, however, by regulations protecting rivers from development and by concerns about the dams' ecological impact.

Big forest-products states, like Georgia, Tennessee, and Oregon, score well on the renewable energy indicators because paper and lumber producers have learned to use wood waste (biomass) as a fuel in their manufacturing processes. Weyerhaeuser and Scott Paper, for example, now satisfy the majority of their energy needs — including heating for buildings — by burning tons of their waste. In fact, Scott Paper gets so much power from its bark-fueled 100-megawatt plant in Mobile that it sells the excess to the Alabama Power Company. In Maine, where non-hydro renewables furnish the largest share of any state's electricity, nine biomass power plants have a combined capacity of 225 megawatts.

Hawaii's vast sugar plantations generate electricity from crushed cane stalks and sell their surplus power to utilities. With the addition of its solar collectors and the world's largest wind-driven turbine, the state ranks third best in non-hydro renewables and fifth overall. Florida scores well on both lists because it leads the nation in turning municipal waste into energy. Just as Hawaii has experimented with wind power to overcome the island's vulnerable dependency on imported oil, so Florida has pursued garbage-to-energy incinerators in response to its specific geological and environmental character. The Sunshine state's shallow water table makes siting landfills for its booming population nearly impossible. But unlike the windmill, the biomass-incinerator solution is causing increasing concern because its pollution creates a new generation of problems (see page 71).

Hydropower and biomass account for 50 percent and 45 percent of all renewable energy sources. Geothermal power adds only 3.7 percent, but that is enough to make the United States the world's leader in producing energy from the steam and hot water below the Earth's crust. Geothermal plants presently provide electricity for three million households in California, mostly drawing on the natural steam of The Geysers north of San Francisco. A new geothermal project in southern California's Mojave Desert could produce 240 megawatts of electricity for Southern California Edison customers. But problems remain with several such large-scale projects in California, including water pollution and well blowouts.

California is by far the nation's leader in developing renewable energy sources other than hydropower. Much of the credit goes to former Governor Jerry Brown, who responded to the oil embargo, lack of in-state coal, and legal restrictions against nuclear power with a package of incentives to promote renewable energy. Chief among these incentives were tax credits, research grants, and a provision that gave independent energy producers better leverage in selling their power to the state's big utilities. Even private developers of geothermal power in Nevada have used this provision to sell their capacity to California-based utilities that serve the Sagebrush state. Inside California, innovators of photovoltaic cells, solar power, and wind energy have relied on these long-term contracts to finance a multiplicity of projects.

A favorable contract with Utah Power & Light (UP&L) allowed a private developer of geothermal power to build a 25.5 megawatt generator. The plant supplies Utah with less than 1 percent of its electricity, but that's enough to make the state the nation's third biggest user of this energy source. A vast geothermal resource remains untapped in Utah, reinforcing UP&L's dependence on the locally produced, relatively low-sulfur coal.

The two states with the least energy derived from renewables are Texas, home of Big Oil, and Kansas, a surprisingly large producer (and consumer) of oil and natural gas. Kansas ranks 40th in the percent of its gross state product derived from energy resource development, 38th in per-capita carbon dioxide emissions, and 43d in per-capita energy consumption. Other states lagging way behind in the development of renewables include Missouri, Indiana, Illinois, and New Jersey — all big consumers of fossil and/or nuclear fuels. Without aggressive development of sustainable energy — from passive solar buildings to tidal power turbines — the sinister web of dependency, pollution, and, inevitably, militarism will continue.

ENERGY PRODUCTION

State	COAL PRODUCTION Million Tons	Rank	OIL PRODUCTION Million Barrels	Rank	NATURAL GAS PRODUCTION Billion Barrels	Rank	GROSS STATE PRODUCT FROM ENERGY %	Rank	PIPELINES IN NON-COMPLIANCE #	Rank	OIL SPILLS IN STATE WATERS 1,000 Gals.	Rank	OIL & GAS INJECTION WELLS #	Rank
Alabama	26.4	39	20.8	35	175.1	37	2.56	36	157	30	39	11	206	24
Alaska	1.7	28	738.1	50	1,933.0	47	30.31	50	na		408	49	266	39
Arizona	12.4	35	0.1	21	0.2	21	0.33	25	3,215	48	>1	3	413	27
Arkansas	0.3	25	13.6	34	190.7	39	2.08	35	186	40	1,240	47	1,128	38
California	0.1	24	354.7	48	451.9	43	1.29	33	220	13	2,355	29	11,201	37
Colorado	15.9	36	32.4	40	212.0	40	2.86	37	85	25	828	40	932	30
Connecticut	0.0	1	0.0	1	0.0	1	0.06	16	227	38	26	9	0	1
Delaware	0.0	1	0.0	1	0.0	1	0.10	19	0	1	29	24	0	1
Florida	0.0	1	7.7	32	8.4	28	0.60	29	244	23	240	14	77	22
Georgia	0.0	1	0.0	1	0.0	1	0.02	10	42	12	519	28	0	1
Hawaii	0.0	1	0.0	1	0.0	1	0.01	9	3	8	165	36	0	1
Idaho	0.0	1	0.0	1	0.0	1	0.10	20	na		>1	5	0	1
Illinois	58.6	46	22.5	36	1.3	24	0.80	30	28	6	806	26	14,147	43
Indiana	31.2	41	3.7	29	0.4	22	0.55	28	18	9	100	13	3,274	40
Iowa	0.3	26	0.0	1	0.0	1	0.03	14	150	34	398	35	0	1
Kansas	0.7	27	58.8	43	577.8	44	3.73	40	269	41	519	38	14,009	48
Kentucky	156.7	49	5.5	30	73.6	33	6.33	41	262	37	145	21	5,399	44
Louisiana	2.9	30	165.0	47	5,248.2	49	21.94	48	648	45	11,641	50	4,212	42
Maine	0.0	1	0.0	1	0.0	1	0.01	6	3	7	43	20	0	1
Maryland	3.2	31	0.0	1	>0.1	20	0.08	18	3	3	102	15	0	1
Massachusetts	0.0	1	0.0	1	0.0	1	0.00	1	57	17	252	23	0	1
Michigan	0.0	1	23.3	37	151.8	34	0.48	27	32	10	268	17	1,631	28
Minnesota	0.0	1	0.0	1	0.0	1	0.02	11	199	32	98	16	0	1
Mississippi	0.0	1	27.6	39	237.2	41	3.59	39	184	36	79	18	936	31
Missouri	4.2	32	0.2	22	>0.1	19	0.11	21	157	28	502	31	275	25
Montana	38.9	43	23.3	38	53.0	31	7.15	42	39	33	6	8	1,449	45
Nebraska	0.0	1	6.0	31	0.9	23	0.28	24	2	4	67	22	624	33
Nevada	0.0	1	3.2	28	0.0	1	0.21	23	73	39	>1	2	8	23
New Hampshire	0.0	1	0.0	1	0.0	1	0.01	7	35	29	1	6	0	1
New Jersey	0.0	1	0.0	1	0.0	1	0.01	8	11	5	927	33	0	1
New Mexico	21.8	38	71.2	44	812.0	46	16.38	47	345	46	0	1	3,913	46
New York	0.0	1	0.6	23	27.5	30	0.07	17	307	20	7,352	45	3,254	29
North Carolina	0.0	1	0.0	1	0.0	1	0.01	4	62	16	747	32	0	1
North Dakota	29.7	40	39.3	42	66.3	32	8.27	43	47	35	91	34	595	41
Ohio	33.8	42	11.7	33	166.7	35	0.87	31	103	15	3,012	43	3,952	32
Oklahoma	2.1	29	128.9	46	2,106.6	48	13.84	45	30	14	859	41	22,579	49
Oregon	0.0	1	0.0	1	4.0	26	0.02	13	55	22	1,846	48	1	20
Pennsylvania	69.6	47	2.8	27	167.1	36	1.26	32	63	11	703	25	4,788	36
Rhode Island	0.0	1	0.0	1	0.0	1	0.02	12	10	18	157	37	0	1
South Carolina	0.0	1	0.0	1	0.0	1	0.01	3	91	26	32	10	0	1
South Dakota	0.0	1	1.7	25	4.3	27	0.14	22	0	1	9	12	40	26
Tennessee	6.4	34	0.6	24	2.1	25	0.39	26	85	21	1,568	44	9	21
Texas	52.3	45	735.5	49	6,918.6	50	12.86	44	4,927	47	4,424	42	49,476	47
Utah	18.2	37	33.0	41	277.9	42	3.14	38	232	44	56	19	664	34
Vermont	0.0	1	0.0	1	0.0	1	0.01	2	74	43	>1	4	0	1
Virginia	45.5	44	>0.1	20	18.7	29	1.34	34	88	19	1,406	39	0	1
Washington	5.2	33	0.0	1	0.0	1	0.06	15	103	24	338	27	0	1
West Virginia	144.4	48	2.6	26	182.0	38	14.83	46	56	27	180	30	760	35
Wisconsin	0.0	1	0.0	1	0.0	1	0.01	5	205	31	15	7	0	1
Wyoming	164.0	50	114.0	45	810.8	45	28.04	49	58	42	227	46	5,749	50
U.S. Total	946.5		2,648.3		20,880.2				13,490		44,824		155,967	

ENERGY USE

State	GROWTH OF CARBON EMISS. 1966-86 %	Rank	CARBON EMISSIONS Per $ GSP Tons	Rank	PER CAPITA ENERGY CONSUMP. Million BTUs	Rank	GROWTH IN PER CAPITA ENERGY CONSUMPTION 1960 to '75 %	Rank	1975 to '87 %	Rank	ENERGY GROWTH VS. POPULATION GROWTH Ratio	Rank	LOW-INCOME HOMES WEATHERIZED %	Rank
Alabama	25.6	19	527	44	381.3	40	63.4	42	-7.0	26	3.6	41	10.2	42
Alaska	321.2	50	407	35	899.0	50	141.7	50	39.6	50	5.2	46	36.5	9
Arizona	178.2	46	285	20	251.3	10	46.2	25	-17.1	6	1.3	8	9.7	43
Arkansas	89.9	42	462	40	297.3	26	70.2	46	-19.3	3	2.5	25	17.6	25
California	18.9	17	160	5	246.1	9	28.3	13	-9.7	18	1.4	9	8.4	46
Colorado	71.3	36	279	19	267.9	13	38.0	18	-18.1	4	1.3	6	36.1	10
Connecticut	-16.3	2	147	2	227.0	5	18.0	4	-1.3	36	1.8	12	12.4	38
Delaware	25.6	20	385	33	344.7	36	6.5	2	1.8	41	1.3	5	16.6	29
Florida	109.5	44	345	28	231.2	8	51.2	33	-1.0	38	1.9	14	2.2	50
Georgia	130.4	45	245	16	309.1	27	85.7	48	5.2	44	3.6	40	9.3	44
Hawaii	55.5	31	228	13	217.0	3	67.8	44	-15.2	10	2.0	17	12.9	37
Idaho	6.2	12	207	10	338.7	35	68.5	45	-25.0	2	1.8	13	53.2	4
Illinois	-11.0	5	263	18	290.0	23	38.9	20	-15.3	9	2.4	22	12.9	36
Indiana	16.1	16	579	46	429.0	45	40.4	23	-5.5	29	3.1	33	17.0	27
Iowa	27.9	21	366	30	309.5	28	58.1	38	-9.5	20	16.7	49	24.4	16
Kansas	46.8	27	429	38	407.9	44	39.3	22	1.3	40	4.5	43	14.7	32
Kentucky	64.3	35	565	45	356.9	38	39.0	21	-2.8	32	2.9	29	16.9	28
Louisiana	77.4	37	695	47	764.4	49	61.8	41	4.9	43	3.6	39	4.9	48
Maine	28.4	22	256	17	277.2	15	47.8	28	-6.6	27	3.1	34	48.3	5
Maryland	-1.8	7	230	14	265.7	12	21.0	7	2.6	42	1.8	11	14.1	33
Massachusetts	-5.6	6	188	7	225.3	4	25.3	10	-8.6	21	2.2	20	55.2	3
Michigan	-0.5	9	308	25	280.7	17	35.0	16	-10.6	17	2.4	24	17.0	26
Minnesota	7.6	14	235	15	284.5	20	57.6	37	-11.7	14	3.0	32	38.5	8
Mississippi	79.4	41	424	37	262.5	11	95.3	49	-17.3	5	4.6	44	13.4	35
Missouri	46.7	26	329	26	283.2	18	48.3	30	-4.7	31	3.7	42	18.9	23
Montana	90.4	43	520	43	396.8	43	38.4	19	-11.6	15	2.4	23	65.8	1
Nebraska	29.4	24	300	23	311.2	29	64.3	43	-12.2	13	5.0	45	20.5	21
Nevada	258.9	49	373	31	334.7	33	34.9	15	-17.0	7	1.2	4	10.3	41
New Hampshire	53.0	29	193	8	229.9	7	47.9	29	-6.2	28	1.9	15	26.6	13
New Jersey	-1.6	8	202	9	293.5	24	20.8	6	15.5	48	2.9	30	10.4	40
New Mexico	78.5	39	509	41	334.0	32	18.9	5	-16.4	8	1.0	3	19.6	22
New York	-29.3	1	137	1	195.0	1	26.9	12	-11.6	16	3.2	35	59.4	2
North Carolina	43.0	25	295	22	286.3	21	60.9	40	7.9	45	3.6	38	7.7	47
North Dakota	218.7	47	968	48	458.3	46	48.7	31	30.9	49	17.7	50	47.2	6
Ohio	0.3	10	382	32	338.1	34	21.4	8	-8.4	22	2.1	18	23.1	18
Oklahoma	78.4	38	429	39	383.3	41	58.3	39	-1.2	37	3.0	31	10.9	39
Oregon	20.9	18	176	6	313.5	30	55.3	35	-13.8	11	2.0	16	25.0	14
Pennsylvania	-16.0	4	357	29	287.4	22	17.4	3	-13.6	12	1.3	7	29.9	12
Rhode Island	-16.0	3	159	4	211.0	2	6.3	1	-7.8	23	0.9	2	24.5	15
South Carolina	58.4	32	330	27	327.6	31	57.2	36	11.1	47	3.5	37	13.6	34
South Dakota	28.9	23	300	23	279.3	16	52.3	34	-2.0	34	14.4	48	30.2	11
Tennessee	54.5	30	397	34	348.7	37	46.2	26	-7.4	25	2.3	21	15.5	30
Texas	78.5	40	510	42	545.1	47	25.8	11	-5.0	30	1.5	10	4.3	49
Utah	61.4	34	412	36	283.9	19	24.2	9	-31.1	1	0.7	1	23.6	17
Vermont	3.1	11	152	3	228.1	6	49.0	32	-2.1	33	2.6	27	47.2	7
Virginia	8.7	15	224	12	297.3	25	35.4	17	10.5	46	2.5	26	8.7	45
Washington	60.7	33	209	11	376.6	39	47.1	27	-1.5	35	2.2	19	15.2	31
West Virginia	49.0	28	1,179	50	386.9	42	30.9	14	-9.5	19	9.0	47	18.6	24
Wisconsin	7.1	13	287	21	269.6	14	41.3	24	-7.5	24	2.7	28	22.4	19
Wyoming	235.2	48	996	49	763.3	48	80.2	47	-0.7	39	3.4	36	21.9	20
Total US	**27.6**				**313.2**		**37.0**		**-5.1**		**2.2**		**18.1**	

NUCLEAR POWER

State	% ELECTRIC CAPACITY IN NUCLEAR POWER	Rank	DECOMMISSION COST FOR NUKE PLANTS Total Mill.$	Per Capita Unpaid	Rank	CITATIONS AT NUCLEAR PLANTS #	Rank	LOW-LEVEL RAD. WASTE SENT FOR DISPOSAL Curies	% U.S. Total	Rank	TOTAL RADIOACTIVE WASTE IN STATE Million Curies	% U.S. Total	Rank	SUMMARY OF NUCLEAR INDICATORS Score	Rank
Alabama	25.7	43	1,102	209.63	45	121	48	979	0.4	28	972.0	5.2	45	209	44
Alaska	0.0	1	0	0.00	1	0	1	0	0.0	1	0.0	0.0	1	5	1
Arizona	25.4	42	523	205.80	44	70	39	976	0.4	27	44.0	0.2	19	171	36
Arkansas	17.7	37	485	185.39	42	86	43	1,529	0.6	32	425.7	2.3	34	188	39
California	12.6	29	1,891	44.12	18	67	37	29,461	10.9	46	548.5	2.9	37	167	35
Colorado	3.1	19	239	66.66	26	0	1	120	0.0	19	0.1	0.0	12	77	17
Connecticut	45.1	50	992	246.44	47	36	30	23,842	8.8	45	939.4	5.0	44	216	46
Delaware	0.0	1	0	0.00	1	0	1	1	0.0	8	0.0	0.0	1	12	5
Florida	11.4	26	1,048	65.70	25	105	46	2,757	1.0	38	1,158.3	6.1	47	182	37
Georgia	12.9	30	863	121.96	37	43	32	1,928	0.7	36	315.6	1.7	31	166	34
Hawaii	0.0	1	0	0.00	1	0	1	7	0.0	14	0.0	0.0	1	18	7
Idaho	0.0	1	0	0.00	1	0	1	4	0.0	12	66.3	0.4	21	36	15
Illinois	38.7	47	2,655	204.78	43	220	50	33,917	12.6	48	2,274.4	12.1	50	238	50
Indiana	0.0	1	0	0.00	1	0	1	35	0.0	16	0.0	0.0	1	20	10
Iowa	6.4	21	311	98.75	32	14	22	1,068	0.4	30	125.4	0.7	26	131	22
Kansas	11.9	27	248	95.40	30	33	29	119	0.0	18	62.1	0.3	20	124	21
Kentucky	0.0	1	0	0.00	1	0	1	40	0.0	17	1.2	0.0	17	37	16
Louisiana	11.9	28	487	108.46	35	64	34	522	0.2	24	75.1	0.4	22	143	26
Maine	35.8	46	206	136.90	40	19	24	229	0.1	20	418.9	2.2	33	163	32
Maryland	17.2	35	343	64.38	24	47	33	688	0.3	25	564.1	3.0	38	155	31
Massachusetts	8.5	24	366	49.51	21	12	21	1,724	0.6	34	320.2	1.7	32	132	23
Michigan	17.8	38	1,094	103.55	33	100	45	4,794	1.8	40	907.7	4.8	43	199	43
Minnesota	17.7	36	646	115.58	36	30	28	1,042	0.4	29	470.6	2.5	35	164	33
Mississippi	16.4	34	290	108.05	34	18	23	1,663	0.6	33	82.8	0.4	23	147	28
Missouri	7.5	22	193	33.32	16	3	18	310	0.1	22	107.4	0.6	24	102	19
Montana	0.0	1	0	0.00	1	0	1	<1	0.0	4	0.0	0.0	1	8	2
Nebraska	23.1	39	482	268.71	48	73	40	907	0.3	26	277.0	1.5	30	183	38
Nevada	0.0	1	0	0.00	1	0	1	<1	0.0	4	3.5	0.0	18	25	12
New Hampshire	0.0	1	273	246.34	46	6	19	3	0.0	11	0.0	0.0	1	78	18
New Jersey	28.6	45	607	71.07	28	66	36	35,940	13.3	49	571.4	3.0	39	197	42
New Mexico	0.0	1	0	0.00	1	0	1	1	0.0	8	1.2	0.0	16	27	13
New York	15.4	33	1,495	68.38	27	84	42	5,060	1.9	41	1,277.5	6.8	48	191	41
North Carolina	23.5	40	1,033	130.85	39	108	47	45,245	16.8	50	836.4	4.4	41	217	48
North Dakota	0.0	1	0	0.00	1	0	1	<1	0.0	4	0.0	0.0	1	8	2
Ohio	7.9	23	505	45.17	20	38	31	309	0.1	21	120.0	0.6	25	120	20
Oklahoma	0.0	1	0	0.00	1	0	1	13	0.0	15	0.0	0.0	1	19	8
Oregon	9.8	25	231	75.03	29	29	27	420	0.2	23	258.2	1.4	29	133	24
Pennsylvania	23.8	41	2,004	154.62	41	94	44	15,673	5.8	44	1,103.8	5.9	46	216	46
Rhode Island	0.0	1	0	0.00	1	0	1	4	0.0	12	0.0	0.0	1	16	6
South Carolina	42.8	48	1,253	324.77	49	128	49	3,286	1.2	39	1,954.1	10.4	49	234	49
South Dakota	0.0	1	25	34.97	17	0	1	0	0.0	1	0.0	0.0	11	31	14
Tennessee	13.5	31	375	55.81	22	65	35	1,984	0.7	37	207.9	1.1	27	152	30
Texas	2.1	18	1,044	61.20	23	68	38	7,028	2.6	42	0.0	0.0	14	135	25
Utah	0.0	1	0	0.00	1	0	1	1	0.0	8	0.0	0.0	13	24	11
Vermont	45.0	49	251	360.53	50	6	19	11,897	4.4	43	222.1	1.2	28	189	40
Virginia	26.5	44	903	128.88	38	78	41	31,042	11.5	47	907.4	4.8	42	212	45
Washington	4.6	20	467	96.71	31	26	26	1,097	0.4	31	526.8	2.8	36	144	27
West Virginia	0.0	1	0	0.00	1	0	1	<1	0.0	4	0.0	0.0	1	8	2
Wisconsin	14.0	32	464	45.11	19	19	24	1,885	0.7	35	701.9	3.7	40	150	29
Wyoming	0.0	1	0	0.00	1	0	1	0	0.0	1	0.0	0.0	15	19	8
U.S. Total	14.0		25,631	89.18		1,976		269,550			18,848.5				

ENERGY USE AND AUTO ABUSE

State	PRICE PER KWH Indus/Resid Ratio	Rank	% ELECTRIC CAPACITY BY FUEL Coal	Rank	Oil & Gas	Rank	Hydro or Other	Rank	GASOLINE USE PER CAPITA Gal.	Rank	MILES PER GALLON GAS CONSUMED Miles	Rank	HIGHWAY DEATHS PER BILLION MILES DRIVEN #	Rank
Alabama	68.0	18	56.2	35	2.5	5	15.6	17	604	40	16.1	17	25.8	34
Alaska	77.2	8	3.7	7	77.4	48	18.9	13	444	6	15.2	28	25.3	31
Arizona	60.0	36	33.0	21	23.3	30	18.4	14	482	16	17.4	4	27.6	41
Arkansas	63.5	27	40.0	23	29.2	32	13.1	20	530	26	12.0	50	31.7	45
California	80.4	4	0.0	1	54.6	42	32.8	7	477	15	16.9	7	22.3	23
Colorado	65.2	22	70.4	40	11.5	18	15.0	18	488	18	16.3	15	17.9	4
Connecticut	74.7	9	5.4	10	46.6	36	2.8	35	463	12	16.6	10	18.6	8
Delaware	57.6	44	52.1	28	47.9	38	0.0	50	535	29	16.4	13	25.6	33
Florida	65.2	23	30.4	16	56.6	45	1.6	38	499	20	16.1	16	29.4	43
Georgia	66.5	20	65.9	38	8.6	14	12.6	21	555	37	14.6	37	26.2	35
Hawaii	70.2	14	0.0	1	99.4	49	0.6	44	342	2	20.0	1	20.1	12
Idaho	54.4	46	0.0	1	2.6	6	97.4	1	519	24	15.1	29	31.6	44
Illinois	53.1	48	45.9	27	15.4	23	0.0	47	550	33	14.1	41	23.7	27
Indiana	59.3	38	94.5	48	5.1	12	0.4	45	616	42	15.6	22	21.6	18
Iowa	54.6	45	76.0	43	15.7	24	1.9	37	641	45	13.1	47	25.4	32
Kansas	64.0	25	52.7	29	35.4	33	0.0	48	584	39	13.6	46	22.8	25
Kentucky	84.3	2	92.0	46	2.7	7	5.3	28	681	50	13.6	45	26.6	36
Louisiana	58.6	41	19.8	15	67.1	47	1.2	41	475	13	14.8	31	26.6	37
Maine	61.5	34	0.0	1	47.8	37	16.4	16	552	34	15.4	24	21.6	17
Maryland	66.0	21	41.3	24	37.0	34	4.5	31	456	11	16.0	18	21.1	13
Massachusetts	80.2	5	17.7	13	53.9	41	19.9	10	435	5	15.8	21	16.9	1
Michigan	73.5	11	53.7	31	18.7	27	9.8	23	530	26	16.5	11	21.8	21
Minnesota	62.1	29	65.3	37	14.8	22	2.2	36	530	26	16.0	19	16.9	2
Mississippi	77.4	7	32.1	18	51.4	39	0.0	50	475	13	14.5	38	32.8	49
Missouri	67.3	19	70.9	41	14.6	21	7.1	26	542	32	14.2	40	24.2	29
Montana	58.6	42	45.6	26	2.4	4	51.9	5	554	36	15.4	25	24.3	30
Nebraska	64.7	24	53.3	30	20.5	28	3.1	34	665	49	14.3	39	21.7	20
Nevada	73.7	10	55.4	34	25.1	31	19.4	11	650	48	12.8	48	31.8	46
New Hampshire	71.0	13	43.0	25	37.6	35	19.4	12	485	17	16.7	9	17.1	3
New Jersey	69.2	16	12.2	11	55.9	44	3.3	33	450	9	15.2	27	17.9	5
New Mexico	58.9	39	75.7	42	23.1	29	1.2	42	627	43	15.2	26	31.9	47
New York	47.2	50	12.5	12	54.9	43	17.3	15	334	1	16.8	8	21.6	16
North Carolina	62.1	30	62.1	36	4.8	11	9.7	24	536	30	15.0	30	27.4	39
North Dakota	78.9	6	85.7	45	2.3	3	12.0	22	613	41	14.0	42	18.0	6
Ohio	53.0	49	85.2	44	5.8	13	1.1	43	556	38	14.6	36	21.3	14
Oklahoma	54.3	47	37.7	22	53.6	40	8.7	25	513	23	16.5	12	19.8	11
Oregon	69.9	15	4.7	8	4.0	10	81.4	3	499	20	15.5	23	26.9	38
Pennsylvania	63.6	26	54.0	32	16.2	25	6.1	27	399	3	14.7	33	23.8	28
Rhode Island	83.3	3	0.0	1	99.6	50	0.4	46	406	4	13.8	44	21.4	15
South Carolina	59.5	37	32.5	19	9.8	15	14.9	19	490	19	17.5	2	32.6	48
South Dakota	69.1	17	18.6	14	12.8	19	68.6	4	642	46	14.6	34	22.2	22
Tennessee	90.5	1	54.7	33	9.8	16	22.0	9	643	47	14.6	35	28.6	42
Texas	58.9	40	31.1	17	65.2	46	1.6	39	541	31	15.9	20	21.7	19
Utah	58.1	43	93.4	47	3.2	9	3.4	32	453	10	14.7	32	22.4	24
Vermont	72.3	12	0.0	1	10.3	17	44.6	6	528	25	17.1	6	23.1	26
Virginia	62.0	31	33.0	20	17.0	26	23.6	8	553	35	16.4	14	18.6	7
Washington	61.6	32	5.3	9	3.2	8	87.0	2	503	22	17.2	5	18.8	9
West Virginia	60.9	35	98.7	50	0.1	1	1.3	40	445	7	13.9	43	33.1	50
Wisconsin	61.6	33	68.0	39	12.8	20	5.2	29	445	7	17.4	3	19.1	10
Wyoming	62.2	28	95.2	49	0.3	2	4.5	30	631	44	12.8	49	27.4	40
U.S. Total	**65.7**		**43.5**		**28.6**		**14.0**		**502**		**15.6**		**24.1**	

ENERGY USE AND AUTO ABUSE 55

TRANSPORTATION

State	PERSONS PER MOTOR VEHICLE #	Rank	CARS PER TRANSIT BUSES #	Rank	DEPENDENCY ON VEHICLE AND RELATED INDUSTRIES for Jobs %	Rank	for Taxes %	Rank	HIGHWAY SPEND. AS % VEHICLE-RELATED REV. %	Rank	MASS TRANSIT SPENDING AS % HIWAY SPEND. %	Rank	MASS TRANSIT USE IN URBAN AREAS Rate	Rank
Alabama	1.06	47	1,453	22	15.4	25	11.7	23	109.1	20	0.0	50	0.76	45
Alaska	1.45	12	191	1	21.0	49	4.2	3	397.6	50	0.0	50	1.99	16
Arizona	1.29	25	1,748	29	14.8	20	13.8	35	131.2	37	1.8	22	1.88	20
Arkansas	1.68	2	19,200	50	16.0	32	14.4	38	111.0	22	0.1	36	0.76	45
California	1.33	21	1,192	17	13.5	7	6.7	5	75.8	6	32.7	4	2.48	11
Colorado	1.13	41	3,456	43	13.9	11	14.3	37	103.4	15	0.0	50	8.25	3
Connecticut	1.22	34	990	12	12.3	4	11.4	22	115.4	25	16.6	10	1.89	19
Delaware	1.29	26	1,197	18	12.9	5	12.6	29	129.9	34	3.5	18	1.39	29
Florida	1.12	43	2,393	38	14.6	17	10.6	14	117.8	26	2.0	21	1.28	31
Georgia	1.22	33	3,215	42	15.7	29	8.7	8	159.8	44	21.0	7	2.68	9
Hawaii	1.56	3	234	2	17.1	41	3.3	1	161.6	45	0.5	27	4.34	6
Idaho	1.07	46	698	6	17.2	42	14.5	39	126.5	32	0.0	50	0.94	40
Illinois	1.48	8	1,217	20	14.1	14	12.2	26	107.9	19	9.8	12	2.78	8
Indiana	1.33	20	728	7	16.9	39	10.0	10	121.9	29	2.9	20	1.53	26
Iowa	1.10	45	1,628	25	15.9	30	16.2	42	83.1	9	1.2	24	1.68	24
Kansas	1.13	42	3,988	47	16.7	37	10.4	13	130.4	36	0.0	50	1.49	28
Kentucky	1.33	18	1,611	24	16.3	34	11.1	19	158.5	42	0.1	35	1.52	27
Louisiana	1.50	6	2,265	37	16.7	37	12.0	25	145.1	41	0.0	50	1.56	25
Maine	1.28	28	4,075	48	14.9	21	11.1	19	103.9	16	0.2	31	0.85	44
Maryland	1.33	19	1,075	14	13.6	8	10.0	10	107.8	18	43.1	3	5.09	5
Massachusetts	1.54	5	965	10	12.0	2	5.7	4	73.0	5	94.4	2	2.65	10
Michigan	1.29	23	2,203	36	20.2	48	10.7	15	51.6	1	21.8	6	1.69	23
Minnesota	1.34	17	1,131	16	14.0	13	11.0	17	87.2	10	4.6	16	3.20	7
Mississippi	1.47	9	1,682	28	16.1	33	14.6	40	103.3	14	0.0	38	0.96	38
Missouri	1.35	15	2,621	40	16.3	34	12.4	28	113.2	23	0.2	30	1.97	17
Montana	1.11	44	1,089	15	18.2	46	18.8	49	118.0	27	0.0	37	1.37	30
Nebraska	1.21	35	1,672	27	17.0	40	16.3	43	106.6	17	0.5	26	1.86	21
Nevada	1.30	22	427	4	13.0	6	13.5	32	122.9	30	0.2	33	0.55	47
New Hampshire	1.17	39	2,120	34	13.6	8	22.9	50	131.2	38	0.0	50	1.03	36
New Jersey	1.35	16	972	11	14.7	18	7.0	6	121.1	28	26.1	5	2.40	12
New Mexico	1.19	38	1,441	21	17.4	44	13.4	31	125.3	31	0.0	50	0.95	39
New York	1.82	1	677	5	12.2	3	3.8	2	109.2	21	125.3	1	9.97	1
North Carolina	1.29	24	1,828	30	14.4	16	12.3	27	71.7	3	0.3	29	1.09	34
North Dakota	1.02	49	3,565	44	19.3	47	15.7	41	135.0	39	0.0	50	0.97	37
Ohio	1.26	30	883	9	15.9	30	11.8	24	80.0	8	3.0	19	1.80	22
Oklahoma	1.27	29	4,722	49	16.6	36	18.0	48	58.7	2	0.2	32	0.86	43
Oregon	1.19	37	1,215	19	15.6	26	17.6	46	99.0	13	3.5	17	5.45	4
Pennsylvania	1.55	4	767	8	13.9	11	9.6	9	173.0	46	18.6	8	2.01	15
Rhode Island	1.48	7	1,935	32	10.9	1	7.7	7	199.4	47	8.2	14	2.40	12
South Carolina	1.44	13	2,031	33	14.1	14	11.1	19	71.8	4	0.0	50	0.94	40
South Dakota	1.03	48	1,462	23	17.8	45	17.7	47	201.2	48	0.0	50	1.04	35
Tennessee	1.16	40	1,907	31	15.6	26	17.2	45	94.7	12	1.3	23	0.92	42
Texas	1.36	14	2,714	41	15.3	24	16.5	44	114.1	24	0.1	34	2.04	14
Utah	1.46	11	2,429	39	15.6	26	10.9	16	158.8	43	9.1	13	1.95	18
Vermont	1.23	32	3,635	46	13.7	10	12.6	29	130.0	35	0.6	25	0.00	50
Virginia	1.29	27	1,667	26	15.0	22	13.8	35	126.5	33	7.9	15	1.09	33
Washington	1.20	36	3,599	45	14.7	18	10.1	12	92.6	11	16.8	9	8.69	2
West Virginia	1.46	10	992	13	17.3	43	13.5	32	139.3	40	0.3	28	1.15	32
Wisconsin	1.24	31	2,128	35	15.2	23	11.0	17	76.5	7	9.9	11	0.24	48
Wyoming	0.99	50	353	3	21.4	50	13.7	34	250.3	49	0.0	50	0.00	50
U.S. Total	1.33		1,260		14.9		10.2		106.8		14.7			

RENEWABLE ENERGY

State	RENEWABLES AS % OF ALL ENERGY %	Rank	RENEWABLES AS % OF ALL ELECTRICITY %	Rank	NON-HYDRO RENEWABLES OF ELECTRIC %	Rank	ENERGY FROM MUNI. WASTE Billion BTUs	Rank	SOLAR COLLECTION SYSTEMS Million	Rank	SUMMARY OF RENEWABLE ENERGY Score	Rank	COMPOSITE OF 38 INDICATORS Score	Rank
Alabama	17.25	9	17.5	12	4.43	10	1,035	27	3.7	29	87	14	1,160	44
Alaska	3.07	40	21.3	11	0.47	33	279	36	0.0	50	170	37	1,078	35
Arizona	8.87	22	15.8	15	0.66	30	0	41	183.0	3	111	21	970	26
Arkansas	16.25	10	9.1	18	1.51	21	611	30	2.0	37	116	24	1,217	46
California	13.44	13	41.7	7	18.22	2	10,860	8	499.7	1	31	1	712	7
Colorado	5.33	26	6.6	25	0.16	39	0	41	37.3	6	137	31	903	20
Connecticut	9.04	21	3.8	35	2.44	18	17,667	5	36.8	7	86	13	714	8
Delaware	4.17	34	0.2	49	0.17	38	5,749	13	1.2	42	176	40	796	16
Florida	5.80	25	4.0	34	3.78	12	34,328	1	205.5	2	74	8	1,011	30
Georgia	15.91	12	8.2	20	3.89	11	1,314	23	4.8	25	91	17	949	24
Hawaii	8.03	23	13.2	16	12.06	3	2,824	18	64.1	4	64	5	542	3
Idaho	46.49	3	99.9	1	2.96	14	644	29	2.0	36	83	12	693	6
Illinois	2.20	46	0.4	48	0.19	37	4,106	14	3.8	27	172	38	1,107	37
Indiana	2.05	47	0.7	46	0.00	48	5	40	2.5	35	216	49	1,013	31
Iowa	3.25	36	3.1	37	0.04	44	591	32	1.0	43	192	46	1,109	38
Kansas	0.28	50	0.0	50	0.01	46	0	41	1.4	39	226	50	1,375	49
Kentucky	6.49	24	5.0	33	0.05	43	1,051	26	0.5	46	172	39	1,105	36
Louisiana	5.31	27	1.5	42	1.48	22	0	41	0.7	45	177	42	1,381	50
Maine	27.00	6	53.3	5	27.77	1	5,913	12	2.9	33	57	3	775	14
Maryland	4.56	32	5.8	30	1.06	27	9,730	10	8.2	21	120	26	719	9
Massachusetts	5.20	29	6.9	23	3.65	13	25,009	3	32.3	8	76	9	458	1
Michigan	4.27	33	3.7	36	1.65	20	10,082	9	19.6	14	112	22	901	19
Minnesota	9.05	20	5.9	29	2.94	15	21,566	4	5.9	22	90	16	724	11
Mississippi	16.02	11	6.6	26	6.59	6	329	35	0.3	48	126	27	1,114	39
Missouri	4.81	30	2.5	39	0.01	47	100	39	0.8	44	199	47	1,070	34
Montana	28.97	5	44.8	6	0.45	34	230	37	5.4	23	105	20	956	25
Nebraska	3.10	39	6.3	27	0.00	49	0	41	2.9	34	190	44	1,142	42
Nevada	9.78	18	16.6	14	4.55	9	2,628	20	8.4	20	81	11	805	17
New Hampshire	20.21	8	30.4	8	9.57	4	2,743	19	3.2	31	70	6	692	5
New Jersey	1.04	48	0.4	47	0.23	35	1,058	24	22.1	12	166	35	819	18
New Mexico	2.96	42	0.9	44	0.02	45	0	41	18.8	15	187	43	1,154	43
New York	10.62	17	22.1	10	1.40	23	31,037	2	45.7	5	57	4	660	4
North Carolina	12.57	14	7.3	21	0.55	31	526	33	10.2	18	117	25	991	28
North Dakota	5.24	28	9.7	17	0.21	36	0	41	0.3	47	169	36	1,193	45
Ohio	2.37	45	1.0	43	0.53	32	11,826	7	4.5	26	153	34	1,025	32
Oklahoma	3.16	38	5.5	32	0.73	28	3,564	16	3.7	30	144	32	1,118	40
Oregon	47.46	2	87.0	3	5.75	7	1,445	22	21.6	13	47	2	720	10
Pennsylvania	2.69	43	2.3	40	0.69	29	6,915	11	25.1	9	132	28	926	23
Rhode Island	4.10	35	8.7	19	5.47	8	460	34	9.0	19	115	23	535	2
South Carolina	11.67	16	6.8	24	1.25	24	723	28	1.3	41	133	29	986	27
South Dakota	29.42	4	84.9	4	0.00	50	138	38	1.8	38	134	30	920	22
Tennessee	12.55	15	17.3	13	1.14	26	3,620	15	24.1	10	79	10	1,031	33
Texas	0.44	49	0.8	45	0.13	41	598	31	22.2	11	177	41	1,272	47
Utah	3.18	37	5.9	28	1.85	19	1,051	25	1.4	40	149	33	908	21
Vermont	22.64	7	28.5	9	6.73	5	0	41	3.1	32	94	18	775	14
Virginia	9.06	19	5.5	31	2.90	16	13,911	6	11.9	16	88	15	1,004	29
Washington	53.54	1	87.6	2	1.20	25	1,918	21	5.4	24	73	7	734	12
West Virginia	2.97	41	1.7	41	0.10	42	0	41	0.2	49	214	48	1,120	41
Wisconsin	4.64	31	7.2	22	2.65	17	3,460	17	11.8	17	104	19	757	13
Wyoming	2.52	44	2.6	38	0.14	40	0	41	3.8	28	191	45	1,352	48
U.S. Total							241,644		1,390.0					

SOURCES FOR ENERGY USE AND AUTO ABUSE INDICATORS

Coal production
Output of coal mines in 1988 in million tons.
Source: "Coal Production, 1988." Published by Energy Information Administration, U.S. Department of Energy, 1990.

Oil production
Crude oil output in 1988 in million barrels, including offshore production attributed to specific states.
Source: "Petroleum Supply, 1988." Published by Energy Information Administration, U.S. Department of Energy, 1990.

Natural gas production
Withdrawals of natural gas in 1988 in billion cubic feet.
Source: "Natural Gas Annual, 1988." Published by Energy Information Administration, U.S. Department of Energy, 1990.

Gross state product from energy industries
Average percent of market value of all goods and services derived from energy industries, including fossil-fuel extraction, for period 1963 through 1986.
Source: Ronald H. Schmidt, "Natural Resources and Regional Growth," *Economic Review*, Fall 1989. Published by Federal Reserve Bank of San Francisco. Additional data furnished by Schmidt.

Pipelines in noncompliance
Number of gaseous and liquid pipelines failing to meet safety standards in 1987.
Source: "Annual Report on Pipeline Safety, 1987." Published by Office of Pipeline Safety, U.S. Department of Transportation, 1989.

Oil spills in state waters
Discharges in navigable waters of solvents, oil, and gasoline (not counting toxic chemicals), including leaks from ship hull and pipeline ruptures. Total gallons in thousands for 1984, 1985, and 1986, ranked on per-capita basis.
Source: "Polluting Incidents In and Around U.S. Waters." Published by U.S. Coast Guard, U.S. Department of Transportation, February 13, 1989.

Oil and gas injection wells
Number of Class II regulated injection wells used by oil and gas operations, 1987.
Source: "Drinking Water: Safeguards Are Not Preventing Contamination From Injected Oil & Gas Wastes." Published by U.S. General Accounting Office, July 1989.

Growth of carbon emissions, 1966 to 1986
Change in pounds of emissions over a 20-year period. Carbon is a standard measure for carbon dioxide releases from fossil fuel plants, the source of about half of greenhouse gases responsible for global warming. Carbon makes up 12/44ths of each pound of carbon dioxide.
Source: "Reducing the Rate of Global Warming: The States' Role," 1988. Published by Renew America, 1400 16th Street, NW, Washington, DC 20036; telephone (202) 232-2252.

Carbon emissions and gross state product
Tons of carbon released per million dollars of gross state product.
Source: "Reducing the Rate of Global Warming: The States' Role," 1988. Published by Renew America.

Energy consumption
> Millions of British thermal units (BTUs, standard measure of heat) consumed from all sources, per capita, 1987.
> *Source:* "State Energy Data Report, Consumption Estimates, 1960-87." Published by Energy Information Administration, U.S. Department of Energy, 1989.

Growth in energy consumption
> Percent change of per-capita energy consumption, an important indicator of energy efficiency, from 1960 to 1975 and from 1975 to 1987.
> *Source:* "State Energy Data Report, Consumption Estimates, 1960-87." Published by Energy Information Administration, U.S. Department of Energy, 1989.

Energy consumption growth versus population growth
> Ratio of change in total energy consumed to change in population, for period 1960 to 1987. Another measure of energy efficiency.
> *Source:* "State Energy Data Report, Consumption Estimates, 1960-87." Published by Energy Information Administration, U.S. Department of Energy, 1989.

Low-income homes weatherized
> Percent of all low-income residences weatherized, from fiscal 1977 through 1988, under the various government-backed weatherization programs.
> *Source:* "Report to Congress on the Present Weatherization Grant Program." Published by Office of Conservation and Renewable Energy, U.S. Department of Energy, August 1989.

Electric capacity from nuclear power
> Percent of total kilowatt generating capability derived from nuclear power plants.
> *Source:* "Electric Power Annual, 1988." Published by Energy Information Administration, U.S. Department of Energy, December 1989.

Cost of decommissioning nuclear power plants
> Total cost in million dollars that utility estimates will be required to safely secure or dispose of radioactive and other material in a nuclear power plant once its useful life ends. Ranking is on per-capita cost still uncollected by utility.
> *Source:* "Payment Due: A Reactor-by-Reactor Assessment of the Nuclear Industry's $25+ Billion Decommissioning Bill," October 1990. Published by Public Citizen's Critical Mass Energy Project, 215 Pennsylvania Avenue, SE, Washington, DC 20003; telephone (202) 546-4996.

Citations at nuclear power plants
> Number of notices of violation issued by Nuclear Regulatory Commission between January 1, 1989 and November 26, 1990. Violations can range from procedural errors to life-threatening accidents or radiation releases.
> *Source:* "The Nuclear Monitor," February 26 and December 3, 1990, based on data from Nuclear Regulatory Commission. Published by Nuclear Information and Resource Service, 1424 16th Street, NW, Washington, DC 20036; telephone (202) 328-0002.

Low-level radioactive waste
> Curies of low-level radioactive waste generated and shipped for disposal in 1987, based on U.S. Department of Energy data; percent this amount represents of U.S. total; and ranking based on state's share of total.
> *Source:* "Nuclear Legacy," September 1989. Published by Public Citizen's Critical Mass Energy Project.

Total radioactive waste in state
> Millions of curies of low- and high-level radioactive waste accumulated inside state as of December 31, 1987, based on U.S. Department of Energy data; percent this amount represents of U.S. total; and ranking based on state's share of total.
> *Source:* "Nuclear Legacy," September 1989. Published by Public Citizen's Critical Mass Energy Project.

Summary of nuclear indicators
> State rankings for previous five indicators were added up, and the lowest total receives the best rank.

Price of electricity for residential versus industrial customers
> Ratio of average price residential customers paid per kilowatt hour to price paid by industrial customers — a partial indicator of wasteful discounts given industrial customers.
> *Source:* "Electric Power Annual, 1988." Published by Energy Information Administration, U.S. Department of Energy, December 1989.

Source of electric generating capacity
> Percent of total kilowatt generating capability derived from coal, oil or natural gas, and hydroelectric or other renewable sources. States with greatest reliance on water and renewable sources rank best; states most dependent on other sources score worst.
> *Source:* "Electric Power Annual, 1988." Published by Energy Information Administration, U.S. Department of Energy, December 1989.

Gasoline use
> Gallons of gasoline consumed per capita, 1988.
> *Source:* "Highway Fact Book, 1990." Published by Highway Users Federation, 1776 Massachusetts Ave., NW, Washington DC 20036; telephone (202) 857-1200.

Miles per gallon of gas
> Gallons of gas consumed divided by total vehicle miles driven for 1988.
> *Source:* "Selected Highway Statistics and Charts, 1988." Published by Federal Highway Administration, U.S. Department of Transportation, 1990.

Highway deaths
> Highway fatalities per billion miles driven, 1988.
> *Source:* "MVMA Motor Vehicle Facts & Figures, 1990." Published by Motor Vehicle Manufacturers Association of the United States, 7430 Second Avenue, Detroit, MI 48202; telephone (313) 872-4311.

Persons per motor vehicle
> Ratio of population to number of motor vehicles (cars, trucks, buses) registered in state, 1988.
> *Source:* "Selected Highway Statistics and Charts, 1988." Published by Federal Highway Administration, U.S. Department of Transportation, 1990.

Cars per transit buses
> Ratio of registered cars to commercial and municipal buses (excluding school buses), 1988.
> *Source:* "MVMA Motor Vehicle Facts & Figures, 1990." Published by Motor Vehicle Manufacturers Association of the United States.

Dependency on motor vehicles for jobs
>Percent of 1987 employment in motor vehicle and parts manufacturing, trucking, sales, servicing, road construction and maintenance, petroleum refining, and related activities.
>*Source:* "MVMA Motor Vehicle Facts & Figures, 1990." Published by Motor Vehicle Manufacturers Association of the United States.

Dependency on motor vehicles for taxes
>Percent of 1989 state revenue from taxes on motor vehicle fuel, vehicle licenses, and operator licenses.
>*Source:* "MVMA Motor Vehicle Facts & Figures, 1990." Published by Motor Vehicle Manufacturers Association of the United States.

Highway spending versus highway revenue
>Percent of highway-related revenues spent for capital and maintenance cost of highways in 1988. Numbers over 100 percent mean more funds were spent than raised.
>*Source:* "MVMA Motor Vehicle Facts & Figures, 1989" and "MVMA Motor Vehicle Facts & Figures, 1990." Published by Motor Vehicle Manufacturers Association of the United States.

Public transit spending versus highway spending
>State financial support for public transportation systems in 1989 represented as percent of what state spent for highways. Includes funds raised through state taxes and retained by local governments for public transit.
>*Source:* "MVMA Motor Vehicle Facts & Figures, 1990." Published by Motor Vehicle Manufacturers Association of the United States. "1989 Survey of State Involvement in Public Transportation." Published by American Association of State Highway and Transportation Officials, 444 N. Capitol Street, NW, Washington, DC 20001; telephone (202) 624-5800.

Mass transit use
>Measure of public transit's carrying capacity based on number of seats per urban mile, 1984.
>*Source:* "The 1989 Development Report Card for the States." Published by the Corporation for Enterprise Development, 1725 K St., NW, Washington DC 20006; telephone (202) 293-7963.

Renewable sources of all energy
>Percent of total energy use supplied by all renewable sources, including biomass, photovoltaics, hydroelectric, geothermal, and solar power.
>*Source:* "The Power of the States: A Fifty-State Survey of Renewable Energy," June 1990. Published by Public Citizen's Critical Mass Energy Project, 215 Pennsylvania Avenue, SE, Washington, DC 20003; telephone (202) 546-4996.

Renewable sources of electricity
>Percent of BTUs of electricity derived from all renewable sources.
>*Source:* "The Power of the States: A Fifty-State Survey of Renewable Energy," June 1990. Published by Public Citizen's Critical Mass Energy Project.

Non-hydro renewable sources of electricity
>Percent of BTUs of electricity derived from all renewable sources, excluding hydroelectric power.
>*Source:* "The Power of the States: A Fifty-State Survey of Renewable Energy," June 1990. Published by Public Citizen's Critical Mass Energy Project.

Energy from municipal solid waste
> Billions of BTUs generated for useful purposes from burning municipal solid waste.
> *Source:* "The Power of the States: A Fifty-State Survey of Renewable Energy," June 1990. Published by Public Citizen's Critical Mass Energy Project.

Solar collection systems
> Number of active solar collection systems, in millions, primarily solar heaters of water and homes.
> *Source:* "The Power of the States: A Fifty-State Survey of Renewable Energy," June 1990. Published by Public Citizen's Critical Mass Energy Project.

Summary for renewable energy
> State rankings for the previous five indicators were added up, and the lowest total receives the best summary rank.

Composite energy and transportation score
> Rankings on the 38 indicators were totaled to produce a composite score. Lowest score

CHAPTER 5

Toxic, Hazardous, and Solid Waste

INDICATORS

Toxic chemical disposal on site
Toxic chemical transfer off site
Total toxic chemical releases
Personal income from chemical industry
Release of cancer-causing poisons
Release of chemicals causing birth defects
Release of neurotoxins
Hazardous waste generated
Hazardous waste managed in state
Number of hazardous waste generators
Number of commercial hazardous waste facilities
Hazardous waste transport accidents
Hazardous sites on military bases
State spending to manage hazardous and solid waste
Number of Superfund sites
Superfund sites being cleaned up
Non-Superfund hazardous sites
"Non-hazardous" waste impoundments
Municipal solid waste generated
Municipal solid waste recycled
Number of curbside recycling programs
Number of open landfills
Waste burned by incinerators

The growth of toxic and hazardous waste parallels the evolution of a society that craves convenience, fears scarcity, glorifies the unrestrained marketplace, and assumes the back alley can absorb unlimited litter. In the island nation of Japan, 70 percent of the solid waste is recycled out of necessity. But in the United States, the mythical abundance of water and land has deceived us into allowing private enterprise to use resources and technology for material gain while dumping the waste in the public's backyard.

Industry continues to generate the bulk of the nation's annual output of noxious, flammable, corrosive, and explosive waste materials. Hazardous substances are produced in smaller yet significant quantities by hospitals, the military, and individuals tossing out paint, household cleaners, oil, pesticides, and the like. Consumers also throw away more non-hazardous solid waste (better known as garbage) than our landfills can hold.

There is no fail-safe method for disposing of hazardous or highly toxic waste. Vehicles carrying it away risk accidents, incineration produces chemical-laden ash and poisonous gases, landfills and underground storage facilities eventually leak. Even household garbage in municipal landfills leaches toxins into groundwater. But instead of using this knowledge to stop waste at its source, we wait until the damage is done, then spend billions of dollars studying the contaminated sites and attempting to clean them up.

The only way to stop the poison is to change the equipment and raw materials that make it a byproduct. According to the congressional Office of Technology Assessment, if industry changed its methods and materials, its annual hazardous waste output could be cut by 50 percent. Instead, the volume steadily grows, jumping by 20 percent between 1980 and 1988.

TOXIC COUNTS

For many years, industries dumped, stored, or burned toxic materials without public accountability. In 1986, Congress passed the Emergency Planning and Right-to-Know provision (Title III of SARA) giving citizens access to information about storage, use, and emissions of toxic chemicals. Under the act, EPA collects data about manufacturers' emissions and transfers of about 300 chemicals, and it publishes the results in the Toxics Release Inventory (TRI).

While the TRI is the most extensive record of industrial toxic emissions, it has serious flaws. Only facilities classified as manufacturers with 10 or more employees and over 50,000 pounds of listed toxins had to report their emissions in 1988 (the minimum for 1989 is 25,000 pounds). One-third of the estimated 30,000 facilities that should have reported emissions did not do so. Moreover, the 300-plus chemicals covered by the TRI represent only a tiny fraction of the more than 60,000 used regularly by industry. Those chemicals left off the TRI list are not necessarily less dangerous; they include suspected carcinogens and ozone depleters, but the toxicity of the vast majority (79 percent) remains unknown because the Environmental Protection Agency refuses to use its authority to press industry for detailed analyses of the chemicals' characteristics, much less a reduction in their releases to the environment.

Taking these shortcomings into consideration, the Office of Technology Assessment estimates that the true figure for total industrial chemical releases and transfers each year is about 400 billion pounds — roughly 1,600 pounds for every man, woman, and child in the United States. That's a far cry from the 22 billion pounds counted by the TRI in 1987, or the 6 billion pounds reported in 1988.

The sharp drop in recorded TRI emissions between 1987 and 1988 (the only years for which the TRI has been published) highlights another problem. EPA officials acknowledge that two-thirds of this decrease was not real. It was due to "phantom reductions" resulting from chemicals being taken off the 1988 list that were counted in 1987, or facilities reclassifying part or all of their operation as "non-manufacturing," or companies changing how they measure their emissions.

For instance, Kennecott Utah Copper, a metals producer in Bingham Canyon, Utah, stopped reporting toxic releases from its mine and mill operations because such operations do not fall under the designation of "manufacturer" and therefore are not subject to reporting requirements. Rexene Products in Odessa, Texas reduced its emissions 84 percent simply by changing methods of measurement, and Kaiser Aluminum in Gramercy, Louisiana reported lower releases because it sold off three manufacturing operations.

Some companies did achieve genuine source reduction. Unocal Chemicals Division in Kenai, Alaska replaced ozone-depleting methyl chloroform with a citrus-based solvent to clean equipment. Under public pressure, an IBM plant in San Jose, California began using soap and water as a cleaner instead of chlorofluorocarbon-113 (Freon). As part of its commitment to reduce toxic emissions 90 percent by 1992, the Upjohn Company in Portage, Michigan cut emissions 16 percent between 1987 and 1988 by using less poisonous chemicals and improving its solvent recovery equipment.

Despite its limitations, the TRI pinpoints the biggest chemical polluters, some of what they release, and where it goes. In previous chapters, we discussed toxins put into the ground, surface water, public sewage systems, and air. The focus here is on what the reporting facilities kept on their site, what they sent away for someone else to handle, and what their total releases add up to.

ON SITE, OFF SITE, OUTTA SIGHT

Toxic chemicals kept on a company's property generally went to lagoons, surface impoundments, or its own landfill; smaller quantities were spread on fields or simply leaked onto the property accidentally. Florida leads the nation in land disposal because its phosphate industry stores phosphoric acid and other toxins on site. By simply reinterpreting the TRI requirements, two of the state's biggest producers — Occidental Chemical Corporation and Royster Company — cut their land disposal from 158 million pounds in 1987 to 49 million in 1988.

By contrast, Inland Steel Company in East Chicago, Indiana and U.S. Steel's Fairless Works in Fairless, Pennsylvania recorded sharp increases of on-site releases, including manganese compounds and carcinogenic chromium. Other heavily industrialized states with large primary metals facilities (Ohio, Michigan, Missouri) join Florida, Indiana, and Pennsylvania in the bottom

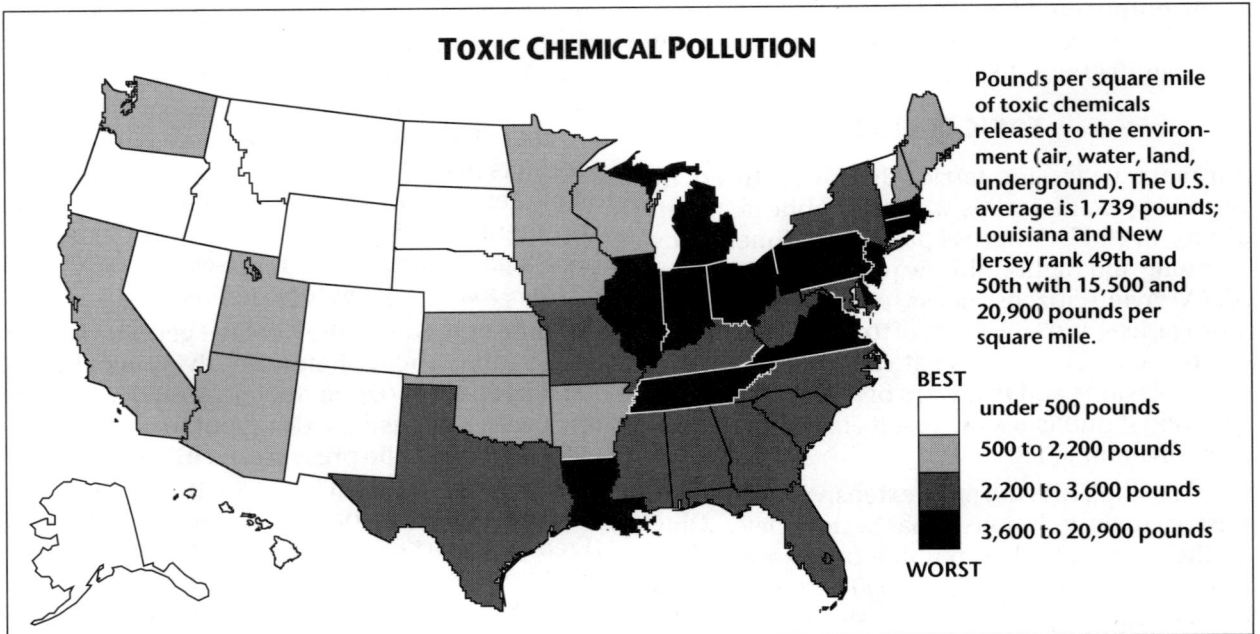

TOXIC CHEMICAL POLLUTION

Pounds per square mile of toxic chemicals released to the environment (air, water, land, underground). The U.S. average is 1,739 pounds; Louisiana and New Jersey rank 49th and 50th with 15,500 and 20,900 pounds per square mile.

BEST
- under 500 pounds
- 500 to 2,200 pounds
- 2,200 to 3,600 pounds
- 3,600 to 20,900 pounds

WORST

dozen for on-site releases. For five Rocky Mountain states with big mine-and-milling operations, land disposal accounts for more than two-thirds of their total TRI releases; in order of their total toxic output, they are Arizona, Montana, New Mexico, Idaho, and Nevada. Because of two companies in Gila County, (Asarco Inc. and Cypus Miami Mining) Arizona ranks 48th in total and per-capita on-site toxic releases.

The big industrial states, especially those bordering the Great Lakes, send the most toxins off site for disposal or treatment. Many firms transfer waste from one site to impoundments or injection wells at another site they own; but two-thirds of the off-site toxins goes to facilities they do not control, mostly to commercial hazardous waste landfills, incinerators, or treatment plants whose emissions are not recorded by the TRI. The majority of those facilities are regulated by another EPA division described below in the hazardous waste section.

Companies in Ohio send the most toxins off site — but 70 percent of the 124 million pounds shipped away stays inside the state. In addition, Ohio receives 69 million pounds from other states, by far the most imported for disposal. Most of the waste comes from Pennsylvania, Michigan, Wisconsin, New Jersey, New York, Illinois, and Indiana — which along with Texas and California make up the 10 biggest states for off-site transfers (excluding toxins sent into sewers).

J & L Specialty Products Corporation in Louisville, Ohio transfers 99.8 percent of the chromium, nickel, and manganese left over from making stainless steel. In 1987 these transfers amounted to just under 6 million pounds, but in 1988 the company reported only 500,000 pounds for the same metals. Rather than reflecting a decrease in toxic byproduct, the change resulted from a TRI loophole that allows manufacturers to omit toxins sent for recycling or reuse.

TOXIC TOTALS

When TRI chemical releases to air, water, land, and off-site are added up, Ohio has the third highest total — 376 million pounds in 1988, more than 1 million pounds a day, or 9,000 pounds per square mile. Only Louisiana and Texas, with their massive petrochemical complexes, generate more toxic waste. Texas ranks 50th in total volume, and edges out Ohio for the greatest releases of both nerve-damaging and ozone-depleting chemicals. Louisiana is 50th on a per-capita basis, with 168 pounds per person, substantially more than the next three states: Wyoming (96 pounds per capita), Utah (81 pounds), and Kansas (70 pounds).

Louisiana's TRI emissions are concentrated in the eight counties (parishes) along the lower Mississippi River's "chemical corridor." PCBs, dioxin, and heavy metals contaminate fish in the river, and area cancer rates are 14 percent above the U.S. average, according to the Greenpeace report, "We All

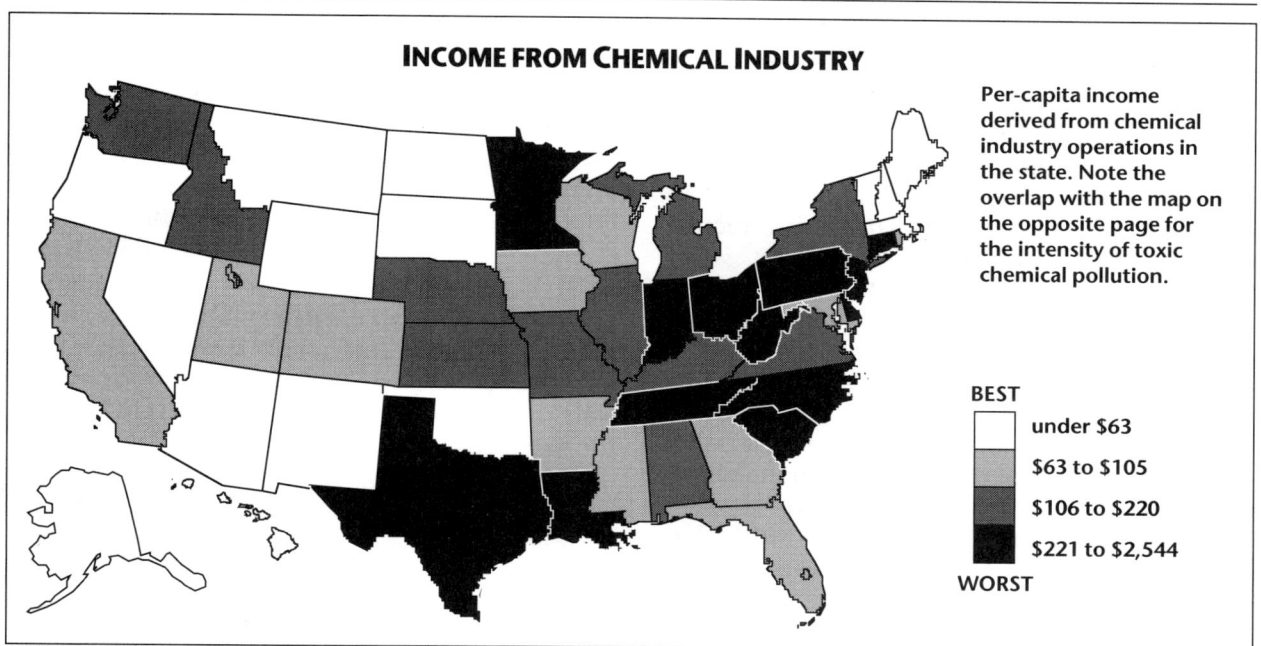

INCOME FROM CHEMICAL INDUSTRY

Per-capita income derived from chemical industry operations in the state. Note the overlap with the map on the opposite page for the intensity of toxic chemical pollution.

BEST
- under $63
- $63 to $105
- $106 to $220
- $221 to $2,544

WORST

Live Downstream." Four of the parishes are among the six counties with the nation's largest releases. Their polluting refineries and factories are owned by the nation's leaders in toxic emissions — DuPont, Monsanto, American Cyanamid, Shell, Exxon, Texaco, and Dow Chemical.

The Dow plant in Freeport, Texas reported the greatest number of different TRI chemicals (86), while DuPont and Monsanto's 111 facilities nationwide pumped out 620 million pounds of toxins, nearly 10 percent of the TRI total. After the chemical industry, which accounts for 46 percent of all releases, the biggest sources of toxins come from the production of primary metals (14 percent), paper products (6 percent of the TRI total), and vehicles (4 percent).

Some states with large releases, such as California (ranked 42d in total volume) and New York (rank 37), fare better when their discharges are measured on a per-capita basis. Just the reverse happens for sparsely populated Alaska (rank 14), Montana (rank 17), and Wyoming (rank 18); on the per-capita ranking, they drop to 46th, 41st, and 49th place respectively. When total emissions are divided by square miles, the low-volume states of Delaware (rank 6) and Rhode Island (rank 7) plunge to the bottom 10. But as the tables show, there is a remarkable overlap in the three ways to grade the best and worse states. For example, Oklahoma ranks 20th in total releases, 18th on the per-capita scale, and 17th per square mile. Oregon is 16th, 12th, and 11th, making it one of eight states ranking in the top third on all three indicators.

The Southern states score poorest when the focus is on producers of the most dangerous chemicals — those that cause either cancer, birth defects, or nerve damage. On a pounds per-capita basis, Alabama, Arkansas, Kentucky, Louisiana, North Carolina, South Carolina, Tennessee, and West Virginia rank 35th or worse for each of the these classes of poisons. In each case, Texas is the biggest producer by volume, but the per-capita scale gives it a boost out of the cellar. Yet another Southern state, Virginia, is dead last in releases of neurotoxins (nerve-damaging chemicals) and 48th for birth-defect agents. Indiana, Ohio, Connecticut, and Delaware also score especially poorly on these three indicators, which are based on an analysis of TRI data by the Citizens Fund in Washington, D.C.

HAZARDOUS REGULATIONS

Each year, government officials track the flow of more than 500 billion pounds of hazardous solid waste to thousands of treatment, storage, and disposal facilities. That amounts to over a ton for each man, woman, and child living in the United States, with more than half of it coming from the chemical and petroleum industries. Two-thirds of these flammable, corrosive, explosive, and health-threatening wastes (including some, but not all, TRI chemicals) are deposited in landfills, stored in pits and lagoons, or injected underground. Twenty-two percent is poured into water, while only 11 percent is recycled or neutralized before discharge.

Although no comprehensive listing like the TRI is available for hazardous substances, the federal government promised to regulate the production, transport, and disposal of hazardous waste through the Resource Conservation and Recovery Act (RCRA), passed in 1976. Subtitle C of the Act directed EPA to regulate waste management with the goal of minimizing environmental damage. But it turns out that many RCRA facilities (like the one at Love Canal) are among the nation's worst polluters, with tons of poisons spewing from their incinerators or leaking from dumps into water supplies. The 1984 RCRA amendments required EPA to evaluate and remedy the hazards posed by 4,615 regulated facilities. Yet as of January 1990, only 1,711 had been assessed, even though 83 percent of that number showed evidence of serious problems. Instead of sounding the alarm, EPA uses its staff shortage to justify its slow work and missed deadlines. So far, only 3 of the 1,711 problem sites have been cleaned up.

Added to the RCRA facilities are the dump sites of illegal waste brokers, plus the abandoned lagoons or landfills of corporate America. As the extent of hazardous waste contamination became obvious, Washington was forced to respond. In 1980, Congress passed the Comprehensive Environmental Response, Compensation and Liability Act (CERCLA) to establish a National Priority List (NPL) of the sites urgently needing cleanup. Known as the Superfund, this program also has been a fiasco. States as varied as Massachusetts and Montana now avoid referring sites to EPA for Superfund listing because the procedure stalls, rather than expedites, remedial action. Ten years after its start, the Superfund has cleaned up only 22 of its 1,214 targeted sites.

Along with Superfund, states are responsible for funding and administering cleanup of 30,500 hazardous waste sites they believe need attention. The 1,200 NPL sites, 30,500 non-Superfund sites, and 4,600 RCRA facilities bring the total number of "hot spots" to just over 36,000. Adding military and other sites not fully assessed easily doubles that figure. Three of the shorter profiles from the National Priority List provide a sobering glimpse at the scope of the problem:

• *Kerr-McGee Corporation*'s plant in Cushing, Oklahoma covers 116 acres in rural Payne County. Various oil and pipeline companies have occupied the site since 1915. Kerr-McGee acquired a refinery in 1956 and also processed uranium in a plant on the site during 1963-65. In 1965 and 1966, it produced thorium metal for the Atomic Energy Commission, then demolished the plant. Soil and wash water containing thorium were placed in an on-site surface impoundment known as Pit 4. Other pits with acid sludges and oily wastes had been filled in prior to 1956.

In 1986, EPA detected uranium, radium, chromium, nickel, zinc, and arsenic in on-site monitoring wells. An estimated 7,800 people obtain drinking water from public and private wells within 3 miles of the site.

• *The Anne Arundel County Landfill* covers 130 acres near an industrial park, homes, and a commercial area in Glen Burnie, Maryland. When the county took over daily operations in 1970, it capped a 30-acre private dump (open since the 1950s) with clay, vegetation, and vents to release methane gas. Diamond Shamrock Corporation of Baltimore deposited about 100 tons of inorganic salts and solids in the landfill in the late 1970s; dozens of other clients used the site until it closed in 1982.

In 1983, EPA detected trichloroethylene, dichloroethylene, and chromium in monitoring wells at the site. The landfill overlies a recharge area that supplies drinking water to nearby municipal and private wells serving 93,000 people.

• *Hi Mill Manufacturing Company* has fabricated aluminum, copper, and brass parts on a 2.5-acres site in Okland County, Michigan since 1946. Until 1981, rinse water from dipping operations was discharged to an on-site unlined lagoon adjacent to a marsh connected to Waterbury Lake, a popular recreational attraction. Rinse waste was also sprayed into the air for disposal. Currently, some is recycled and the rest is neutralized with caustic acid, stored in underground tanks, and then sent off-site.

In 1982, Michigan regulators detected copper in nearby wells; heavy metals also contaminate the marsh and lake. About 13,500 people use drinking water from private wells within 3 miles of the site. The company has shipped the sludge and soil from its lagoon to a RCRA-waste facility, and continues work on cleaning up the site.

THE NATION'S DUMPING GROUND

Any sane president who reviewed the catalog of contaminated sites might announce a national emergency and declare a "war on waste." If unlimited resources can go to wage war in the Persian Gulf or bail out bankers, why can't the funds — and the

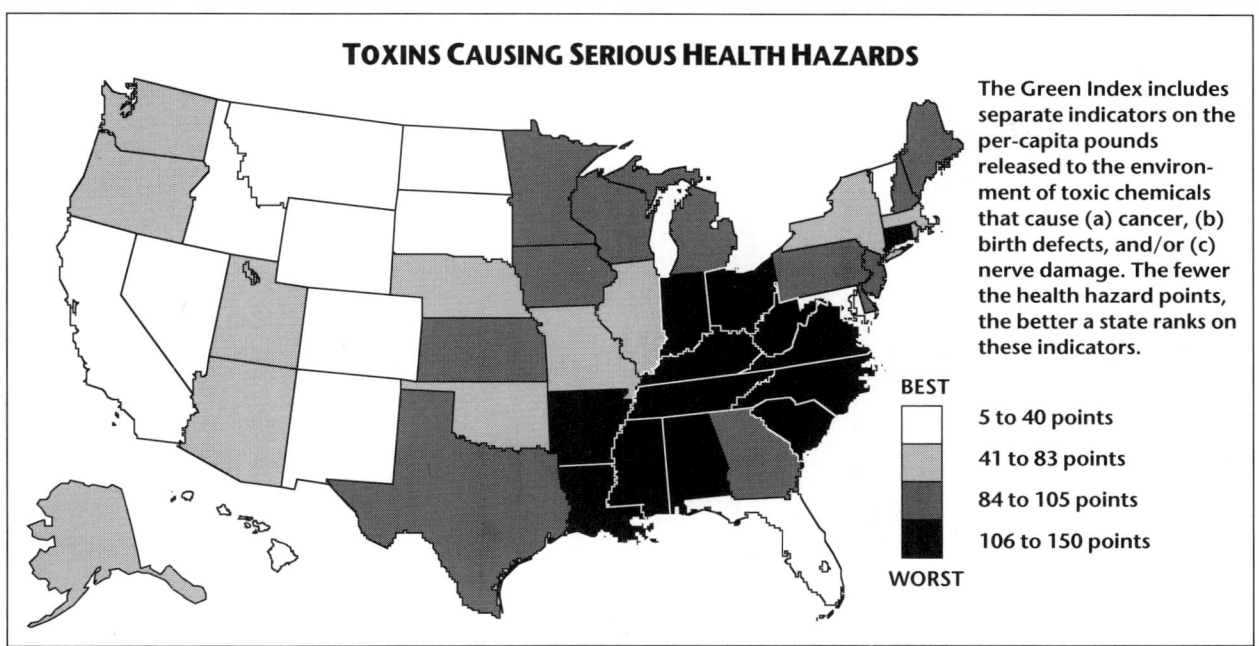

TOXINS CAUSING SERIOUS HEALTH HAZARDS

The Green Index includes separate indicators on the per-capita pounds released to the environment of toxic chemicals that cause (a) cancer, (b) birth defects, and/or (c) nerve damage. The fewer the health hazard points, the better a state ranks on these indicators.

BEST
- 5 to 40 points
- 41 to 83 points
- 84 to 105 points
- 106 to 150 points

WORST

courage — be found to stop hazards at their source? Instead, state and federal officials act as if simply counting the pounds of discharge is a major victory. In fact, in the case of RCRA hazardous waste, EPA has not issued new data since it added up the volume generated and managed by each state in 1985.

Like the TRI, the RCRA data can be deceptive; for example, some states counted the weight of the water carrying waste in their totals, while most did not. The numbers are still useful, however, for uncovering trends. In most states, for example, the top 100 hazardous waste generators produce 90 percent or more of the waste. And, as with carcinogens and neurotoxins, the South leads the nation in the per-capita pounds of RCRA waste generated and managed, while such non-industrial states as New Mexico, the Dakotas, Vermont, Idaho, Hawaii, and Alaska score best.

Tennessee is the country's biggest producer, with nearly 7 tons of hazardous waste per resident coming from Union Camp, Chemical Products Corporation, Eastman Kodak, Lockheed Aeronautical Systems, General Electric, Whirlpool, and 550 other generators. With 6 tons per capita, Georgia and West Virginia are close behind. Georgia also ranks 50th in total waste managed, 50th in state spending per ton of managed waste, and 43d in the percent of its Superfund sites with cleanup completed or underway.

The only non-Southern state among the 10 biggest per-capita generators of hazardous waste is Pennsylvania (rank 45). On other per-capita indicators, the Quaker state ranks 48th in RCRA-waste generators, 48th in waste management facilities, 39th in Superfund sites, and 42d in non-Superfund waste sites. But unlike most Southern states, Pennsylvania spends above the national average to manage its waste problems. By contrast, seven of the dozen states that spend the least per capita are in the South; three of the non-Southern misers — Missouri, Nebraska, and Oklahoma — also have sizable waste problems.

Taken together, the 13 Southern states generate 66 percent of the nation's 500 billion pounds of RCRA hazardous waste. After adjusting for non-hazardous wastewater, the region's treatment, storage, and disposal facilities manage an even larger proportion, about 73 percent. Most hazardous waste is managed on the same property where it is generated, but about 30 percent is handled by facilities that import all or part of their material. California, New York, Delaware, Minnesota, and Nebraska all ship a substantial portion of their RCRA waste out of state. Three of the states that import more than 1 billion pounds — Arkansas, Kentucky, and Louisiana — have commercial incinerators that burn RCRA waste to the detriment of nearby residents.

More commonly, the waste is shipped in drums or by the truckload to landfills. The nation's biggest hazardous waste dump — located in Emelle, Alabama — receives shipments totaling over 1 billion pounds a year from as far away as Puerto Rico.

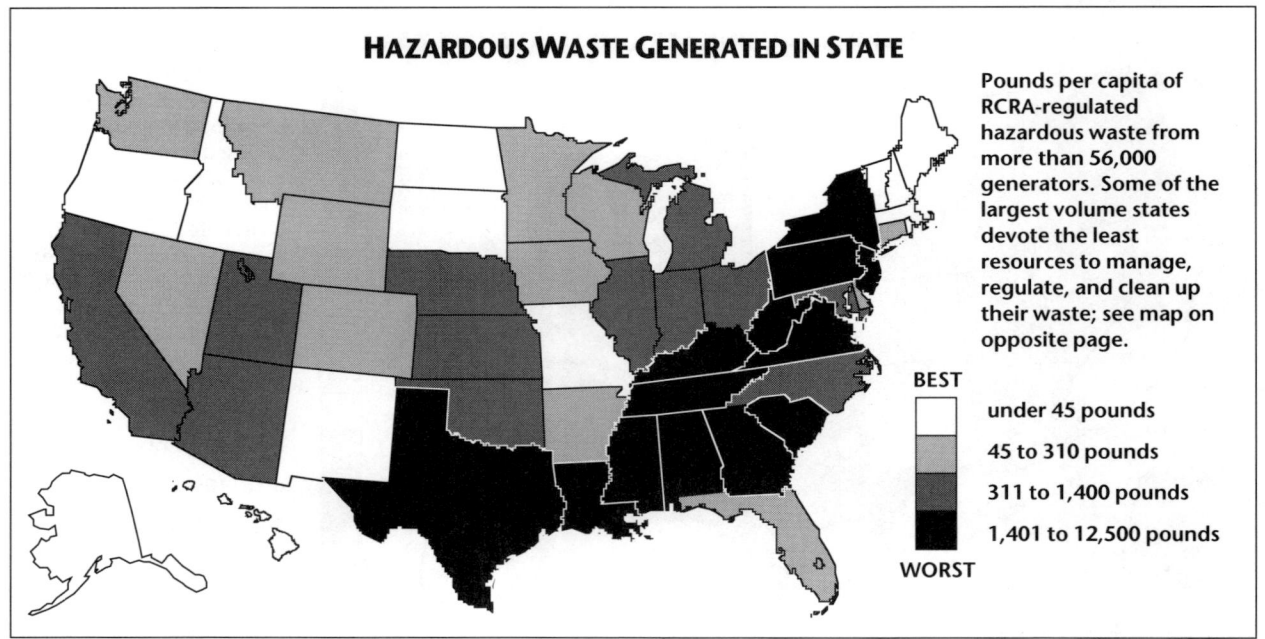

Its 2,400 customers include the Pentagon, General Motors, Exxon, IBM, General Electric, DuPont, Phillip Morris, and many state governments eager to transfer their waste burden to someone else. In 1989, for example, Texas shipped 94 million pounds of PCB-contaminated soil from a closed oil refinery to Emelle, earning Chemical Waste Management, the dump's owner, $16.1 million.

Other poisons buried at Emelle include cyanide, arsenic acid, cadmium, nickel, lead, and heptachlor. Because of repeated leaks, truck accidents, fires, and spills, state officials are asking when, not if, the toxins will reach the aquifer that supplies nearby towns with water. Under pressure from the public, the governor declared a moratorium on out-of-state waste, but federal courts have recently ruled that such bans violate the U.S. Constitution's protection of interstate trade. Efforts in Congress to grant states the right to restrict trade in waste foreshadow a fractious fight between exporting and importing states, industrial polluters, and neighborhood activists.

People have good reason to be nervous about hazardous waste traffickers. Because of human error and poor equipment, accidents causing millions of dollars in damage are common. In Texas, nearly 900 accidents involving the transport of hazardous materials by trucks, trains, ships, or planes occurred in 1987 and 1988; the cleanup and recovery cost hit $8.7 billion. Even North Dakota, ranked best on this indicator, experienced 14 accidents and $12 million in damages. With its huge chemical industry, Delaware ranks 50th in per-capita damage, 50th in per-capita Superfund sites, 49th in non-Superfund sites, and 44th in hazardous sites on military bases. Perhaps as a consequence, DuPont's home state winds up 50th in cancer deaths and 2d in spending per person to manage and clean up its waste.

GOVERNMENT POISONS

The pricetag for cleaning up our toxic mess will easily rival the much publicized bill for the S&L bailout, and federal policy is equally to blame. The cost just to remedy leaks at the Department of Energy's Hanford Nuclear Reservation in southeastern Washington state is now estimated at a staggering $57 billion. About 100 federal installations are already on the Superfund NPL, and the military alone has 20,000 more sites whose cleanup will consume well over $100 billion. The wastes range from tons of aviation fuel contaminating an aquifer under New Jersey's Lakehurst Naval Air Station, to byproducts from chemical and nerve munitions polluting waters near Maryland's Aberdeen Proving Ground, to explosive compounds littering Indiana's Jefferson Proving Ground, to PCBs and radioactive waste contaminating 167 separate sites at California's McClellan Air Force Base.

California hosts the largest number of military waste sites (twice the number found in Virginia), including two on the Superfund list from the San Francisco Bay area. California also leads in the to-

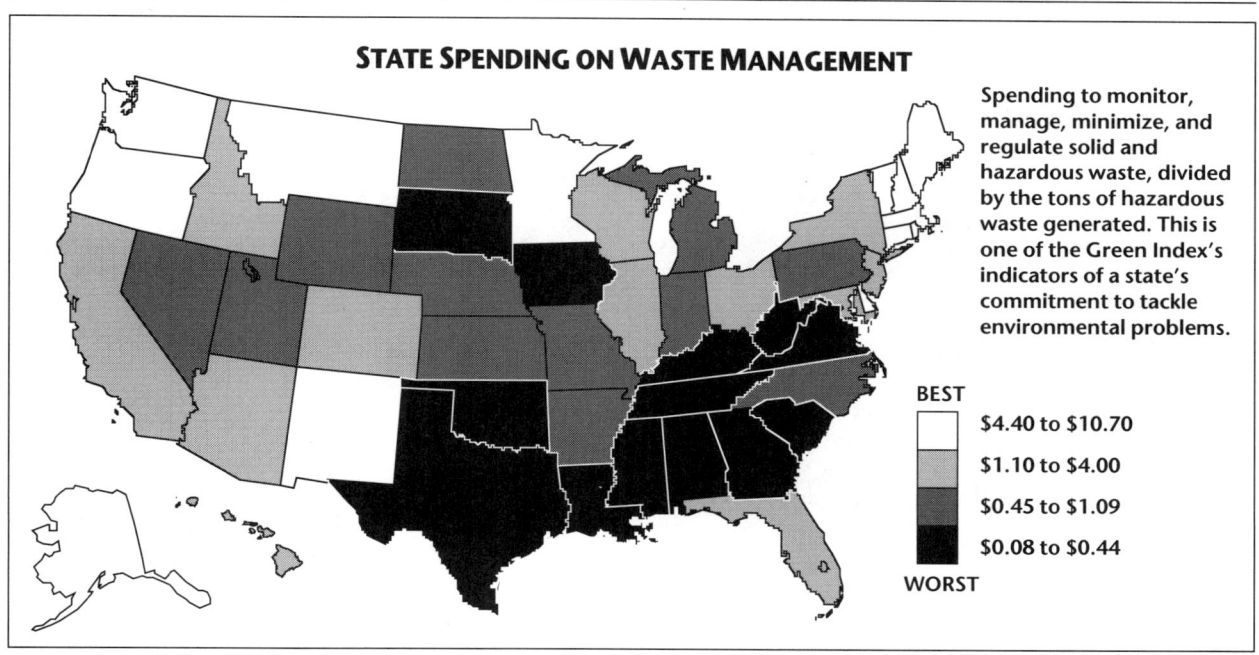

tal number of non-military waste sites, with many in the backyards of defense contractors. Silicon Valley, for example, has the nation's largest concentration of Superfund sites. On a per-capita basis, Alaska (rank 50), New Mexico, and Hawaii rank the worst in military waste sites — and their native populations suffer accordingly. At Mountainview, New Mexico, for example, a low-income Hispanic community has been engaged in a protracted struggle with nearby Kirtland Air Force Base over nitrate-contaminated well water traced to nitroaromatic compounds used in explosives.

Not far from Sante Fe, New Mexico, the Los Alamos National Laboratory designs nuclear warheads and blends two grades of plutonium for shipment to the Rocky Flats Plant in Colorado. Studies show that the plutonium has migrated into the Rio Grande and onto neighboring Indian lands. Radioactive contamination plagues dozens of other communities that surround facilities tied to the production of nuclear weapons, the source of 70 percent of radioactive waste by volume. (See page 44 for more on radioactive waste.) The Department of Energy owns many of these properties and has its own list of contaminated properties to add to the Pentagon's. Slowly, the lethal fallout from the military-nuclear-industrial complex is coming into focus. "In the name of protecting our national security and well-being, we are poisoning ourselves," conclude the authors of "Deadly Defense," a guide to nuclear bomb plants written by the Radioactive Waste Campaign of New York.

The fact that the New Mexico communities mentioned above are populated by brown, red, and poor people is no coincidence. The pattern is the same nationwide. The communities most endangered by poisoned water from nuclear facilities at Oak Ridge, Tennessee or the Savannah River Plant in South Carolina are black and poor. The greatest concentration of hazardous waste sites in the country is in Chicago's South Side, a predominantly black and ethnic area of the city. Three of the five largest commercial landfills — including the one at Emelle, Alabama — are located in majority black or Hispanic areas. According to an exhaustive study by the United Church of Christ called "Toxic Wastes and Race," communities with hazardous waste facilities have twice the proportion of non-whites as other towns.

The same study determined that about half of the nation's population live in cities with uncontrolled hazardous waste sites (those abandoned or closed for health reasons). But people of color face a even higher risk: Waste facilities are more often located in their neighborhoods, yet they often lack the economic power to move away or the political clout to force a site cleanup. As a consequence, 60 percent of blacks and Hispanics live in areas with uncontrolled waste sites.

GARBAGE IN, GARBAGE OUT

Municipal solid waste — garbage — is not as lethal as toxic and hazardous waste, but its disposal is reaching the point of crisis in many cities. Much of

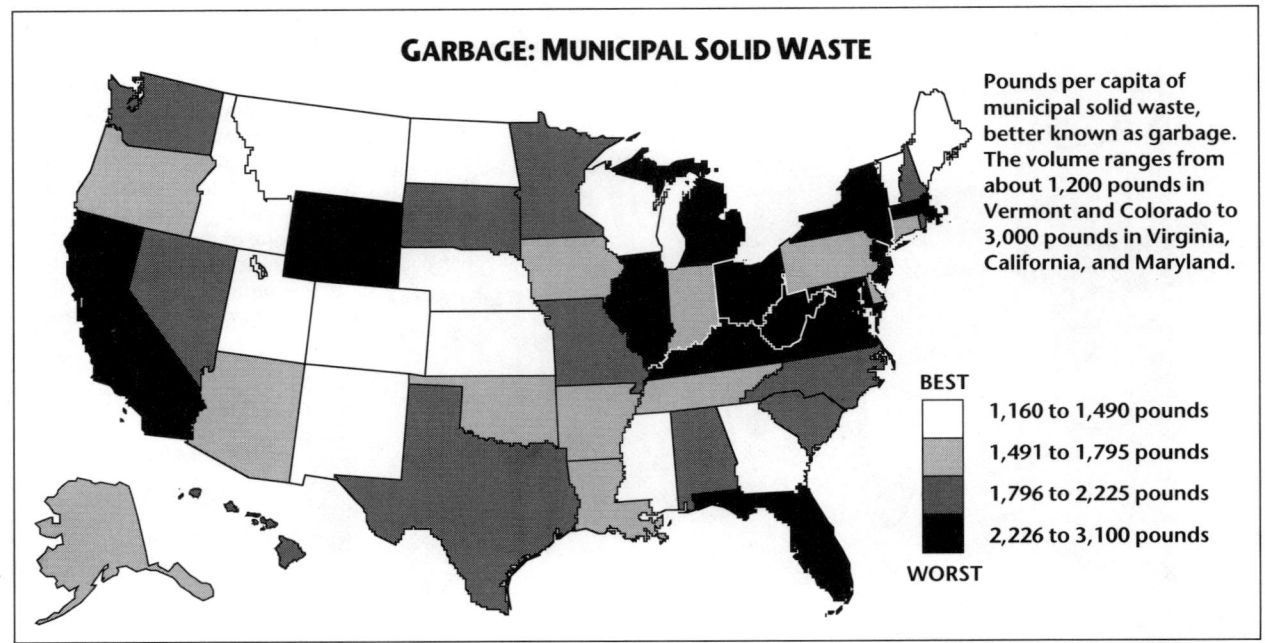

the 20,000 tons New York City produces each day is taken to Fresh Kills Landfill. This gigantic waste mound on Long Island, covering 3,000 acres, leaches 2 million gallons of toxic fluid into the ground and surface water daily. Facing mounting costs and environmental problems, New York City has decided to phase in mandatory recycling.

New York's solid waste problems reflect a national trend. Since 1960, the volume of garbage has almost doubled, with packaging now making up one-third of the wastestream. *BioCycle* magazine estimates our output now tops 500 billion pounds a year, or 6 pounds per person each day. Only 9 percent of this waste — chiefly paper, bottles, cans, yard trash, and food — is recycled or composted. Another 8 percent is incinerated, leaving 83 percent destined for landfills.

In the past decade, about three-quarters of the nation's landfills have closed, and 2,000 of the remaining 7,300 will reach saturation point in the next 5 years. On a per-capita basis, such rural states as Alaska, Wyoming, Montana, Wisconsin, Maine, and Nevada lead in landfills; however, the biggest problems are in the population centers of the Mid-Atlantic, New England, and South. Each day, 200 trucks loaded with garbage from New York and New Jersey roll into dumps in Scranton, Pennsylvania. Dump operators collect as much as $1.5 million a week, but leaching lead and toxic chemicals have taken a toll. Residents nearby suffer above-average rates of cancer, birth defects, seizures, and learning disabilities.

"I am concerned about the serious first-trimester anomalies and the falling birth weights," says Kenneth Lilik, a Scranton pediatrician and neurologist. "Something unhealthy is going on." David Anderson, a Texas environmental consultant, reviewed the area's dumps, toxic sites, and mine wastes and concluded that in 15 years, "I've never encountered such a complex conglomeration of land-based pollution sources as in Lackawanna Valley." But Mark McClellan, deputy secretary for the Pennsylvania Department of Environmental Resources, cautions that "we've seen no data to support those conclusions" of health problems caused by landfills.

Pennsylvania, a major producer of fossil-fuel wastes, also has the most "non-hazardous" landfills and impoundments regulated under Subtitle D of RCRA. Other fossil-fuel producers — West Virginia, Louisiana, Arkansas, New Mexico, and Alaska — host thousands of Subtitle D waste sites. Municipal landfills and many industrial facilities fall under this section's lax regulations, too. But EPA tests confirm that at least 10 percent of these "non-hazardous" industrial landfills actually handle dangerous chemicals (such as arsenic) and one-fourth of those violate state groundwater standards. As a consequence, Congress directed EPA in 1984 to establish new controls for Subtitle D facilities by 1988. EPA has proposed revisions that require liners and monitoring for municipal landfills, but according to an April 1990 report from the U.S. General Accounting Office, the agency "has made little progress" regarding industrial landfills and "does not have a strategy in place to guide its assessment and revision effort."

Because of such regulatory cowardice in the face of health problems like those found in Scranton, citizens throughout the nation have increasingly fought the siting of landfills, drawing on help from the Citizens Clearinghouse on Hazardous Waste, the National Toxics Campaign, and other organizations. As an alternative, some public officials have embraced trash incinerators. Maine, Connecticut, Delaware, Massachusetts, New Hamsphire, Florida, New York, Ohio, Tennessee, Oklahoma, Minnesota, and Maryland (the state with the most garbage per person) now burn from 13 to 57 percent of their garbage.

Although burning reduces the volume of waste, the remaining ash and toxic emissions contain dangerous levels of mercury, lead, dioxin, furans, and cadmium. As much as 12 pounds of hydrogen chloride, which can corrode metal and cause respiratory problems, is produced for each ton of trash burned. Newer incinerators are equipped with acid scrubbers, but some of the larger ones, including a massive facility in Detroit, have none. And those with emission controls, like five in Florida that are not properly monitored, still release thousands of pounds of mercury into the air. Neighbors of incinerators from Rock Hill, South Carolina to Oswego County, New York report chronic breathing problems. Also, burning waste, even for conversion to energy, is not cheap. A small, 200-ton-per day incinerator can cost $200 million — and its investment discourages resource recovery. Instead, 80 percent of the waste that could be recycled is burned to keep the incinerator fueled and economically viable for its operators.

The states doing the best job of recycling municipal solid waste include two that are its biggest producers (New Jersey and California), the two with the least per-capita volume (Vermont and Colorado), and four with about average trash output (Washington, Oregon, Minnesota, and Rhode Island). Delaware has chosen to invest heavily in solid waste composting. More typically, three of the largest waste producers — Virginia, Florida, and Michigan — are expanding recycling programs at the same time that they pour millions of dollars into building new incinerators.

Meanwhile, stopping waste at its source gets little attention. "Recycling may be the best form of waste management, but that is not the same thing as not producing waste to begin with," concludes the congressional Office of Technology Assessment. "The bad news is that the nation's pollution prevention efforts are scattered and uncoordinated, lack permanent institutional support, lack strong funding, and, for the most part, pale in comparison to the established pollution control culture."

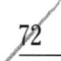

1991–1992 GREEN INDEX

TOXIC WASTE

State	TOXIC CHEMICAL RELEASES TO THE LAND						TOXIC CHEMICAL TRANSFERS OFF SITE					
	Total Pounds	Rank	Pounds Per Capita	Rank	Pounds Per Square Mile	Rank	Total Pounds	Rank	Pounds Per Capita	Rank	Pounds Per Square Mile	Rank
Alabama	4,597,573	28	1.1	30	88.9	22	15,474,062	31	3.7	32	299.3	27
Alaska	1,467	3	0.0	3	0.0	2	202,310	6	0.4	7	0.3	2
Arizona	53,764,405	48	15.5	48	471.6	46	1,578,483	13	0.5	8	13.8	10
Arkansas	1,938,400	22	0.8	27	36.4	18	7,941,692	25	3.3	29	149.3	20
California	18,163,490	41	0.6	24	114.4	24	41,237,250	41	1.5	17	259.8	26
Colorado	2,621,705	24	0.8	26	25.2	12	5,415,112	19	1.6	19	52.0	14
Connecticut	1,676,468	20	0.5	21	334.1	42	17,722,091	32	5.5	41	3,531.7	48
Delaware	251,208	9	0.4	18	122.9	27	2,722,103	15	4.1	35	1,331.8	42
Florida	82,552,586	50	6.7	42	1,407.2	49	14,789,622	30	1.2	14	252.1	25
Georgia	9,178,212	33	1.4	33	155.8	32	24,472,111	38	3.8	33	415.4	31
Hawaii	179,745	7	0.2	10	27.8	14	13,682	1	0.0	1	2.1	7
Idaho	10,173,306	34	10.2	45	121.7	26	136,595	5	0.1	3	1.6	5
Illinois	10,469,190	35	0.9	29	185.8	36	55,444,122	45	4.8	38	984.0	40
Indiana	63,043,385	49	11.3	46	1,742.3	50	51,466,382	43	9.2	46	1,422.3	43
Iowa	240,030	8	0.1	7	4.3	6	7,467,635	23	2.6	24	132.7	19
Kansas	482,324	11	0.2	11	5.9	7	54,398,454	44	21.9	50	661.2	37
Kentucky	5,736,357	30	1.5	34	142.0	31	31,787,074	40	8.5	44	786.6	39
Louisiana	2,019,803	23	0.5	20	42.3	20	21,897,335	37	5.0	39	458.6	33
Maine	955,633	16	0.8	25	28.7	15	1,282,633	11	1.1	12	38.6	12
Maryland	2,666,276	25	0.6	23	254.9	39	5,574,470	20	1.2	15	532.9	35
Massachusetts	906,657	14	0.2	8	109.4	23	21,628,310	36	3.7	31	2,610.9	46
Michigan	17,593,984	40	1.9	36	300.6	40	95,848,610	49	10.3	48	1,637.7	44
Minnesota	889,448	13	0.2	13	10.5	8	5,913,230	21	1.4	16	70.1	17
Mississippi	9,000,495	32	3.4	41	188.7	37	7,693,365	24	2.9	27	161.3	21
Missouri	40,182,059	47	7.8	43	576.5	47	14,113,097	29	2.7	25	202.5	23
Montana	32,910,607	46	40.9	50	223.8	38	46,370	2	0.1	2	0.3	1
Nebraska	55,018	5	0.0	4	0.7	4	3,841,681	16	2.4	23	49.7	13
Nevada	3,490,521	27	3.3	40	31.6	17	639,396	9	0.6	10	5.8	9
New Hampshire	428,868	10	0.4	19	46.2	21	2,098,561	14	1.9	20	226.2	24
New Jersey	2,874,575	26	0.4	14	369.2	44	68,514,999	46	8.9	45	8,798.6	50
New Mexico	22,267,882	43	14.7	47	183.1	35	210,780	7	0.1	4	1.7	6
New York	1,141,102	18	0.1	6	23.2	11	50,430,010	42	2.8	26	1,026.9	41
North Carolina	19,607,668	42	3.0	39	372.3	45	20,725,143	34	3.2	28	393.5	30
North Dakota	752	2	0.0	2	0.0	3	101,287	3	0.2	5	1.4	4
Ohio	30,202,247	44	2.8	38	730.8	48	124,322,305	50	11.4	49	3,008.0	47
Oklahoma	1,787,909	21	0.5	22	25.6	13	11,690,367	26	3.6	30	167.1	22
Oregon	1,032,032	17	0.4	16	10.6	9	5,313,630	18	1.9	21	54.7	15
Pennsylvania	16,424,639	39	1.4	31	362.5	43	83,798,182	47	7.0	43	1,849.5	45
Rhode Island	157,968	6	0.2	9	130.3	30	4,321,293	17	4.3	36	3,565.4	49
South Carolina	1,306,263	19	0.4	15	42.0	19	13,970,376	28	4.0	34	449.0	32
South Dakota	1	1	0.0	1	0.0	1	421,384	8	0.6	9	5.5	8
Tennessee	13,210,057	36	2.7	37	313.5	41	21,581,214	35	4.4	37	512.1	34
Texas	30,837,047	45	1.8	35	115.6	25	88,110,657	48	5.3	40	330.2	28
Utah	15,360,002	38	9.1	44	180.9	34	1,546,165	12	0.9	11	18.2	11
Vermont	24,341	4	0.0	5	2.5	5	645,139	10	1.2	13	67.1	16
Virginia	5,059,278	29	0.8	28	124.1	29	13,480,493	27	2.2	22	330.7	29
Washington	914,424	15	0.2	12	13.4	10	7,330,715	22	1.6	18	107.6	18
West Virginia	710,117	12	0.4	17	29.3	16	18,747,276	33	10.0	47	773.7	38
Wisconsin	6,944,824	31	1.4	32	123.7	28	30,749,287	39	6.3	42	547.6	36
Wyoming	15,274,367	37	32.4	49	156.2	33	101,526	4	0.2	6	1.0	3
U.S. Total	561,306,715		2.3		155.1		1,078,958,066		4.4		298.2	

HAZARDOUS, TOXIC AND SOLID WASTE

TOXIC WASTE

State	TOTAL TOXIC CHEMICAL RELEASE TO ENVIRONMENT						SUMMARY OF 9 TOXIC INDICATORS		PERSONAL INCOME FROM CHEMICAL INDUSTRY		
	Total Pounds	Rank	Pounds Per Capita	Rank	Pounds Per Square Mile	Rank	Score	Rank	% All Income	$ Per Capita	Rank
Alabama	126,962,842	32	30.8	36	2,455.5	28	266	31	0.8	106	26
Alaska	26,476,465	14	51.6	46	44.8	4	87	5	0.2	37	9
Arizona	74,657,306	27	21.5	29	654.9	14	243	28	0.3	39	10
Arkansas	72,272,458	26	29.8	34	1,358.8	21	222	23	0.6	73	18
California	201,568,789	42	7.2	7	1,270.1	20	242	27	0.5	101	24
Colorado	21,132,981	10	6.4	6	203.0	7	137	9	0.6	96	21
Connecticut	53,449,946	21	16.5	21	10,651.6	48	294	37	1.4	323	46
Delaware	10,692,005	6	16.2	20	5,230.9	42	214	20	14.4	2,544	50
Florida	208,977,798	43	16.9	23	3,562.3	37	313	39	0.4	66	16
Georgia	131,410,860	33	20.5	25	2,230.7	26	284	34	0.7	100	22
Hawaii	2,964,331	3	2.7	2	458.1	12	57	3	0.1	12	2
Idaho	15,105,613	8	15.1	16	180.8	5	147	12	1.1	137	31
Illinois	251,302,153	46	21.8	31	4,460.1	40	340	44	1.2	214	36
Indiana	276,346,921	47	49.6	44	7,637.1	44	412	50	1.6	242	42
Iowa	58,668,674	23	20.7	26	1,042.5	19	155	15	0.5	73	17
Kansas	174,468,243	38	70.2	47	2,120.5	25	270	32	0.7	113	27
Kentucky	115,319,338	30	31.0	37	2,853.8	33	318	40	1.1	139	32
Louisiana	741,206,814	49	167.7	50	15,522.3	49	320	41	2.4	291	45
Maine	21,965,123	11	18.2	24	660.3	15	141	11	0.1	22	3
Maryland	33,340,174	15	7.2	8	3,187.4	35	215	22	0.5	103	25
Massachusetts	66,381,565	25	11.3	11	8,013.2	45	239	26	0.6	126	29
Michigan	231,681,301	44	24.9	33	3,958.5	38	372	48	1.2	204	35
Minnesota	65,506,519	24	15.2	17	776.1	18	147	12	1.7	283	43
Mississippi	120,820,916	31	46.0	42	2,533.5	29	284	34	0.7	82	19
Missouri	184,627,555	39	35.9	40	2,649.0	32	325	42	1.4	218	37
Montana	35,467,330	17	44.1	41	241.2	8	205	18	0.2	24	5
Nebraska	22,649,337	12	14.1	15	292.8	10	102	6	0.9	128	30
Nevada	4,874,292	5	4.6	5	44.1	3	125	7	0.1	24	4
New Hampshire	15,171,504	9	13.8	14	1,635.0	23	154	14	0.2	40	11
New Jersey	162,741,774	36	21.1	28	20,899.2	50	339	43	3.2	701	49
New Mexico	24,398,821	13	16.2	19	200.7	6	180	16	0.1	11	1
New York	172,106,105	37	9.6	9	3,504.6	36	226	24	0.8	149	33
North Carolina	136,857,071	34	21.0	27	2,598.4	30	309	38	1.6	231	39
North Dakota	1,394,580	1	2.1	1	19.7	1	22	1	0.5	62	14
Ohio	375,989,294	48	34.6	39	9,097.2	46	409	49	1.6	242	41
Oklahoma	51,720,309	20	15.9	18	739.3	17	189	17	0.3	33	7
Oregon	33,604,243	16	12.3	12	346.2	11	135	8	0.2	26	6
Pennsylvania	201,102,129	41	16.7	22	4,438.6	39	350	46	1.4	221	38
Rhode Island	12,568,955	7	12.6	13	10,370.4	47	214	20	0.6	101	23
South Carolina	82,177,534	28	23.5	32	2,641.3	31	238	25	2.9	374	47
South Dakota	3,059,629	4	4.3	4	39.7	2	38	2	0.5	62	13
Tennessee	249,417,227	45	50.7	45	5,918.2	43	353	47	2.1	284	44
Texas	824,477,706	50	49.1	43	3,090.2	34	348	45	1.6	235	40
Utah	137,472,389	35	81.3	48	1,619.2	22	255	30	0.5	63	15
Vermont	2,374,596	2	4.3	3	247.0	9	67	4	0.2	34	8
Virginia	196,619,903	40	32.8	38	4,823.0	41	283	33	1.1	194	34
Washington	50,338,221	19	10.9	10	738.8	16	140	10	0.7	113	28
West Virginia	57,901,379	22	30.7	35	2,389.6	27	247	29	3.7	436	48
Wisconsin	105,049,429	29	21.6	30	1,870.8	24	291	36	0.5	84	20
Wyoming	45,464,978	18	96.5	49	464.8	13	212	19	0.3	42	12
U.S. Total	6,292,305,425		25.7		1,738.8					180	

TOXIC WASTE

State	CANCER-CAUSING CHEMICALS RELEASED TO ENVIRONMENT			BIRTH DEFECT TOXINS RELEASED TO ENVIRONMENT			NERVE DAMAGING TOXINS RELEASED TO ENVIRONMENT			SUMMARY FOR HEALTH-HAZARD TOXINS	
	Pounds	Pounds Per Capita	Rank	Pounds	Pounds Per Capita	Rank	Pounds	Pounds Per Capita	Rank	Score	Rank
Alabama	10,787,924	2.61	40	36,694,696	8.89	46	23,488,756	5.69	45	131	47
Alaska	474,927	0.93	13	351,939	0.69	3	2,085,235	4.06	34	50	15
Arizona	2,504,054	0.72	11	10,904,090	3.15	16	4,653,756	1.34	14	41	14
Arkansas	6,200,280	2.56	38	20,543,422	8.48	42	11,995,276	4.95	43	123	44
California	23,679,142	0.84	12	53,380,413	1.90	10	21,590,363	0.77	11	33	12
Colorado	3,451,633	1.05	14	5,449,303	1.66	8	2,275,463	0.69	10	32	11
Connecticut	11,135,408	3.44	46	23,117,564	7.13	37	11,037,040	3.41	32	115	39
Delaware	1,646,617	2.49	37	3,996,109	6.05	27	2,864,625	4.34	37	101	35
Florida	7,757,864	0.63	10	17,165,060	1.39	5	14,811,799	1.20	12	27	8
Georgia	14,267,342	2.23	33	25,750,652	4.02	19	43,356,454	6.77	46	98	32
Hawaii	115,345	0.11	3	354,190	0.32	1	2,250	0.00	1	5	1
Idaho	1,119,760	1.12	15	1,583,761	1.59	7	563,134	0.56	8	30	10
Illinois	22,135,826	1.92	30	70,116,380	6.07	28	31,118,737	2.70	25	83	25
Indiana	31,759,346	5.70	49	74,846,502	13.43	50	23,335,305	4.19	35	134	48
Iowa	6,295,652	2.22	32	24,241,219	8.55	43	8,812,469	3.11	28	103	36
Kansas	4,353,597	1.75	26	15,390,249	6.19	29	7,860,932	3.16	30	85	27
Kentucky	9,651,106	2.59	39	25,770,645	6.93	35	18,170,240	4.88	42	116	40
Louisiana	23,931,423	5.41	48	44,951,542	10.17	47	38,307,929	8.67	48	143	49
Maine	2,265,742	1.88	28	8,213,193	6.81	33	3,192,557	2.65	24	85	27
Maryland	2,629,288	0.57	9	8,271,630	1.78	9	8,599,061	1.85	17	35	13
Massachusetts	8,491,397	1.45	20	24,938,652	4.25	20	11,197,451	1.91	19	59	17
Michigan	25,531,483	2.75	41	65,825,654	7.08	36	27,870,594	3.00	27	104	37
Minnesota	5,405,456	1.26	16	37,402,053	8.69	44	19,768,728	4.59	38	98	32
Mississippi	6,512,528	2.48	36	23,276,616	8.86	45	8,917,457	3.39	31	112	38
Missouri	8,864,314	1.72	25	32,404,872	6.31	31	11,757,367	2.29	22	78	24
Montana	292,869	0.36	7	1,233,800	1.53	6	218,278	0.27	4	17	3
Nebraska	2,605,140	1.63	22	8,428,559	5.26	24	3,203,316	2.00	20	66	19
Nevada	79,515	0.08	2	3,678,004	3.47	18	501,262	0.47	5	25	7
New Hampshire	3,189,705	2.91	44	7,128,397	6.50	32	2,430,234	2.22	21	97	31
New Jersey	9,851,296	1.28	17	38,701,629	5.01	23	43,694,906	5.66	44	84	26
New Mexico	85,493	0.06	1	855,861	0.57	2	32,168	0.02	2	5	1
New York	35,674,339	1.99	31	50,971,376	2.85	15	29,958,887	1.67	16	62	18
North Carolina	17,989,674	2.76	42	49,569,183	7.60	39	30,391,706	4.66	40	121	42
North Dakota	243,636	0.37	8	734,143	1.11	4	335,147	0.51	6	18	4
Ohio	31,141,636	2.86	43	87,447,167	8.04	41	52,834,798	4.86	41	125	45
Oklahoma	6,127,464	1.88	27	14,650,944	4.49	21	6,115,167	1.87	18	66	19
Oregon	4,723,684	1.72	24	7,474,786	2.73	14	11,870,297	4.33	36	74	23
Pennsylvania	27,246,604	2.27	34	68,150,644	5.67	25	32,979,631	2.74	26	85	27
Rhode Island	1,635,375	1.64	23	4,712,224	4.74	22	2,336,679	2.35	23	68	22
South Carolina	8,577,509	2.46	35	27,517,312	7.88	40	24,212,095	6.93	47	122	43
South Dakota	171,070	0.24	6	1,542,052	2.16	11	395,301	0.55	7	24	6
Tennessee	17,880,308	3.63	47	60,894,214	12.38	49	48,476,487	9.85	49	145	50
Texas	51,707,413	3.08	45	95,113,468	5.67	26	52,973,017	3.16	29	100	34
Utah	2,445,091	1.45	19	11,675,872	6.90	34	2,200,919	1.30	13	66	19
Vermont	122,961	0.22	5	1,445,632	2.60	13	363,062	0.65	9	27	8
Virginia	7,675,038	1.28	18	68,803,795	11.47	48	73,949,873	12.33	50	116	40
Washington	6,749,598	1.46	21	14,773,838	3.20	17	6,417,213	1.39	15	53	16
West Virginia	10,884,294	5.78	50	13,649,411	7.24	38	8,683,158	4.61	39	127	46
Wisconsin	9,313,636	1.92	29	30,473,810	6.27	30	18,932,900	3.90	33	92	30
Wyoming	97,557	0.21	4	1,026,734	2.18	12	86,454	0.18	3	19	5
U.S. Total	497,478,359	2.03		1,325,593,261	5.41		811,225,933	3.31			

HAZARDOUS, TOXIC AND SOLID WASTE

HAZARDOUS WASTE

State	HAZ. WASTE GENERATED Pounds Per Capita	Rank	HAZARDOUS WASTE STAYS IN STATE Pounds Per Capita	Rank	HAZ. WASTE RCRA GENERATORS #	Rank	HAZARDOUS WASTE MGMT. FACILITIES #	Rank	HAZARDOUS MATERIALS TRANSPORT ACCIDENTS #Incidents	Million $ Damage	Rank	MILITARY HAZARDOUS SITES #	Rank
Alabama	3,685	42	3,778	42	217	28	66	35	216	652	31	470	43
Alaska	10	4	5	5	9	3	5	9	18	32	6	498	50
Arizona	536	29	582	31	160	25	98	46	100	557	32	292	33
Arkansas	49	14	614	32	114	22	35	31	201	1,127	46	221	37
California	733	32	283	26	3,972	44	348	23	676	3,665	26	1,713	22
Colorado	182	22	173	20	90	9	34	14	157	237	10	346	42
Connecticut	112	19	110	17	364	40	138	49	89	198	7	91	2
Delaware	304	25	88	16	25	16	15	42	22	2,183	50	87	44
Florida	147	20	127	18	273	6	72	4	324	1,269	19	487	9
Georgia	12,498	49	12,496	50	330	29	91	33	419	597	16	458	29
Hawaii	14	7	12	9	26	7	12	18	8	106	18	176	48
Idaho	4	2	9	7	24	5	11	16	36	169	33	68	28
Illinois	371	27	408	29	760	34	295	45	880	1,286	20	368	6
Indiana	916	34	681	33	395	37	133	43	384	425	12	240	15
Iowa	84	18	66	15	123	20	46	34	359	393	28	166	24
Kansas	1,082	36	1,082	35	131	27	35	28	238	1,164	45	242	40
Kentucky	4,110	43	4,424	43	187	23	44	20	186	421	21	338	36
Louisiana	6,097	46	6,555	47	302	35	67	32	290	1,198	42	152	8
Maine	12	6	4	4	69	30	17	29	42	379	44	62	19
Maryland	318	26	274	25	206	21	44	11	260	835	37	479	41
Massachusetts	39	12	186	21	1,013	45	52	7	193	792	27	190	5
Michigan	898	33	1,219	37	542	31	126	26	361	1,187	25	152	1
Minnesota	157	21	45	13	291	36	41	10	211	543	24	212	17
Mississippi	1,919	39	1,875	39	109	18	47	36	146	209	14	153	23
Missouri	27	10	14	10	191	14	96	37	377	399	13	213	12
Montana	61	16	60	14	17	4	9	15	30	201	41	77	38
Nebraska	678	31	6	6	65	17	8	3	59	37	4	119	31
Nevada	202	24	206	22	34	12	8	6	65	204	38	174	47
New Hampshire	40	13	1	2	102	39	9	8	15	104	17	51	16
New Jersey	2,378	40	2,375	40	1,480	47	284	47	367	1,319	35	332	14
New Mexico	12	5	10	8	56	15	16	17	110	227	30	241	49
New York	1,798	38	1,151	36	652	13	132	5	454	1,164	8	533	3
North Carolina	411	28	452	30	384	32	78	21	395	4,495	48	264	11
North Dakota	9	3	247	23	8	2	7	12	14	12	1	62	39
Ohio	556	30	717	34	688	33	251	40	908	1,237	22	340	4
Oklahoma	960	35	1,310	38	118	11	46	27	95	295	15	270	35
Oregon	23	8	21	11	505	46	13	2	146	106	5	146	21
Pennsylvania	5,278	45	5,256	45	2,607	48	464	48	989	819	9	593	18
Rhode Island	24	9	139	19	403	50	13	24	15	21	3	71	30
South Carolina	3,180	41	3,175	41	171	26	83	44	127	588	34	267	32
South Dakota	3	1	0	1	4	1	2	1	15	103	29	45	27
Tennessee	13,932	50	384	28	556	41	50	13	447	877	36	248	20
Texas	4,731	44	5,055	44	2,450	43	1,153	50	880	8,733	47	658	10
Utah	1,381	37	5,812	46	220	42	39	41	112	495	43	230	46
Vermont	37	11	3	3	124	49	7	22	20	123	40	19	7
Virginia	8,769	47	8,760	48	532	38	67	19	214	723	23	812	45
Washington	199	23	292	27	188	19	60	25	194	344	11	408	34
West Virginia	12,476	48	12,443	49	57	10	39	38	78	370	39	112	26
Wisconsin	52	15	44	12	240	24	70	30	305	94	2	208	13
Wyoming	62	17	259	24	14	8	11	39	41	484	49	28	25
U.S. Total	2,276		1,996		21,728		4,944		12,288	43,197		14,401	

HAZARDOUS WASTE

State	STATE SPENDING TO MANAGE SOLID & HAZARDOUS WASTE				SUPERFUND NPL SITES		CLEANUP OF NPL SITES UNDERWAY OR COMPLETED			NON-SUPERFUND WASTE SITES		NON-HAZARDOUS SUBTITLE D IMPOUNDMENTS	
	$ Per Capita	Rank	$ Per Ton	Rank	#	Rank	#	%	Rank	#	Rank	#	Rank
Alabama	0.52	45	0.18	48	12	11	5	41.7	5	543	27	4,560	37
Alaska	5.23	8	6.09	5	6	44	0	0.0	47	203	50	1,806	46
Arizona	1.35	29	1.18	25	11	12	2	18.2	26	450	24	864	18
Arkansas	0.73	39	0.80	30	10	22	1	10.0	40	108	1	26,321	49
California	6.26	4	3.54	15	88	10	11	12.1	36	2,400	6	1,170	2
Colorado	1.18	32	1.70	20	16	29	6	37.5	6	387	18	6,723	42
Connecticut	4.42	13	4.64	11	15	25	4	26.7	14	567	37	337	6
Delaware	7.58	2	7.66	3	50	50	4	20.0	22	215	49	92	7
Florida	4.31	14	3.24	16	51	20	11	21.2	20	916	4	3,022	17
Georgia	0.55	43	0.08	50	13	4	1	7.7	43	777	20	961	9
Hawaii	3.29	17	3.63	14	7	30	0	0.0	49	109	11	268	16
Idaho	1.83	24	2.46	18	9	41	1	11.1	37	173	36	422	24
Illinois	4.58	12	3.09	17	37	16	6	15.8	32	1,258	15	2,356	11
Indiana	1.16	33	0.97	27	35	31	8	22.9	19	1,375	47	2,622	26
Iowa	0.33	50	0.39	39	21	37	4	19.0	24	417	33	1,547	27
Kansas	1.11	34	0.94	28	11	24	2	18.2	26	365	32	8,366	45
Kentucky	1.08	35	0.32	41	17	26	5	29.4	11	503	29	233	3
Louisiana	1.18	31	0.30	44	11	6	5	45.5	4	533	26	20,635	47
Maine	7.93	1	10.70	1	9	36	1	11.1	37	149	21	854	33
Maryland	2.38	22	1.41	23	10	5	3	30.0	8	327	2	1,161	19
Massachusetts	5.15	9	4.40	12	25	21	7	28.0	13	731	23	906	10
Michigan	1.36	28	0.76	31	78	40	10	12.7	35	1,491	34	3,394	22
Minnesota	4.76	10	4.91	9	42	43	8	19.0	24	389	8	1,010	15
Mississippi	0.42	48	0.26	47	2	1	0	0.0	45	348	28	2,332	35
Missouri	0.58	42	0.58	35	24	28	6	25.0	15	1,073	44	138	1
Montana	7.57	3	9.77	2	10	46	3	30.0	8	175	45	506	30
Nebraska	0.63	41	0.74	32	6	19	0	0.0	47	297	40	3,067	40
Nevada	0.47	46	0.47	37	1	2	0	0.0	44	139	17	647	31
New Hampshire	5.57	6	6.09	4	16	49	4	25.0	15	135	22	333	21
New Jersey	3.78	15	1.57	22	109	47	25	22.9	18	1,309	35	1,119	8
New Mexico	3.73	16	5.65	6	10	33	3	30.0	8	282	39	17,343	50
New York	3.06	18	1.65	21	83	27	17	20.5	21	1,458	7	1,506	5
North Carolina	0.67	40	0.59	34	22	17	4	18.2	26	785	19	1,328	12
North Dakota	0.75	38	1.01	26	2	14	1	50.0	2	58	9	1,036	39
Ohio	2.10	23	1.32	24	33	13	6	18.2	26	1,001	10	7,990	34
Oklahoma	0.44	47	0.31	43	11	18	2	16.7	30	569	38	7,584	43
Oregon	4.66	11	5.52	7	8	8	2	25.0	15	287	12	740	20
Pennsylvania	2.88	20	0.85	29	95	39	28	28.9	12	2,363	42	36,257	44
Rhode Island	5.26	7	5.04	8	11	45	1	9.1	42	249	48	74	4
South Carolina	0.76	37	0.28	46	23	32	3	13.0	34	396	16	2,029	29
South Dakota	0.33	49	0.32	42	3	23	0	0.0	46	72	13	723	36
Tennessee	1.42	27	0.32	40	14	9	2	14.3	33	714	31	5,989	38
Texas	0.55	44	0.16	49	28	3	14	48.3	3	2,324	30	9,168	28
Utah	1.30	30	0.53	36	12	35	2	16.7	30	186	14	391	13
Vermont	2.60	21	4.40	13	8	48	0	0.0	50	112	43	211	23
Virginia	1.66	25	0.28	45	20	15	4	20.0	22	460	5	2,499	25
Washington	5.97	5	4.91	10	45	42	5	11.1	37	608	25	1,060	14
West Virginia	3.03	19	0.40	38	5	7	3	60.0	1	341	41	19,947	48
Wisconsin	1.46	26	1.91	19	39	38	4	10.0	40	337	3	9,298	41
Wyoming	0.77	36	0.62	33	3	34	1	33.3	7	110	46	336	32
U.S. Total	2.82		1.71		1,197		245	20.3		30,574		223,281	

HAZARDOUS, TOXIC AND SOLID WASTE

SOLID WASTE

State	MUNICIPAL SOLID WASTE GENERATED			MUNICIPAL WASTE RECYCLED		CURBSIDE RECYCLING PROGRAMS		OPEN MUNICIPAL LANDFILLS		MUNICIPAL INCINERATION			COMPOSITE FOR 30 WASTE INDICATORS	
	Million Tons	Pounds Per Capita	Rank	%	Rank	#	Rank	#	Rank	Units	#Tons Per Day	Rank	Score	Rank
Alabama	4.4	2,137	35	5	20	6	24	107	25	1	225	23	944	41
Alaska	0.5	1,708	22	5	20	0	48	740	50	2	100	18	581	8
Arizona	3.1	1,744	23	na		3	30	100	28	0	0	1	730	24
Arkansas	1.8	1,496	14	5	20	3	25	85	32	3	160	20	837	31
California	44.0	3,028	49	12	9	103	11	423	12	3	2,500	42	668	20
Colorado	2.0	1,206	2	14	6	5	23	150	36	0	0	1	522	6
Connecticut	2.9	1,791	25	na		47	5	60	16	7	5,700	47	815	30
Delaware	0.6	1,783	24	20	3	0	48	3	2	1	600	30	798	27
Florida	16.0	2,525	44	4	29	42	13	170	11	10	9,200	49	669	21
Georgia	4.4	1,367	8	na		6	29	191	30	1	500	28	904	35
Hawaii	1.0	1,799	26	4	29	0	48	17	14	1	600	29	454	2
Idaho	0.8	1,479	11	3	31	1	28	110	44	1	50	15	608	12
Illinois	15.0	2,573	46	6	18	65	9	126	8	1	1,200	35	839	32
Indiana	4.5	1,609	18	5	20	3	36	83	13	3	3,000	43	1,075	50
Iowa	2.3	1,620	19	8	13	2	33	82	29	1	125	19	737	25
Kansas	1.6	1,273	3	5	20	3	26	130	39	0	0	1	871	33
Kentucky	4.6	2,468	42	na		2	35	83	21	0	0	1	927	39
Louisiana	3.5	1,597	17	2	32	5	27	41	6	0	0	1	959	44
Maine	0.9	1,473	10	6	18	3	18	185	46	5	1,400	39	621	14
Maryland	7.2	3,068	50	na		12	16	41	5	4	5,000	46	654	18
Massachusetts	6.6	2,232	39	7	16	18	14	160	26	10	8,600	48	675	22
Michigan	11.7	2,523	43	na		26	15	71	4	3	1,250	36	985	46
Minnesota	4.0	1,838	30	15	5	185	2	87	19	11	2,000	41	615	13
Mississippi	1.8	1,374	9	na		na		102	34	1	200	21	913	36
Missouri	5.1	1,977	31	7	16	8	22	84	15	3	50	16	801	29
Montana	0.6	1,489	13	na		0	48	140	48	1	70	17	636	16
Nebraska	1.1	1,366	7	9	12	3	21	39	24	0	0	1	574	7
Nevada	1.0	1,800	27	5	20	0	48	150	45	0	0	1	621	14
New Hampshire	1.0	1,807	28	5	20	6	10	56	38	17	910	34	604	11
New Jersey	9.5	2,456	41	18	4	452	1	90	9	1	400	27	922	38
New Mexico	1.0	1,309	5	1	35	0	48	130	41	0	0	1	592	10
New York	20.0	2,228	38	10	11	na		217	10	12	9,877	50	654	18
North Carolina	6.0	1,826	29	na		5	32	124	17	2	250	24	920	37
North Dakota	0.5	1,364	6	1	35	0	48	70	43	0	0	1	395	1
Ohio	13.9	2,549	45	5	20	26	19	103	7	7	3,750	44	1,003	47
Oklahoma	2.7	1,675	21	2	32	2	34	122	33	3	1,250	37	799	28
Oregon	2.4	1,667	20	22	2	106	3	94	31	2	650	31	468	3
Pennsylvania	9.2	1,528	15	2	32	245	4	72	3	2	700	32	958	43
Rhode Island	1.0	2,004	32	13	7	14	6	4	1	0	0	1	641	17
South Carolina	3.9	2,221	37	8	13	1	37	79	22	2	800	33	961	45
South Dakota	0.8	2,098	34	1	35	0	48	36	37	0	0	1	499	5
Tennessee	3.9	1,579	16	na		4	31	110	20	4	1,450	40	1,050	49
Texas	17.8	2,095	33	8	13	3	38	934	40	8	200	22	1,029	48
Utah	1.1	1,289	4	na		0	48	40	23	1	350	25	878	34
Vermont	0.3	1,164	1	12	9	5	8	60	42	0	0	1	493	4
Virginia	9.0	2,952	48	10	11	15	17	257	35	7	4,000	45	946	42
Washington	5.2	2,184	36	29	1	16	12	95	18	4	370	26	586	9
West Virginia	2.5	2,693	47	na		0	48	51	27	0	0	1	940	40
Wisconsin	3.6	1,479	12	na		65	7	775	47	8	1,300	38	797	26
Wyoming	0.6	2,316	40	5	20	1	20	113	49	0	0	1	723	23
U.S. Total	**268.6**	**2,170**				**1,517**		**7,392**		**153**	**68,787**			

SOURCES FOR TOXIC, HAZARDOUS, AND SOLID WASTE INDICATORS

Toxic chemical release left on site
>   Total pounds, pounds per capita, and pounds per square mile of toxins left in drums, impoundments, landfills, etc., on the facility's property. Discharges in 1988 reported by manufacturing facilities using or releasing at least 50,000 pounds of 322 chemicals, including 123 carcinogens.
>   *Source:* "Toxics in the Community: The 1988 Toxic Release Inventory National Report," September 1990. Published by Office of Toxic Substances, U.S. Environmental Protection Agency, Washington.

Toxic chemicals sent off site
>   Total pounds, pounds per capita, and pounds per square mile of toxins transferred to other facilities for waste disposal.
>   *Source:* "Toxics in the Community: The 1988 Toxic Release Inventory National Report," September 1990. Published by Office of Toxic Substances, U.S. Environmental Protection Agency, Washington.

Total toxic chemical release to environment
>   Total pounds, pounds per capita, and pounds per square mile of total volume of toxins released to air, water, or land and transferred to other facilities or public sewage systems. Based on 1988 reports from manufacturers using or releasing at least 50,000 pounds of 322 chemicals.
>   *Source:* "Toxics in the Community: The 1988 Toxic Release Inventory National Report," September 1990. Published by Office of Toxic Substances, U.S. Environmental Protection Agency, Washington.

Summary of 9 Toxic Indicators
>   Ranks for previous nine indicators are totaled and the lowest total receives the best (lowest) summary ranking.

Personal income from chemical industry
>   Per-capita personal income derived from the chemical industry, with ranking; also, percent of all personal income in the state derived from the chemical industry activities.
>   *Source:* "Growing Employment, Salaries Push Up Chemical Industry Compensation," *Chemical & Engineering News*, October 23, 1989.

Release of cancer-causing poisons
>   Total pounds, ranked on per-capita basis, of 106 chemicals on the Toxic Release Inventory that are (a) classified as positive or suspected human or animal carcinogens by the International Agency for Research on Cancer, (b) classified as possible, probable, or positive carcinogens by U.S. Environmental Protection Agency, or (c) evaluated by GENETOX as inducing tumors or showing an indication of causing tumors.
>   *Source:* "Poisons in Our Neighborhoods: Toxic Pollution in the United States," June 1990. Published by Citizens Fund, 1300 Connecticut Avenue, NW, Washington, DC 20036; telephone (202) 857-5168.

Release of chemicals causing birth defects
>   Total pounds, ranked on per-capita basis, of 63 chemicals on the Toxic Release Inventory that exhibit embryotoxicity, fetotoxicity, or teratogenicity, which distort developmental progress for fetuses.
>   *Source:* "Poisons in Our Neighborhoods: Toxic Pollution in the United States," June 1990. Published by Citizens Fund, Washington.

HAZARDOUS, TOXIC AND SOLID WASTE

Release of neurotoxins
Total pounds, ranked on per-capita basis, of 25 chemicals on the Toxic Release Inventory that cause damage to nerves or nerve tissue from exposure to very small doses (no more than 1 g/kg per day) over a sustained period (at least 90 days).
Source: "Poisons in Our Neighborhoods: Toxic Pollution in the United States," June 1990. Published by Citizens Fund, Washington.

Summary score for health-hazard toxins
Each state's rank on previous three indicators (chemicals causing cancer, birth defects, or nerve damage) was totaled; lowest score receives best summary rank for release of toxins posing serious health hazards.

Hazardous waste generated
Pounds per capita of RCRA-regulated hazardous waste produced in the state. Based on data from state reports covering more than 56,000 generators in 1985, as required by Resource Conservation and Recovery Act (RCRA). Some states include waste-laden water in total pounds, others did not; excludes domestic sewage, industrial wastewater regulated under the Clean Water Act, and radioactive waste.
Source: "1985 National Biennial Report of Hazardous Waste Generators & Treatment, Storage and Disposal Facilities Regulated Under RCRA," December 1988. Prepared for U.S. Environmental Protection Agency, Office of Solid Waste, by DPRA Inc., 200 Research Drive, Manhattan, KS 66502; telephone (913) 539-3565.

Hazardous waste managed in state
Pounds per capita of RCRA-regulated hazardous waste treated, stored, disposed, or otherwise "managed" in the state. Based on data from state reports covering about 4,800 treatment, storage, and disposal facilities in 1985, as required by Resource Conservation and Recovery Act (RCRA) for regulated waste. Some states include waste-laden water in total pounds, others did not; excludes domestic sewage, industrial wastewater regulated under the Clean Water Act, and radioactive waste.
Source: "1985 National Biennial Report of Hazardous Waste Generators & Treatment, Storage and Disposal Facilities Regulated Under RCRA," December 1988. Prepared for U.S. Environmental Protection Agency, Office of Solid Waste, by DPRA Inc., Manhattan, KS.

Number of RCRA hazardous waste generators
Facilities producing RCRA-regulated hazardous waste in 1985.
Source: "1985 National Biennial Report of Hazardous Waste Generators & Treatment, Storage and Disposal Facilities Regulated Under RCRA," December 1988. Prepared for U.S. Environmental Protection Agency, Office of Solid Waste, by DPRA Inc., Manhattan, KS.

Number of commercial hazardous waste facilities
RCRA-regulated commercial facilities which treated, stored, disposed, or otherwise "managed" hazardous waste in 1985.
Source: "1985 National Biennial Report of Hazardous Waste Generators & Treatment, Storage and Disposal Facilities Regulated Under RCRA," December 1988. Prepared for U.S. Environmental Protection Agency, Office of Solid Waste, by DPRA Inc., Manhattan, KS.

Hazardous materials transport accidents
Accidents during transport of hazardous materials by truck, rail, ship, or plane during 1987 and 1988. Data provided for total number of incidents over two years and value in million dollars of damage from accidents, ranked on a per-capita basis.
Source: "Annual Report on Hazardous Materials Transportation, 1987" (also 1988 edition). Published by Research and Special Programs Administration, U.S. Department of Transportation, Washington.

Hazardous waste sites on military installations
> Number of sites as of September 30, 1989, ranked on per-capita basis. Many bases have multiple sites. About 100 sites are also on the NPL Superfund list.
> *Source:* "Department of Defense Environmental Restoration Report to Congress for Fiscal Year 1989," U.S. Department of Defense, Washington.

State spending on solid and hazardous waste
> Per-capita spending in fiscal 1988 to monitor, manage, minimize, and regulate solid and hazardous wastes. Includes state, federal, and other funds (fines, licenses, etc.) that pass through state budgetary process. Excludes funds raised and spent by municipal and county governments for garbage or waste management.
> *Source:* "Resource Guide to State Environmental Management," second edition, 1991. Published by Council of State Governments, P.O. Box 11910, Lexington, KY 40578; telephone (606) 231-1939.

Number of Superfund sites
> National Priorities List (NPL) sites, final and proposed, ranked on per-capita basis. NPL sites are eligible for possible remedial action financed by the Superfund. Generally, they are sites where uncontrolled hazardous waste poses a significant threat to public health or cleanup requires considerable federal assistance. The NPL list totalled 1,207 as of August 1990, but the 10 sites in Puerto Rico are excluded here; hence the total is 1,197.
> *Source:* "National Priorities List, Supplementary Lists and Supporting Materials, August 1990," document number HW-10.14S, August 1990. Published by Office of Emergency & Remedial Response, U.S. Environmental Protection Agency, Washington.

Number of non-Superfund hazardous sites
> Sites identified by local, state, and federal authorities as needing attention, ranked on per-capita basis.
> *Source:* "Superfund Progress Report, May 1990." Prepared by Office of Solid Waste and Emergency Response, U.S. Environmental Protection Agency, Washington.

Superfund site cleanup
> Number of sites with cleanup actually underway (not simply planned) or certified as completed by EPA, including several that were simply dropped from the NPL because they did not merit federal priority attention. Also, percent this number represents of total number on NPL list, with ranking based on state's percentage.
> *Source:* "Superfund Progress Report, May 1990." Prepared by Office of Solid Waste and Emergency Response, U.S. Environmental Protection Agency, Washington.

Non-hazardous waste impoundments
> Impoundments, landfills, and other sites handling waste classified as non-hazardous under Subtitle D of RCRA, chiefly oil and gas exploration waste that includes low levels of toxic substances; ranked on a per-capita basis.
> *Source:* "Census of State and Territorial Subtitle D Non-Hazardous Waste Programs," October 1988. Prepared by Office of Solid Waste, U.S. Environmental Protection Agency, Washington.

Municipal solid waste generated
> Millions of tons, per-capita pounds, and ranking per capita of municipal solid waste disposed of in 1989. Generally excludes sewage sludge (except some in California and Louisiana), demolition waste (except some in California, Florida, New Hampshire, Oregon, Texas, and Virginia), and industrial waste.
> *Source:* Jim Glenn, "The State of Garbage in America," *BioCycle* magazine, March 1990. Published by The JG Press, P.O. Box 351, Emmaus, PA 18049; telephone (215) 967-4135.

HAZARDOUS, TOXIC AND SOLID WASTE

Municipal solid waste recycled
> Estimated percent of municipal solid waste recycled or composted in 1989, based on state-by-state survey.
> *Source:* "The State of Garbage in America," *BioCycle* magazine, March 1990. Published by The JG Press, Emmaus, PA.

Number of curbside recycling programs
> Voluntary and mandatory programs involving curbside pickup in 1989.
> *Source:* Data from Jim Glenn, The JG Press, Emmaus, PA.

Number of open landfills
> Municipal landfills and open dumps in 1989, ranked on a per-capita basis.
> *Source:* "The State of Garbage in America," *BioCycle* magazine, March 1990. Published by The JG Press, Emmaus, PA.

Municipal incinerators
> Number of incinerators burning municipal waste in 1989 and their total tons of daily capacity.
> *Source:* "The State of Garbage in America," *BioCycle* magazine, March 1990. Published by The JG Press, Emmaus, PA.

Composite waste score
> Each state's rank for the 30 indicators was totaled to produce a composite score. Lowest score receives best composite rank for toxic, hazardous, and municipal waste.

CHAPTER 6

Community and Workplace Health

INDICATORS

Cancer cases
Cancer deaths and rate per capita
Rate of premature deaths
Death from nine diseases
Doctors delivering patient care
Population in medically underserved areas
Population without any insurance
State spending for public health
State resources committed to health and welfare
Rating of state Medicaid program
Homes without adequate plumbing
Infant mortality rate
Health rating by Northwestern National Life Insurance
Occupational deaths
Workers in jobs with high risk of disabling diseases
Workers in five industries with most toxic releases
Workers in five industries with highest injury rates
Workers directly involved with hazardous waste
Maximum total disability payment
Maximum unemployment insurance benefits
Unemployed workers with unemployment insurance
Unemployment rate
Workers covered by workplace insurance
Manufacturing workers in unions
State laws for worker rights and workplace safety

When the environment is sick, people get sick. Despite our efforts to create walls between ourselves and our waste, pollution seeps in. The chemicals in our factories and farms permeate the air we breathe, the water we drink, and eventually, our body tissues.

The people hardest hit are often the poorest. They tend to live in areas downstream or downwind of dirty industries, or in areas that lack adequate plumbing, sewage disposal, and public health programs. Conduct a survey in your community: Are waste dumps, heavily polluting industries, low property values, and poor or working class neighborhoods concentrated on the same side of the tracks (often the southern or southeastern part of town), while wealthy neighborhoods are located upwind, in the northwest section? Money flows in the opposite direction of pollution.

Now conduct a survey of the town's workforce: Are the most hazardous jobs in a factory held by people of color, by those with the least education, and/or by contract or temporary workers with few benefits or protections?

Nationally, miners face the highest fatality rate: 32 deaths per 100,000 workers, four times the rate for all workers. Thanks to the strength of their union and the inability of companies to move coal seams the way they move cotton mills, miners have managed to extract relatively good wages and health benefits from their employers. But from West Virginia to Montana, their communities still suffer the blight of poor schools, severe pollution, poverty, high unemployment, and weak enforcement of safety regulations. The result is a vicious cycle: Unsafe mines cripple undereducated miners who have few workplace options, while government inspectors count the bodies and pass out meager fines.

In September 1989, 10 miners died in a methane explosion at Pyro Mining Company's mine in Webster County, Kentucky. In the previous year, the Mine Safety and Health Administration (MSHA) had cited the mine 60 times for methane-related ventilation problems. In fact, the explosion resulted from blockage in a makeshift ventilation system installed after the mine was shut down in June for serious problems with its original system. Altogether, inspectors had cited the mine for 312 serious safety violations in the first nine months of 1989 — yet it continued to operate.

"There is a saying that dead miners are the force that causes mine safety to be enforced," said J. Davitt McAteer, director of the Occupational Safety and Health Law Center, a private watchdog group based in Shepardstown, West Virginia. "It's horrible and the worst part is we know how to prevent them."

In the investigation that followed the explosion, federal agents discovered that Pyro had failed to report a dozen serious injuries in the previous year. One MSHA official said the underreporting was typical of Kentucky mines and helped the state maintain an official injury rate 20 percent below the national average.

DISPOSABLE LIVES

How a company or a state regards the safety of its working and poor people says a great deal about its commitment to environmental health. Not only is their environment shaped by high-risk jobs and communities at the end of the waste stream, working and poor people are also the first to feel the effects of inept policies that allow individual actions to become public hazards. Like the canaries once sent into the mines to test the air, their pain and sickness should sound the alarm for all of us.

The 23 indicators we chose to measure a state's community and workplace health emphasize this relationship between public policy, pollution, living conditions, and human health. The results are distressing — the nation's community and workplace health is ailing and no state can claim a clean record. Not a single state ranked in the top half in all indicators. Even Massachusetts and Minnesota, respectively first place winners in workplace health and community health, had significant weaknesses. Massachusetts ranks 39th for cancer deaths; Minnesota ranks 36th in public health spending and 27th in homes without adequate plumbing.

At the other extreme, Alabama and Arkansas rank below average on nearly every indicator. Pennsylvania scores in the bottom half on most factors related to dangerous jobs and disease, even ranking 40th in infant mortality, but it is among the best 15 for health services, insurance coverage, and disability payments. Five Farmbelt states (Iowa, Nebraska, Kansas, Wisconsin, and Minnesota) scored in the top 12 states on the composite community health index, thanks largely to their low cancer and premature death rates and the high percentage of their people covered by private medical insurance. The same states, however, vary widely in public support for health care, laws protecting worker safety, disability payments, and overall workplace health.

On a national scale, the health data suggest that workers and the poor are considered disposable:

• One in seven of the nation's nonelderly population — 33 million people — had no medical insurance coverage in 1988, either through a private plan or Medicaid. The proportion jumps to one in five for African American children and almost two in five (38 percent) for Latino children, trends that translate into fewer doctor visits. Regardless of race, families with incomes under $25,000 are only one third as likely to have insurance coverage for their children as families earning over $40,000.

• Each day in America, more than 100 babies under age one die — 39,500 babies in 1989. The nation's infant mortality rate of 9.6 deaths per 1,000 live births is the second highest in the industrialized Western Hemisphere. At the same time, 11 percent of the gross national product goes for medical care, a larger share than any other developed nation.

• Using federal health data, the National Safe Work Institute in Chicago estimates that 70,000 workers are permanently disabled each year and more than 71,000 people die from occupational diseases annually. Yet the share of the federal budget that goes to the agencies regulating workplace health has dropped by a third since 1981.

• On top of fatal diseases like black lung and asbestosis, the National Safety Council says 10,500 people die from worksite injuries and accidents each year. In addition, in 1988 the Bureau of Labor Statistics counted about 11,000 workers *each day*

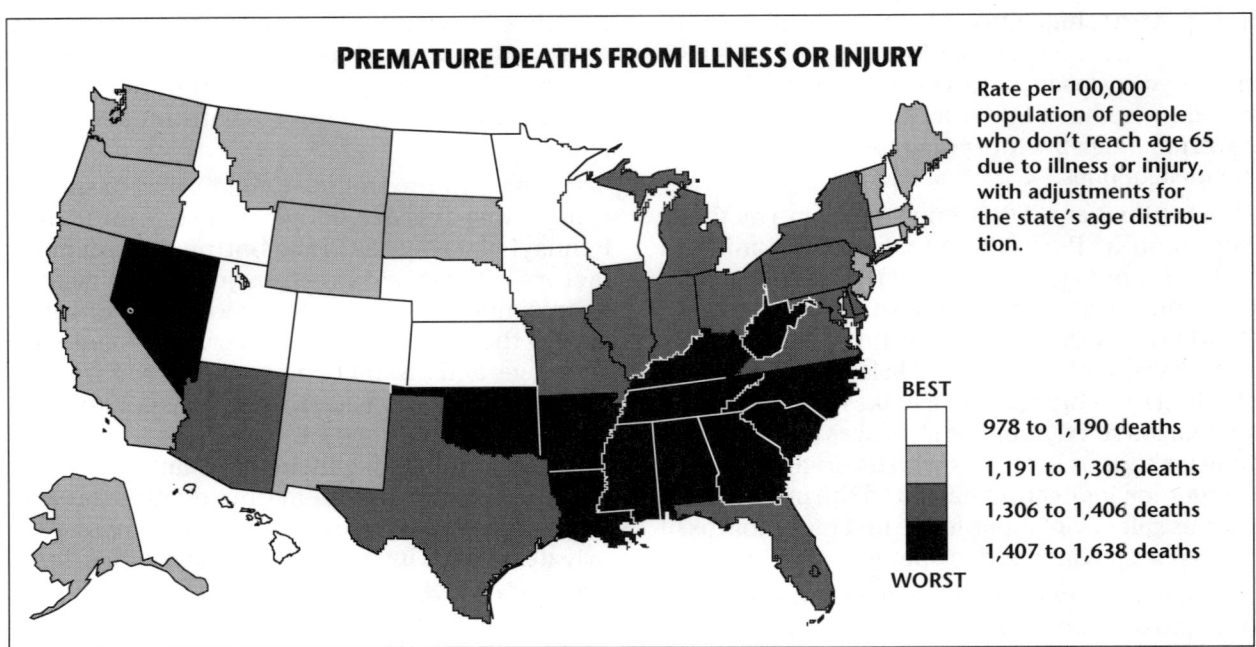

who were injured seriously enough to lose work time or to be put on restricted work duty. The rate of lost-time injuries has increased by 39 percent since 1974.

While several studies point out that these numbers understate the problem, they are stark enough to indict America's health care system in general and workplace safety regulators in particular. In reviewing the performance of the Occupational Safety and Health Administration (OSHA), the U.S. General Accounting Office concluded that (a) "even employers in high-hazard, targeted industries are rarely inspected," (b) sanctions by OSHA "provide limited deterrence to employer noncompliance" since the average assessed penalty for a serious violation was only $261 in 1988, (c) OSHA relies on employer reports to verify compliance rather than conducting its own follow-up inspections, and (d) "safety and health standards fail to cover existing hazards or keep up with new ones."

By contrast, the management consultant firm, Grant Thornton, calls laws to limit pollution an "encumbrance to manufacturers" and praises states that offer the *cheapest* disability compensation for injured workers. Indiana, it notes, has led the nation for five years in this regard. On our set of indicators, Indiana stands out in the Midwest as the state with the lowest number of doctors per capita, and it shows up with below average rankings in all the policy areas (state health spending, Medicaid program, worker rights laws, disability payments, unemployment compensation). The consequences may be short-term savings for companies, but they are devastating for ordinary people.

An Auburn, Indiana iron foundry, for example, has a fatality rate that is five times that of mining. Auburn Foundry officials call their record "indefensible" and say they are making safety the plant's number one priority. But the union president says he was dismissed for pushing safety-and-health issues. The state-administered OSHA program fined the company only $1,000 after the most recent death. Under pressure from the union, the agency raised the seriousness of the citation and hiked the fine to $10,000 — an action the company has protested. In 1989, the company paid a $40,000 fine to EPA for dumping foundry sand on wetlands. Across the street from Auburn Foundry, five more workers died at Bastian Plating Company in a 1988 hydrogen cyanide gas accident. "We refer to Auburn as the industrial death capital of the United States," says William R. Groth of the Foundation for Advancement of Industrial Research in Indianapolis.

A new study from Bloomington, Indiana, where Westinghouse used PCBs between 1957 and 1977 to make electrical equipment, shows that employees from that period are dying with brain cancers at twice the normal rate. Men are getting melanoma skin cancer at seven times the normal rate;

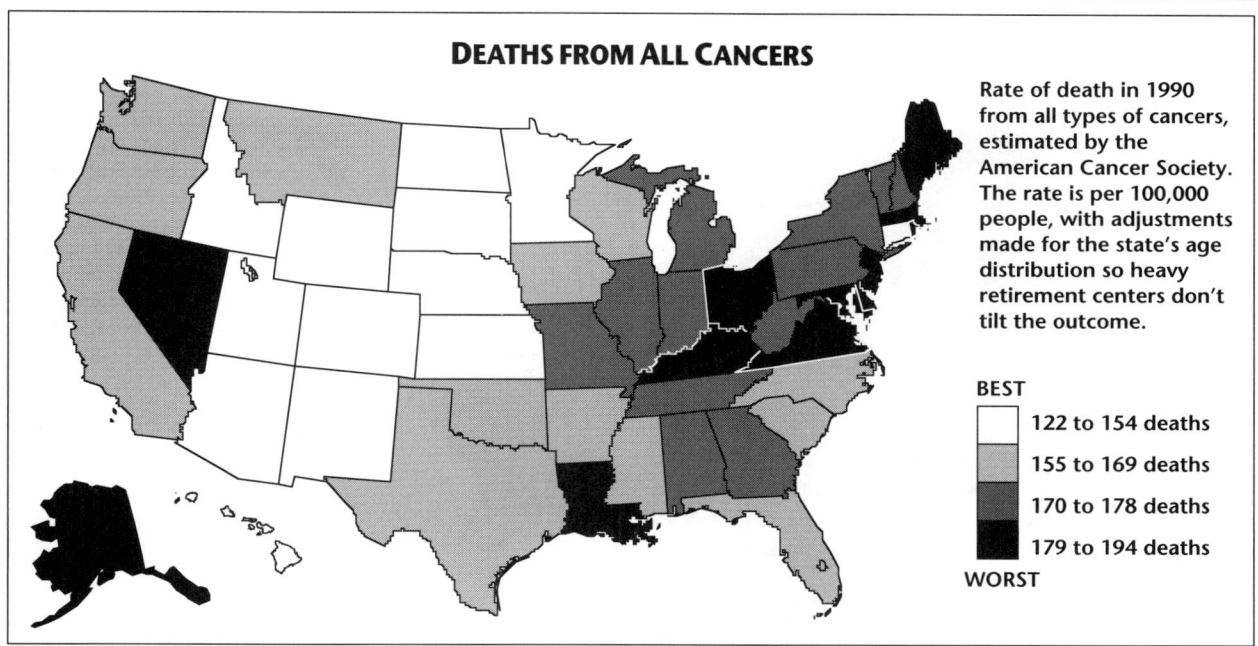

DEATHS FROM ALL CANCERS

Rate of death in 1990 from all types of cancers, estimated by the American Cancer Society. The rate is per 100,000 people, with adjustments made for the state's age distribution so heavy retirement centers don't tilt the outcome.

BEST
- 122 to 154 deaths
- 155 to 169 deaths
- 170 to 178 deaths
- 179 to 194 deaths

WORST

women contract the disease 12 times more often. County residents also remain at risk from six sites contaminated with the PCBs.

The interplay between health policy and conditions varies state by state, region by region, but at the community level the high correlation between a company's regard for its employees' health and its respect for pollution standards means people on both sides of the factory walls have a self-interest in protecting one another.

CANCER BY REGION

In Plaquemine, Louisiana, a small town 30 miles down the Mississippi River from Baton Rouge, Etta Lee Gulotta discovered 40 cancer cases in a five block radius. Her husband died of lung cancer even though he never smoked. In nearby St. Gabriel, Kay Gaudet noticed that women were having miscarriages at about twice the state's average rate. Gaudet discovered that vinyl chloride gas, emitted by chemical companies around St. Gabriel, is a known carcinogen and a suspected embryotoxin. Next door in Geismar, a predominantly black town with some homes only a few hundred yards from factories emitting dangerous gases, 9 of every 10 children had regular respiratory problems.

For residents of these towns along Louisiana's "Chemical Corridor" from Baton Rouge to New Orleans, the connection between pollution and health problems could hardly be more clear. Cancer death rates are already well above the national average (rank 46), and an unusually large share of Louisiana's workforce are in jobs with a high risk of contracting serious diseases (rank 48), as well as jobs in the most toxic industries (rank 46). Indeed, the proportion of Louisiana citizens who do not reach age 65 because of illness or injury — the premature death rate — is one of the highest in the nation (rank 47). At the same time, private employers furnish only half the state's workers with insurance (rank 49) and per-capita spending on public health is barely 40 percent of the national average (rank 43).

Compared to Louisiana, cancer rates are higher or nearly as high in such older industrial states as Maryland, Delaware, New Jersey, Ohio, and Rhode Island. But Maryland and Delaware are leaders in public health spending, the other three are leaders in workplace insurance coverage, and all five have vastly better Medicaid programs for the health care of their poor than does Louisiana. Perhaps as a consequence, their overall premature death rates rank among the middle tier of states instead of at the bottom.

The West Coast states (California, Oregon, Washington) rank in the top half for cancer and premature death rates and in the top 10 for their Medicaid programs. But Oregon ranks last in state public health spending and Washington ranks 42d. Hawaii ranks second best in low cancer and premature death rates, and best in jobs with the high-

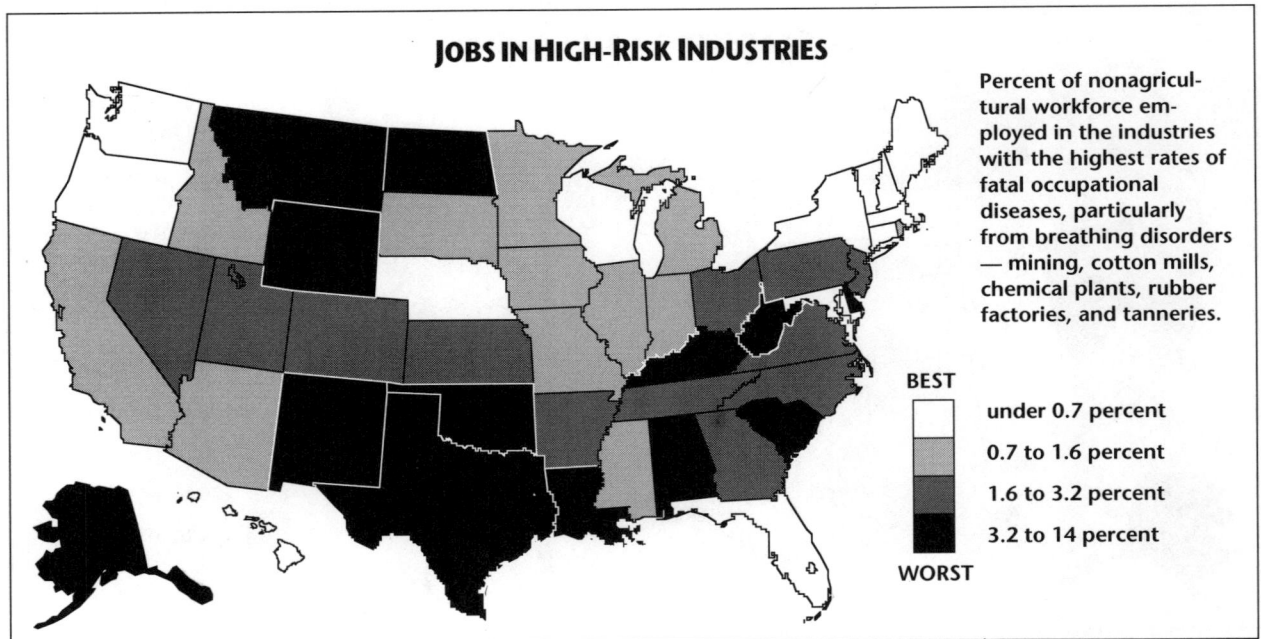

est risk of fatal diseases. Yet, because of its sugar and other food processors, Hawaii ranks 43d for its share of industrial jobs with twice the national injury rate. Washington, home of Boeing aircraft and numerous lumber companies, ranks 49th on the same indicator. Alaska is 50th in high-injury jobs and workplace death, and 49th in cancer deaths.

The states that rank best on cancer indicators stretch across the Rocky Mountains and include Utah, Colorado, Wyoming, Idaho, and New Mexico. Most of them host none or only one of the plants emitting the most high-risk carcinogenic chemicals. But in recent years each state has become home to a booming mining industry. Consequently, their occupational death rates have shot up, ranking them among the worst states for workplace fatalities. Interestingly, Nevada — home of nuclear bomb testing — has the region's highest cancer death rate, ranking it 44th nationally.

Like the South, most of these Mountain states follow the philosophy that the less government interferes with business, the better. Utah, Idaho, and Wyoming are among the worst dozen states for enacting laws to protect workers, and they offer relatively little financial support for totally disabled workers. They are also generally stingy when it comes to devoting state funds to public health programs. Fortunately for their citizens, lower levels of urban stress and pollution combine with higher rates of private insurance coverage to improve overall life expectancy. The Mountain states join several in the Farmbelt to enjoy the nation's lowest premature death rates, as well as relatively low infant mortality rates, even though the same group falls to the bottom half of the list for doctors per capita.

INFANTS AND MEDICAL ACCESS

Humphries County, Mississippi, has an infant mortality rate of 33.2 deaths per 1,000 live births — a ratio surpassing many Third World nations. Nine of the 10 lowest-ranking states for premature deaths and 7 of the worst 10 for infant mortality are in the South. Factors associated with poverty, including poor nutrition and inadequate health care, figure into the numbers, but the deaths are still higher than normal for poor rural areas. The correlation of a state's high minority population to its high infant and premature death rates reinforces the conclusion that race plays a major role in isolating people from resources needed for a healthy life. If you're not part of the "good ole boy" network, you're relegated to the margins of society, which is also where the waste dumps, landfills, and Superfund sites are often found (see page 69).

Mississippi has pulled its infant mortality ranking up over the past few years, but it is still among the worst 10 states, ranking 41st. With one out of four of its citizens lacking insurance, it also ranks last in this crucial indicator of health care accessibility. The worst state for infant mortality, according to 1989 figures, is South Carolina with a rate of

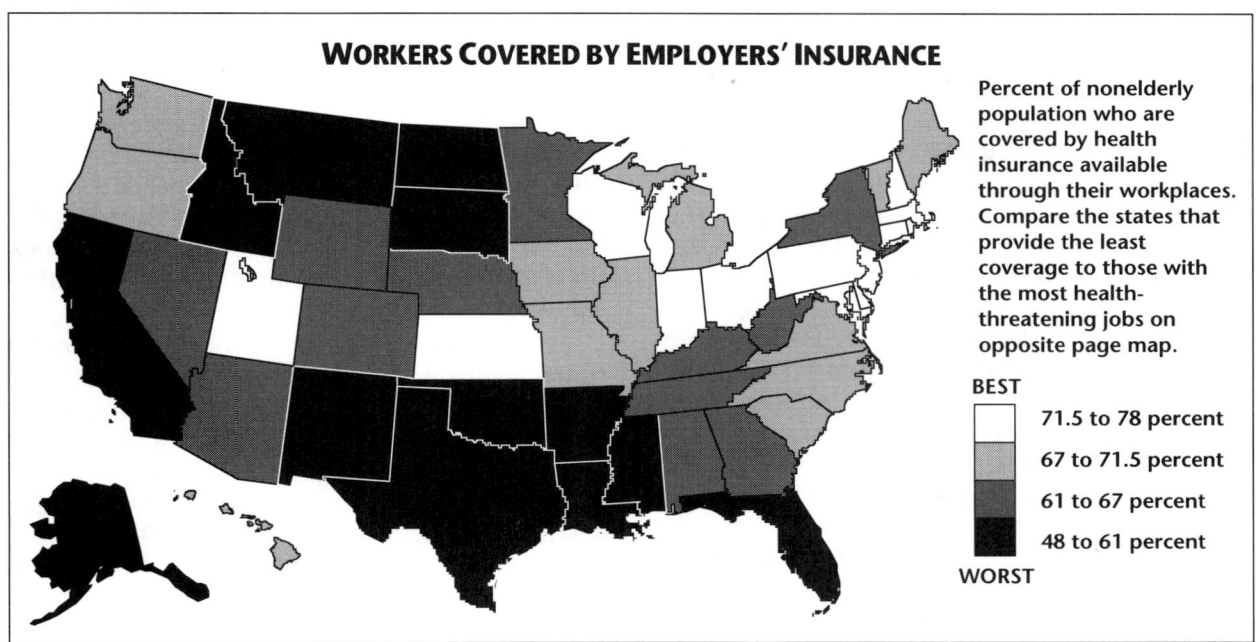

WORKERS COVERED BY EMPLOYERS' INSURANCE

Percent of nonelderly population who are covered by health insurance available through their workplaces. Compare the states that provide the least coverage to those with the most health-threatening jobs on opposite page map.

BEST
- 71.5 to 78 percent
- 67 to 71.5 percent
- 61 to 67 percent
- 48 to 61 percent

WORST

12.5 deaths per 1,000 live births. The Palmetto state hosts more than its share of radioactive and hazardous waste. It also ranks 50th for premature deaths, 48th for people without insurance, and 39th for doctors per capita. Like 7 other Southern states (along with Maine and Alaska), it ranks among the bottom 10 in homes that lack kitchen facilities, toilets, or hot water.

Several states with low infant mortality rates (Rhode Island, Vermont, Massachusetts, Maine, Minnesota, Iowa) also do well in rankings on insurance coverage and Medicaid programs. In all but one case, these same states are among the top 15 for maximum disability payments and for the percent of unemployed receiving benefits, indicating a general progressive tilt toward public programs serving the truly needy.

In contrast to these and other states in the Northeast and Midwest, the South trails in benefits for the disabled and in passing laws to protect workers' rights, even though 6 of the 12 states with the largest share of their workforces in high-risk jobs are in the region. The South also has 7 of the 12 states with the most people lacking insurance coverage and 6 of the 12 with the lowest compensation for unemployed workers. West Virginia — the notable exception in each area — leads the South in union members, public health spending, and disability benefits. But with its dependency on coal mining, West Virginia also leads in unemployment and occupational deaths.

A WORKER'S LOBBY

We include the manufacturing workforce's rate of union membership as a relevant indicator of the workplace environment because unions often act as health-and-safety lobbies and because several studies show that the rise of non-union, contract labor has worsened the job safety records of various industries.

The Oil, Chemical and Atomic Workers Union (OCAW) found that workers for subcontractors of petrochemical firms experienced an injury rate that is two-and-a-half times the rate for the major firms. The increasing use of non-union, inexperienced contract workers has led to several disasters, including 17 deaths at ARCO Chemical in Houston in 1990. An explosion at Phillip Petroleum's Pasadena, Texas refinery in 1989 killed 23 workers and injured 232, making it the worst accident in OSHA's 20-year history.

In another study, Detroit's daily newspaper determined that while half of Michigan's autoworkers are employed in supplier plants, they experience two-thirds of the industry's serious workplace injuries and fatalities. According to the *Detroit Free Press*, the Big Three automakers have relatively fewer incidences than their suppliers because they have less turnover and a more unionized, better trained workforce. By not allowing employers to cut corners at the expense of their health and safety, union members protect their job environment.

In Northfield, Minnesota, a maker of electronic circuitry and laminated products continued to emit methylene chloride even after it was listed as a carcinogen by the National Institute of Occupational Safety and Health (NIOSH) in 1987. The company, Sheldahl, sidestepped NIOSH's recommendation that the chemical be eliminated from worksites by pointing out that OSHA's standard allowed up to 500 parts per million. Through their union, concerned workers began educating themselves about the chemical and pressed the company for changes. Then data from the Toxic Release Inventory revealed that Sheldahl had been releasing 600 tons of methylene chlorine a year into the air. With new pressure from the community and media, the company reduced its use of the chemical by 80 percent in two years and formed a joint labor-community-company taskforce to monitor further progress.

Employers who pollute their host communities and cripple their workers abound throughout America. Unfortunately, many are not as responsive to pressure as Sheldahl. In Virginia, Perdue Farms has repeatedly exceeded standards for the discharge of its poultry waste into a creek near its giant Accomac processing plant; inside the factory, where chickens whiz by on disassembly lines at up to 91 birds a minute, conditions mirror those at other Perdue plants cited for crippling workers with repetitive trauma disorders, the fastest growing occupational disease in the United States.

In Maine, where Boise Cascade pours tons of carcinogenic chloroform into the air and dioxin into the water, federal OSHA fined the company $1.6 million a record for paper-pulp firms — for willful neglect of its 1,600 workers' health. "Many of the hazardous conditions had been identified in Boise Cascade's own safety audit of the mill," said Alan C. McMillan of OSHA, but the problems were never corrected. "They had been cited in the past for similar violations at this and other locations."

UNEVEN STANDARDS

While OSHA parallels EPA in monitoring environmental health problems, it has only one-twentieth the budget and lacks many of EPA's enforcement tools. Like EPA, its regional offices vary greatly in their pursuit of a safe environment. The offices in Texas, for example, are among the nation's weakest when it comes to penalizing companies for workplace deaths. (Brown & Root, the giant Houston-based contractor, paid a mere $16,285 for OSHA violations related to 22 deaths between 1974 and 1988.)* In addition, North Carolina and several other states that set up their own agencies to preempt OSHA have never been fully certified by the federal government because those agencies lack the staff or funding to enforce the Act's minimum standards.

The failure of the federal government to set tough health standards is even more apparent in the area of workers' compensation, the employer-financed insurance programs that shield companies from negligence suits while paying the victims — injured workers — reasonable substitute wages and health benefits. The hodgepodge of compensation systems breeds inequities between the states and, within a state, between the treatment of different injuries and illnesses. The lack of consistent standards also fosters constant maneuvering in the state legislatures to change rules of evidence or to trade this benefit for that cost. Even so-called progressive states like New York and California provide crippled workers with the worst benefits. For a partially disabled worker, New York's plan pays the lowest compensation in the nation, and California ranks 43rd in total disability payments.

A study by the *Orlando Sentinel* documented problems in Florida's system that are common to many states: Insurers and employers harass those who file claims, send them to company doctors (often to be misdiagnosed), drag cases out, stall or terminate payments arbitrarily, cut off medical reimbursement, and pressure workers to settle for less money. Many workers are never even told they're entitled to worker compensation, but are instead paid from the company's cheaper medical insurance policy.

The answer to such alarming regulatory failures is not simply better enforcement and more compensation for these victims of an unhealthy environment. As with other forms of pollution, the answer is prevention — stopping the causes of disease, injury, infant mortality, and occupational death; setting standards that eliminate hazards; and delivering medical and educational resources that serve prevention rather than remediation.

---

* While Texas OSHA has targeted construction companies like Brown & Root, it has largely overlooked the petrochemical industry. Phillip's lethal refinery in Pasadena was not inspected from 1975 to 1989, and regional administrator Gilbert Saulter admitted he "was surprised" to learn that an average of 40 workers a year were dying from accidents in the chemical industry.

COMMUNITY HEALTH

State	CANCER CASES & DEATHS, 1990				PREMATURE DEATHS		DEATH FROM NINE DISEASES		DOCTORS DELIVERING PATIENT CARE		POPULATION IN UNDER-SERVED AREAS		POPULATION WITHOUT INSURANCE	
	# Cases	# Deaths	Rate per 100,000 Pop.	Rank	Rate	Rank	Rate	Rank	Rate	Rank	%	Rank	%	Rank
Alabama	18,300	9,000	175	31	1,579	48	439.6	23	14.0	41	7.5	38	19.7	39
Alaska	1,100	500	190	49	1,218	17	413.8	16	12.7	47	12.1	44	20.9	41
Arizona	13,700	6,700	153	10	1,311	27	396.2	8	17.8	18	5.1	28	21.6	42
Arkansas	11,300	5,600	165	21	1,412	40	407.1	13	13.5	43	6.6	34	22.3	44
California	105,000	51,200	168	24	1,233	19	439.9	24	21.7	6	3.5	18	20.5	40
Colorado	9,700	4,700	144	3	1,105	6	400.3	10	18.3	16	2.4	8	15.5	30
Connecticut	14,800	7,200	173	29	1,161	11	420.2	18	25.7	4	1.8	5	10.3	8
Delaware	3,000	1,500	190	48	1,376	34	494.2	45	17.7	19	2.8	9	11.2	13
Florida	68,000	33,400	162	16	1,366	33	428.6	19	18.7	13	5.6	30	22.2	43
Georgia	24,000	11,500	171	28	1,530	46	471.5	33	15.4	34	7.9	40	18.6	38
Hawaii	3,400	1,700	140	2	1,013	2	326.8	1	20.7	9	1.6	4	13.0	23
Idaho	3,500	1,800	146	6	1,186	12	394.9	7	11.5	50	14.8	49	17.4	35
Illinois	49,700	24,500	176	34	1,376	35	487.9	41	18.9	12	7.6	39	11.8	16
Indiana	24,400	12,000	176	33	1,365	32	490.6	42	14.0	41	3.6	20	12.7	21
Iowa	12,900	6,400	158	13	1,088	5	420.0	17	13.1	45	3.5	18	9.0	3
Kansas	10,200	5,000	152	8	1,157	10	400.5	11	15.7	31	1.3	2	10.9	12
Kentucky	16,800	8,300	180	41	1,455	42	497.2	46	15.1	37	5.2	29	18.1	37
Louisiana	18,600	9,100	186	46	1,558	47	470.1	30	16.8	24	9.2	42	25.7	48
Maine	5,700	2,800	179	40	1,212	16	474.7	34	16.0	29	4.8	26	11.3	14
Maryland	20,000	9,800	194	50	1,399	36	470.7	31	26.7	3	2.9	10	10.6	11
Massachusetts	28,400	14,000	179	39	1,193	14	444.0	26	27.0	1	3.0	11	9.7	5
Michigan	37,900	18,600	176	35	1,405	37	517.6	50	16.4	26	4.5	25	8.3	2
Minnesota	16,900	8,300	154	11	1,056	4	388.4	6	19.3	11	1.5	3	10.4	9
Mississippi	11,000	5,300	166	23	1,627	49	468.9	29	11.9	49	13.1	47	22.4	45
Missouri	23,500	11,600	170	26	1,321	28	440.9	25	17.1	23	5.8	31	13.3	24
Montana	3,300	1,600	160	15	1,242	20	403.6	12	14.4	40	8.4	41	17.4	35
Nebraska	6,700	3,300	154	12	1,144	9	398.3	9	15.5	32	3.4	15	12.6	20
Nevada	4,400	2,200	182	44	1,468	43	481.6	37	14.7	38	6.8	36	23.9	47
New Hampshire	4,700	2,200	177	36	1,139	8	455.8	27	17.2	22	2.0	6	12.8	22
New Jersey	37,700	18,500	185	45	1,302	25	482.0	39	21.1	8	0.9	1	10.5	10
New Mexico	4,700	2,300	145	4	1,273	22	382.0	4	15.5	32	18.4	50	28.1	50
New York	80,000	39,000	177	37	1,406	38	508.5	48	26.9	2	3.2	14	12.5	19
North Carolina	26,000	12,600	164	18	1,478	44	481.7	38	16.1	27	6.3	33	14.8	27
North Dakota	2,800	1,400	151	7	978	1	361.1	2	15.8	30	14.3	48	11.5	15
Ohio	49,000	24,200	182	43	1,359	31	501.2	47	17.5	20	3.8	21	10.1	7
Oklahoma	14,300	7,000	165	22	1,407	39	471.0	32	13.4	44	3.4	15	23.6	46
Oregon	12,300	6,000	165	20	1,273	23	438.1	21	18.1	17	6.6	34	16.9	34
Pennsylvania	61,000	30,000	178	38	1,347	30	478.9	35	20.4	10	2.0	6	9.5	4
Rhode Island	5,200	2,600	181	42	1,259	21	491.0	43	21.8	5	5.0	27	7.7	1
South Carolina	13,200	6,500	169	25	1,638	50	493.2	44	14.5	39	7.4	37	15.3	28
South Dakota	3,200	1,600	152	9	1,289	24	409.8	15	13.0	46	12.8	46	16.0	33
Tennessee	21,100	10,400	170	27	1,446	41	481.1	36	17.3	21	5.8	31	15.4	29
Texas	55,600	27,300	158	14	1,308	26	387.6	5	15.3	35	4.2	22	26.9	49
Utah	3,600	1,800	122	1	1,024	3	361.7	3	16.1	27	3.4	15	13.3	24
Vermont	2,300	1,200	176	32	1,211	15	460.9	28	21.5	7	3.1	13	11.6	17
Virginia	24,500	12,000	189	47	1,346	29	487.3	40	18.6	14	3.0	11	14.0	26
Washington	18,000	8,800	164	19	1,191	13	429.0	20	18.5	15	4.3	24	12.2	18
West Virginia	9,600	4,600	174	30	1,517	45	512.5	49	15.2	36	12.1	44	15.9	32
Wisconsin	20,300	10,000	162	17	1,132	7	438.5	22	16.7	25	4.2	22	9.7	5
Wyoming	1,400	700	146	5	1,222	18	408.2	14	12.6	48	11.3	43	15.7	31
U.S. Total	1,036,700	508,300	171				457.6		18.9				15.7	

COMMUNITY HEALTH

State	PUBLIC HEALTH SPENDING $ Per Capita	Rank	RESOURCES TO HEALTH, WELFARE Rate	Rank	STATE MEDICAID PROGRAM Grade	Rank	HOUSEHOLDS WITHOUT PLUMBING %	Rank	INFANT MORTALITY Rate	Rank	HEALTH RATING BY NWNI Score	Rank	COMPOSITE COMMUNITY HEALTH Score	Rank
Alabama	7.5	38	1.34	34	45	47	4.2	43	12.2	49	93	39	470	48
Alaska	47.6	8	0.87	48	53	31	10.4	50	8.7	20	84	50	421	45
Arizona	29.0	10	1.08	43	42	48	2.1	27	9.6	33	93	39	333	31
Arkansas	11.8	24	1.09	42	46	45	4.2	43	8.9	24	93	39	412	42
California	17.8	14	2.12	5	70	6	1.2	3	8.7	21	103	22	202	9
Colorado	7.2	41	1.73	15	56	23	1.3	8	9.7	34	113	10	204	10
Connecticut	9.6	29	2.35	2	71	5	1.3	8	7.6	8	116	5	132	3
Delaware	53.3	6	1.06	44	53	32	1.7	18	9.5	31	100	26	325	26
Florida	15.1	18	1.36	31	55	29	1.1	2	9.8	36	90	44	314	24
Georgia	16.6	15	2.08	6	56	25	3.2	38	12.1	48	96	34	385	39
Hawaii	99.7	4	1.94	10	62	16	2.2	30	8.6	19	118	4	124	2
Idaho	6.4	44	1.27	36	48	42	1.4	11	7.5	7	97	33	332	30
Illinois	7.3	40	1.67	18	62	17	1.7	18	11.1	44	96	34	348	34
Indiana	11.2	26	1.69	17	55	26	1.6	15	9.8	35	104	20	328	28
Iowa	8.7	31	1.63	22	63	11	1.7	18	7.6	9	114	7	199	7
Kansas	5.9	46	1.38	30	59	20	1.2	3	8.1	14	113	10	197	6
Kentucky	11.5	25	1.11	41	56	23	6.5	49	8.6	18	94	38	426	46
Louisiana	6.6	43	1.21	38	50	38	2.4	32	11.3	45	88	45	478	49
Maine			1.67	18	63	11	4.9	46	6.7	3	110	12	272	20
Maryland	120.4	3	1.77	14	63	13	1.9	24	9.1	27	101	24	246	16
Massachusetts	37.6	9	2.62	1	72	4	1.5	14	7.5	6	114	7	137	4
Michigan	15.0	19	2.16	3	64	10	1.3	8	11.0	43	102	23	281	21
Minnesota	7.6	36	2.06	7	75	1	2.1	27	6.7	4	120	1	120	1
Mississippi	5.9	45	1.27	36	38	50	5.9	48	10.8	41	87	47	509	50
Missouri	8.2	34	1.52	26	45	46	2.1	27	11.4	47	100	26	363	37
Montana			0.92	47	57	22	2.3	31	8.5	17	106	18	325	27
Nebraska	3.3	49	1.55	25	60	19	1.2	3	8.1	16	116	5	214	11
Nevada	8.3	33	1.31	35	48	43	1.2	3	7.9	13	87	47	419	44
New Hampshire	9.7	28	2.16	3	51	36	2.5	33	7.0	5	119	3	229	14
New Jersey	8.7	31	1.87	13	67	7	1.6	15	7.8	10	108	16	220	12
New Mexico	52.6	7	1.01	46	51	36	3.6	39	8.1	15	88	45	350	35
New York	26.2	11	1.94	10	74	3	2.5	33	10.5	39	96	34	288	22
North Carolina	13.3	22	1.36	31	51	35	4.1	41	11.4	46	98	32	394	40
North Dakota	7.6	37	1.17	39	54	30	2.5	33	7.9	12	110	12	266	18
Ohio	3.4	48	1.92	12	55	26	1.7	18	9.8	37	105	19	329	29
Oklahoma	10.2	27	1.36	31	49	40	1.4	11	9.1	25	100	26	358	36
Oregon	2.6	50	1.02	45	65	9	1.4	11	7.9	11	91	43	318	25
Pennsylvania	11.8	23	1.63	22	61	18	1.8	23	10.8	40	104	20	269	19
Rhode Island	18.3	13	1.98	9	63	14	1.7	18	10.1	38	107	17	248	17
South Carolina	21.7	12	1.64	21	52	33	4.1	41	12.5	50	93	39	419	43
South Dakota	4.4	47	0.86	50	47	44	2.7	36	9.1	26	101	24	400	41
Tennessee	15.2	17	1.49	28	52	34	3.7	40	11.0	42	96	34	380	38
Texas	9.4	30	1.17	39	49	39	1.9	24	9.5	30	99	30	343	33
Utah	8.0	35	1.72	16	58	21	0.9	1	8.8	22	120	1	169	5
Vermont	13.8	21	1.42	29	63	14	2.7	36	5.9	1	110	12	225	13
Virginia	13.9	20	1.67	18	49	41	4.2	43	9.5	32	109	15	336	32
Washington	7.0	42	1.60	24	65	8	1.2	3	9.1	28	99	30	244	15
West Virginia	60.0	5	0.87	48	55	26	5.7	47	9.2	29	85	49	440	47
Wisconsin	7.4	39	2.03	8	75	2	1.9	24	8.8	23	114	7	201	8
Wyoming	16.0	16	1.52	26	40	49	1.6	15	6.3	2	100	26	293	23
U.S. Total	16.5				57				9.6		100			

WORKPLACE HEALTH

State	WORKPLACE DEATHS PER 100,000 Rate	Rank	WORKERS IN HIGH-RISK JOBS %	Rank	WORKERS IN MOST TOXIC INDUSTRIES % Mfg.	Rank	WORKERS IN HIGH-INJURY INDUSTRIES % Mfg.	Rank	HAZ. WASTE WORKERS PER 10,000 Pop.	Rank	MAX. TOTAL DISABILITY BENEFITS $/week	Rank	MAXIMUM UNEMPLOYMENT BENEFITS $/week	Rank
Alabama	8.4	25	3.58	40	29.7	32	37.8	32	9.0	22	358	26	150	47
Alaska	34.2	50	6.59	47	5.6	5	78.1	50	18.6	43	700	1	260	10
Arizona	5.9	11	1.15	20	8.3	6	17.3	3	7.8	13	276	38	155	46
Arkansas	11.8	34	1.88	31	24.5	25	45.0	41	4.9	2	226	48	215	24
California	7.1	18	0.77	16	28.0	30	33.9	24	10.1	26	266	42	190	33
Colorado	10.5	31	2.09	34	20.8	15	31.9	21	11.7	31	371	22	224	20
Connecticut	1.6	1	0.70	13	45.8	45	40.5	34	16.9	40	693	2	302	3
Delaware	7.0	17	3.46	39	60.7	50	27.7	13	21.8	46	281	37	225	19
Florida	10.0	29	0.59	11	26.9	27	33.7	23	3.9	1	382	20	200	28
Georgia	12.4	38	1.66	27	23.3	22	30.6	18	8.3	17	175	50	175	39
Hawaii	6.7	15	0.03	1	>1.0	1	47.0	43	7.7	12	383	19	256	11
Idaho	18.2	47	1.52	25	15.3	11	58.6	48	17.2	41	301	31	200	27
Illinois	7.1	18	1.18	21	31.1	35	32.0	22	8.0	15	611	4	260	9
Indiana	8.2	23	1.20	22	40.0	43	42.2	39	12.4	33	274	40	161	43
Iowa	9.6	28	0.86	17	21.4	17	39.0	33	10.9	27	684	3	222	21
Kansas	10.2	30	1.74	29	38.7	42	49.1	44	6.1	6	271	41	216	23
Kentucky	14.0	40	4.08	42	27.7	28	30.3	17	8.2	16	353	27	186	35
Louisiana	12.2	36	6.61	48	45.9	46	41.0	37	11.8	32	276	39	181	36
Maine	8.2	23	0.34	7	34.1	39	35.8	28	28.5	50	472	8	270	8
Maryland	6.4	12	0.33	6	27.9	29	30.7	19	6.2	7	432	9	205	26
Massachusetts	2.4	2	0.67	12	22.8	20	19.0	7	18.1	42	474	7	408	1
Michigan	5.5	9	0.96	18	56.0	49	55.6	46	8.5	19	427	10	275	7
Minnesota	4.6	6	0.71	14	24.0	23	29.5	15	7.4	9	413	13	255	12
Mississippi	14.9	43	1.50	24	22.1	19	36.5	30	9.1	23	213	49	145	48
Missouri	5.7	10	1.13	19	37.1	40	40.7	35	12.7	36	290	35	160	45
Montana	22.6	48	3.12	38	5.5	4	55.0	45	12.6	35	318	29	190	32
Nebraska	11.7	33	0.49	9	17.2	14	43.3	40	5.7	4	245	44	134	50
Nevada	12.3	37	2.37	37	14.2	9	16.5	2	11.5	30	369	24	194	31
New Hampshire	5.1	7	0.20	2	15.8	13	17.9	5	19.6	44	600	5	162	42
New Jersey	3.7	5	1.69	28	33.9	38	19.7	8	26.3	49	370	23	279	6
New Mexico	14.0	40	3.83	41	12.6	8	28.7	14	5.9	5	292	34	170	40
New York	2.7	3	0.35	8	21.8	18	20.8	10	7.8	14	300	32	245	13
North Carolina	7.9	22	2.08	33	15.8	12	18.1	6	8.4	18	390	15	236	17
North Dakota	14.2	42	6.17	46	14.6	10	40.9	36	9.8	25	313	30	187	34
Ohio	5.2	8	2.15	36	43.0	44	41.5	38	8.9	20	419	11	291	4
Oklahoma	7.8	21	6.00	45	26.9	26	35.2	27	7.6	11	231	47	197	30
Oregon	11.9	35	0.28	4	21.2	16	57.6	47	7.4	10	389	17	238	15
Pennsylvania	6.6	14	1.64	26	32.5	37	34.8	26	13.4	38	419	12	288	5
Rhode Island	3.1	4	0.74	15	24.5	24	22.5	11	13.4	37	386	18	323	2
South Carolina	7.0	16	4.61	43	23.0	21	17.4	4	11.2	29	350	28	165	41
South Dakota	15.3	44	1.41	23	>1.0	2	23.0	12	9.2	24	289	36	140	49
Tennessee	8.5	26	1.98	32	29.7	33	29.6	16	6.3	8	252	43	160	44
Texas	13.2	39	4.70	44	32.2	36	34.4	25	15.1	39	238	46	217	22
Utah	15.5	45	2.11	35	38.4	41	46.9	42	12.5	34	295	33	214	25
Vermont	7.2	20	0.25	3	11.0	7	20.3	9	25.4	48	544	6	178	37
Virginia	11.3	32	1.80	30	28.2	31	31.4	20	5.1	3	393	14	176	38
Washington	8.8	27	0.31	5	50.9	48	63.7	49	11.1	28	389	16	237	16
West Virginia	17.2	46	11.03	49	48.3	47	36.8	31	19.9	45	368	25	245	14
Wisconsin	6.5	13	0.53	10	30.7	34	36.1	29	8.9	21	378	21	225	18
Wyoming	32.5	49	13.73	50	>1.0	3	>10.0	1	25.2	47	243	45	200	29
U.S. Total	7.9		1.86		31.0		34.2		10.5		368		216	

WORKPLACE HEALTH

State	UNEMPLOYED WITH UNEMPL. INSURANCE %	Rank	UNEM- PLOYMENT RATE %	Rank	POP. WITH WORKPLACE INSURANCE %	Rank	UNIONS AMONG MFG. WORKERS %	Rank	LAWS FOR WORKER SAFETY #	Rank	COMPOSITE WORKPLACE INDICATORS Score	Rank	COMPOSITE PUBLIC HEALTH Score	Rank
Alabama	23.7	37	7.0	27	62.2	36	14.5	27	0.0	50	374	46	844	48
Alaska	51.5	3	6.7	26	56.0	46	24.7	12	11.5	17	284	22	705	37
Arizona	20.4	42	5.2	16	63.6	33	3.7	48	6.5	43	303	27	636	28
Arkansas	29.8	26	7.2	29	56.4	44	11.3	33	8.0	34	342	38	754	45
California	44.1	8	5.1	15	58.9	40	22.4	16	15.0	1	254	20	456	13
Colorado	24.6	35	5.8	20	66.5	28	9.6	37	10.5	23	297	25	501	19
Connecticut	40.9	13	3.7	4	77.9	1	15.4	26	12.5	9	187	8	319	4
Delaware	39.8	14	3.5	3	73.8	8	19.4	21	10.5	23	287	23	612	25
Florida	17.3	50	5.6	18	58.8	41	9.0	39	8.0	34	303	28	617	27
Georgia	20.1	44	5.5	17	63.3	34	11.8	32	8.5	28	349	40	734	41
Hawaii	41.9	10	2.6	1	69.6	17	41.4	3	11.0	20	152	4	276	2
Idaho	42.2	9	5.1	15	61.1	38	7.4	43	7.0	41	361	44	693	36
Illinois	27.6	31	6.0	22	70.1	15	29.8	7	12.5	9	186	7	534	20
Indiana	20.1	44	4.7	13	71.8	12	37.0	6	8.0	34	339	36	667	33
Iowa	27.5	33	4.3	9	67.5	24	18.6	22	8.5	28	253	19	452	12
Kansas	32.6	20	4.0	6	73.1	9	11.0	35	10.5	23	302	26	499	18
Kentucky	21.3	40	6.2	23	63.1	35	21.5	17	11.5	17	314	30	740	43
Louisiana	20.2	43	7.9	31	50.0	49	19.5	20	5.0	46	432	50	910	49
Maine	41.3	12	4.1	7	67.9	23	18.3	23	14.5	2	223	17	472	15
Maryland	25.1	34	3.7	4	74.5	6	29.3	9	13.5	5	162	5	408	8
Massachusetts	57.3	2	4.0	6	73.0	10	19.7	19	13.5	5	127	1	264	1
Michigan	33.2	19	7.1	28	71.2	14	51.7	1	11.0	20	212	12	493	17
Minnesota	36.2	17	4.3	9	65.8	29	16.7	24	14.0	4	166	6	286	3
Mississippi	22.8	38	7.8	30	53.4	48	7.8	42	0.0	50	414	49	923	50
Missouri	30.9	24	5.5	17	67.1	25	29.8	8	6.0	45	322	32	685	35
Montana	30.6	25	5.9	21	56.0	46	22.8	15	10.5	23	340	37	638	29
Nebraska	29.5	27	3.1	2	63.9	32	8.7	40	8.5	28	321	31	535	21
Nevada	31.4	22	5.0	14	64.9	31	5.4	45	10.0	27	295	24	714	40
New Hampshire	19.1	47	3.5	3	76.0	2	6.7	44	13.0	8	219	16	448	11
New Jersey	47.8	5	4.1	7	75.5	3	24.4	13	12.5	9	187	9	407	7
New Mexico	22.6	39	6.7	26	48.3	50	9.4	38	11.5	17	326	34	676	34
New York	46.2	6	5.1	15	67.0	26	47.2	2	13.5	5	137	2	425	9
North Carolina	32.3	21	3.5	3	68.6	22	4.5	47	6.5	43	256	21	650	32
North Dakota	34.2	18	4.3	9	60.8	39	9.7	36	8.0	34	350	42	616	26
Ohio	28.4	28	5.5	17	72.5	11	39.8	4	12.0	14	218	14	547	23
Oklahoma	18.7	49	5.6	18	56.3	45	16.0	25	8.5	28	354	43	712	39
Oregon	39.4	15	5.7	19	69.0	20	20.4	18	11.0	20	217	13	535	22
Pennsylvania	41.6	11	4.5	11	74.3	7	39.3	5	12.5	9	190	11	459	14
Rhode Island	72.0	1	4.1	7	75.0	4	11.1	34	14.5	2	152	3	400	6
South Carolina	28.1	29	4.7	13	69.6	17	3.0	49	2.0	48	325	33	744	44
South Dakota	20.6	41	4.2	8	56.6	43	2.3	50	7.5	38	362	45	762	46
Tennessee	31.2	23	5.1	15	61.7	37	12.9	30	7.5	38	330	35	710	38
Texas	19.4	46	6.7	26	57.0	42	13.9	28	8.5	28	395	48	738	42
Utah	28.1	29	4.6	12	71.8	12	4.5	46	7.0	41	383	47	552	24
Vermont	50.2	4	3.7	4	69.8	16	8.0	41	8.5	28	219	15	444	10
Virginia	18.9	48	3.9	5	69.2	19	11.9	31	5.0	46	312	29	648	31
Washington	44.9	7	6.2	24	68.7	21	25.4	11	12.0	14	242	18	486	16
West Virginia	23.8	36	8.6	32	65.3	30	28.4	10	12.0	14	347	39	787	47
Wisconsin	39.1	16	4.4	10	75.0	4	23.1	14	12.5	9	189	10	390	5
Wyoming	27.6	31	6.3	25	66.9	27	13.8	29	7.5	38	349	41	642	30
U.S. Total	**31.5**		**5.3**		**65.8**		**18.3**		**9.6**					

SOURCES FOR COMMUNITY AND WORKPLACE HEALTH INDICATORS

Cancer cases
Incidence of all cancers from all causes, 1990 estimate. No ranking is provided for this indicator.
Source: "Cancer Facts and Figures, 1990." Published by American Cancer Society, 1599 Clifton Road, NE, Atlanta, GA 30329.

Cancer deaths and cancer death rate
Estimated deaths from all causes for 1990, based on mortality data for 1982-1986. The cancer death rate per 100,000 people was calculated by the American Cancer Society, with adjustments for age distribution using the 1970 Census of Population.
Source: "Cancer Facts and Figures, 1990." Published by American Cancer Society.

Premature deaths
Rate per 100,000 people in state who do not reach age of 65 because of ill health or injury, calculated from mortality tables in U.S. Public Health Service's "Vital Statistics of the United States, Volume II, 1986."
Source: "The NWNL State Health Rankings, 1989." Published by Northwestern National Life Insurance Company, 20 Washington Avenue, South, Minneapolis, MN 55401; telephone (612) 342-3750.

Deaths from nine diseases
Deaths per 100,000 age-adjusted population from coronary heart disease, stroke, diabetes, chronic obstructive pulmonary disease, lung cancer, breast cancer, cervical cancer, colorectal cancer, or cirrhosis in 1986.
Source: Data from Centers for Disease Control, Public Health Service, U.S. Department of Health and Human Services. Published in *New York Times*, January 21, 1990.

Doctors per capita
Number of doctors of medicine engaged in patient care in 1987, per 10,000 people in state. Excludes doctors in medical teaching, administration, research, and other nonpatient care activities.
Source: "Health, United States, 1989," Table 84. Published by National Center for Health Statistics, Public Health Service, U.S. Department of Health and Human Services, Hyattsville, MD, 1990.

Population in underserved areas
Estimated percent of population that lacks access to primary medical care due to economic or geographic causes.
Source: "The NWNL State Health Rankings, 1990." Published by Northwestern National Life Insurance Company, Minneapolis, MN.

Population without health insurance
Percent of state's nonelderly population lacking insurance through private, public, or Medicaid coverage for 1988.
Source: "Uninsured in the United States, 1988," September 1990. Published by Employee Benefit Research Institute, 2121 K Street, NW, Washington, DC 20005; telephone (202) 659-0670. Estimates for five states were made by Institute for Southern Studies.

Public health-care spending
> Per-capita state funds spent by state health agencies; does not include federal or local funds, or fee income.
> *Source:* "Public Health Agencies, 1990: An Inventory of Programs & Block Grant Expenditures," June 1989. Published by Public Health Foundation, 1220 L Street, NW, Washington, DC 20005; telephone (202) 659-5600.

Resources for health, welfare
> A measure of state and local financial resources committed to health and welfare services in relation to portion of population with an income below $7,500.
> *Source:* "The NWNL State Health Rankings, 1990." Published by Northwestern National Life Insurance Company, Minneapolis, MN.

Medicaid program
> Grade given state's Medicaid program based on an evaluation of its eligibility restrictions, scope of services, availability of health-care providers, quality of service, and reimbursement system. A grade of 100 is best; the higher the grade, the better the chance a poor person has of receiving quality health care through the Medicaid program.
> *Source:* "Poor Health Care For Poor Americans: A Ranking of State Medicaid Programs," 1987, second printing 1988. Published by Public Citizen Health Research Group, 2000 P Street, NW, Washington, DC 20036; telephone (202) 872-0320.

Homes without plumbing
> Percent of year-round occupied housing units lacking complete plumbing (kitchen facilities, toilet, or hot water).
> *Source:* "General Housing Characteristics, U.S. Summary, 1980, U.S. Census of Population." Published by U.S. Bureau of Census, Washington.

Infant mortality rate
> Number of deaths of babies under age 1 year per 1,000 live births for 1989.
> *Source:* "Monthly Vital Statistics Report," August 30, 1990, Tables 1 and 3. Published by National Center for Health Statistics, Public Health Service, U.S. Department of Health and Human Services, Hyattsville, MD.

Health ratings by NWNL
> Northwestern National Life Insurance Company graded states on 17 components that measure population lifestyle, access to health care, disability, disease, and mortality. The median score is 100, with higher scores receiving a higher overall ranking for better health conditions and policies.
> *Source:* "The NWNL State Health Rankings, 1990." Published by Northwestern National Life Insurance Company, 20 Washington Avenue, South, Minneapolis, MN 55401; telephone (612) 342-3750.

Composite of community health indicators
> Each state's rank for the 12 indicators above was totaled; lowest score receives best composite rank for community health.

Workplace deaths
> Rate of traumatic deaths caused by work, per 100,000 workers, for 1980-85.
> *Source:* "National Traumatic Occupational Fatalities, 1980-85," September 1989. Published by National Institute for Occupational Safety and Health, Centers for Disease Control, U.S. Department of Health and Human Services, 944 Chestnut Ridge Road, Morgantown, WV 26505; telephone (304) 291-4812.

Workers in jobs with high-risk of disease
   Percent of 1988 nonagricultural workforce in the six industries with highest rates of occupational diseases, particularly lung diseases from fumes or dust, as identified by an expert in U.S. Occupational Safety & Health Administration; the six are mining, cotton weaving mills, manufacturers of other cotton products, chemical and allied products, rubber and miscellaneous products, and leather tanning and manufacturing.
   Source: "The Climate for Workers in the United States," 1990. Published by Southern Labor Institute, Southern Regional Council, 60 Walton Street, NW, Atlanta, GA 30303; telephone (404) 522-8764.

Workers in most toxic industries
   Percent of 1989 manufacturing workforce employed in five major industrial sectors that released most toxic chemicals. According to U.S. Environmental Protection Agency's "Toxic Release Inventory," the five industries accounted for 74 percent of all releases in 1988: chemicals (46.2 percent); primary metals (13.8 percent); paper products (5.9 percent); transportation (4.2 percent); and fabricating metals (3.5 percent).
   Source: "Toxics in the Community, 1988: National & Local Perspectives." Published by U.S. Environmental Protection Agency, 1990. And, for employment data, U.S. Department of Labor, Bureau of Labor Statistics printout of current employment for 1989.

Workers in high-injury industries
   Percent of 1989 manufacturing workforce in major industries (two-digit SICs) with illness and injury rates at least twice the national average for all private employers — 8.6 cases per 100 full-time workers. The five industries are lumber and wood products (19.5 cases); primary metals (19.4 cases); fabricated metals (18.8 cases); food and kindred products (18.5 cases); and transportation equipment (17.7 cases).
   Source: "Occupational Injuries and Illnesses in the United States by Industry, 1988." Published by Bureau of Labor Statistics, U.S. Department of Labor, August 1990.

Hazardous waste workers
   Number of workers per 100,000 residents who package, dispose, or transport RCRA-regulated hazardous waste or who are involved in cleanups of Superfund waste sites.
   Source: Joseph T. Hughes, "An Assessment of Training Needs for Worker Safety and Health Programs: Hazardous Waste Operations and Emergency Response," *Applied Occupational & Environmental Hygiene*, February 1991. Additional state-by-state data supplied by the author.

Total disability benefits
   Maximum weekly benefits paid by state workers' compensation system to workers whose injuries make them permanently and totally disabled.
   Source: "State Workers' Compensation Laws," Table 7, for 1990. Published by Office of Workers' Compensation Programs, Employment Standards Administration, U.S. Department of Labor, July 1990.

Unemployment benefits
   Maximum dollars of unemployment benefits paid per week, 1990.
   Source: Employment and Training Administration, U.S. Department of Labor, Washington.

Unemployed with unemployment insurance
   Percent of unemployed who received unemployment benefits during 1988.
   Source: "Unprotected: Unemployment Insurance and Jobless Workers in 1988," August 1989. Published by Center for Budget and Policy Priorities, 236 Massachusetts Avenue, NE, Suite 305, Washington, DC 20002; telephone (202) 544-0591.

Unemployment rate
>Percent of all civilian workers unemployed in 1989. Rank is not included in summary or composite scores.
>*Source:* "Employment and Earnings," May 1990. Published by Bureau of Labor Statistics, U.S. Department of Labor.

Population covered by workplace insurance
>Percent of nonelderly population in 1988 who received insurance coverage through their employer.
>*Source:* "Uninsured in the United States, 1988," September 1990. Published by Employee Benefit Research Institute, 2121 K Street, NW, Washington, DC 20005; telephone (202) 659-0670.

Union membership
>Percent of manufacturing workers who belong to unions, 1988.
>*Source:* Source: "Grant Thornton Manufacturing Climates Study," June 1989. Published by Grant Thornton, One Prudential Plaza, Chicago, IL 60601; telephone (312) 856-0001.

Workplace laws
>Grade given by the Southern Labor Institute based on the weighted grouping of 15 possible state laws that protect a worker's rights and access to health information.
>*Source:* "The Climate for Workers in the United States," 1990. Published by Southern Labor Institute, Southern Regional Council, 60 Walton Street, NW, Atlanta, GA 30303; telephone (404) 522-8764.

Composite of workplace indicators
>Rankings on 11 work-related indicators — all except the one for unemployment rates — were added together, and lowest score receives lowest (best) rank for workplace health.

Composite score for public health
>Rankings on 23 community and work-related indicators were totaled to produce a composite score. Lowest score receives best composite rank for community and workplace health.

CHAPTER 7

Farms, Forests, Fish, and Fun

INDICATORS

Number of farms	Commercial fish landings
Farms lost or gained	Drop from record fish landings
Farmland in state	Number of fishing licenses
Average farm size	Number of fishers and hunters
Fertilizer use	Spending by fishers and hunters
Herbicide use	Number of registered motor boats
Pesticide use	Inland waters
Pesticide-tainted groundwater	Miles of coastline
Excessive nitrates in wells	Acres of land
Cropland irrigated	Land owned by federal government
Cropland erosion	Land owned by U.S. Fish and Wildlife Service
Use of conservation tillage	Visits to national parks
Acres in Conservation Reserve Program	Land in state parks and recreational areas
Gross state product from agriculture	Visitors to state parks
Value added by forest products	State funds for parks
Forests owned by timber companies	Local funds for parks and recreation
Forests owned by federal government	Spending for tourism and travel
Forestland lost or gained	Gross state product from natural resources
Number of private tree farms	Population density
Gross state product from lumber goods	Population change, 1970–1990
Paper and pulp mills	Population in rural areas
Wetlands lost	Quality of life in metropolitan areas
Shellfish waters limited for fishing	Memberships in conservation organizations

The renewable resources that we get from the land — including food and lumber — provide the basic necessities for nourishment and shelter, as well as jobs and income for millions of Americans. With proper stewardship, these resources are replenished and can continue sustaining wildlife and human life.

Yet much of our land is poorly managed. Farm practices that stress high yields of a single crop also strip the land of nutrients, breed pests and pesticide dependency, and lead to devastating erosion. Clearcutting disrupts the forest ecosystem, ruins recreation areas, promotes erosion, and increases water contamination problems. Development in coastal areas threatens delicate habitats, pollutes fishing waters, and speeds the loss of wetlands.

At the same time, the Great Outdoors — our land, waterways, mountains, and forests — still give Americans immense pleasure, asking remarkably little in return. If we respect these resources, they will keep giving. By being greedy, we risk total loss.

CHEMICAL FARMS

The Dakotas, Nebraska, and Iowa lead the nation in the share of their economies that depend on agriculture; each derive over 12 percent of their gross state product from the fruits of the soil. But to maximize production, farmers use enormous amounts of chemicals to fertilize their crops, control weeds, and kill pests. The chemicals mix with rain or irrigation water, wash into streams or seep into groundwater, contaminating wells and reservoirs. The end result is that these are also the states where

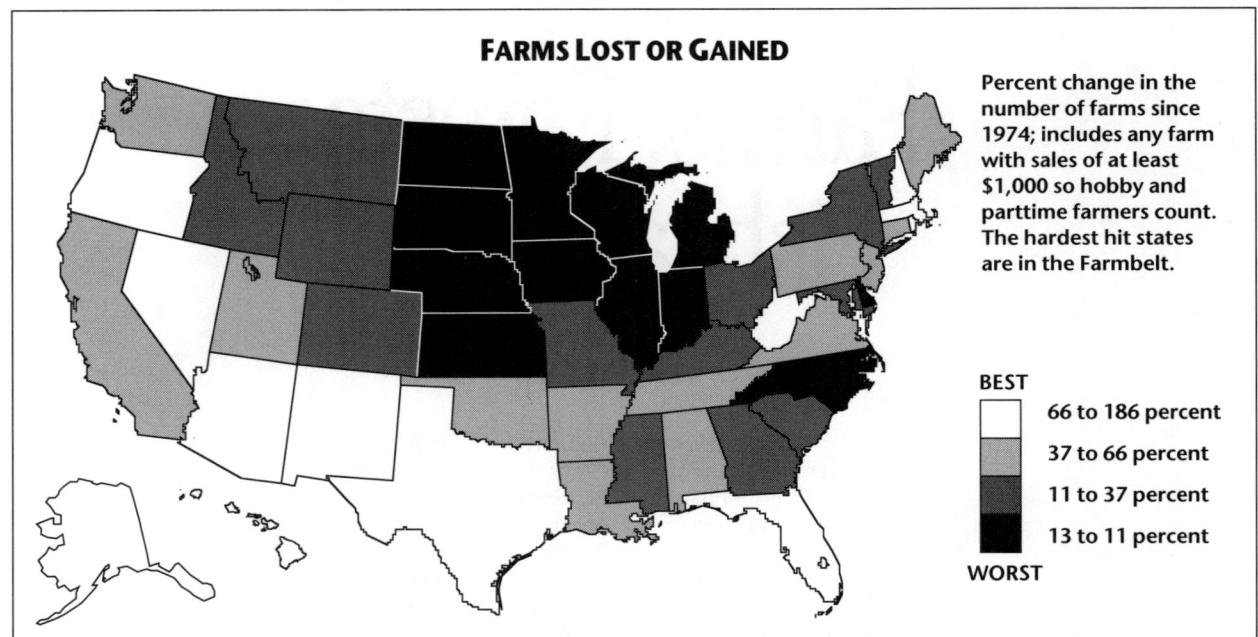

America's style of intensive chemical farming has taken its greatest toll on the environment.

In the Central Loess Plains of Nebraska, farmers dump 378 million pounds of nitrogen fertilizer on 1.6 million acres of corn. Overall, Nebraska consumes 109 tons of fertilizer per person, more than any other state. Because of nitrogen seepage into its groundwater and nitrates detected in its wells, Nebraska is one of eight states targeted for a five-year federally funded project to encourage reduced chemical use and more efficient irrigation practices.

Nebraska also ranks 48th in its use of pesticides per capita, and one study showed that 70 percent of the state's wells are tainted with pesticides. Iowa ranks 48th in herbicide use per acre of cropland, 50th in pesticides per capita, and 50th in pesticide-contaminated groundwater. Weed-killing herbicides, the most common form of pesticide, are potent groundwater contaminants; in Topeka, Kansas, the herbicide Atrazine, which may cause cancer in humans, has been found in the city's drinking water.

An estimated 37 percent of the groundwater in Kansas is potentially contaminated by pesticides, ranking it 46th. Kansas is also a huge consumer of fertilizer — and one of 10 states where the addition of hobby farmers has not outpaced the decline of the traditional farm family since 1974. In fact, 9 of the 15 states with a net loss or only a small gain in their farm population also rank among the 15 most intensive users of fertilizer and pesticides.

Nationwide, Americans used 1.1 billion pounds of pesticides in 1988 at a cost of $7.4 billion. Although herbicides and pesticides have only been in use for about 40 years, we assume that growing food is impossible without them. But bugs develop a tolerance for chemicals, so farmers still lose about a third of their crop to insect infestation — the same proportion they lost 40 years ago. Some research shows that chemical farming is more profitable than low-input or organic farming, but those calculations exclude the costs to society of diminishing water and soil quality, farmworker health, and food safety.

MOUNTING COSTS, LOST LAND

Under the current methods of intensive farming, up to a third of the nation's cropland is eroding at an annual rate of 4.4 tons per acre and a cost of $2 billion. Two-thirds of the erosion is caused by water, while a third is due to wind. In the West, where water is a scarce commodity, tax-subsidized projects encourage wasteful irrigation practices. Several dry states, such as Nevada, Arizona, and New Mexico, rank near the bottom on our indicators for both irrigation and erosion; much of the water pumped to their fields runs off, carrying away valuable topsoil, along with herbicides and pesticides. To make up for lost soil, farmers overload the land with more fertilizer.

Many farmers recognize the problems with chemical-intensive agriculture, but until very recently they've received little help from their gov-

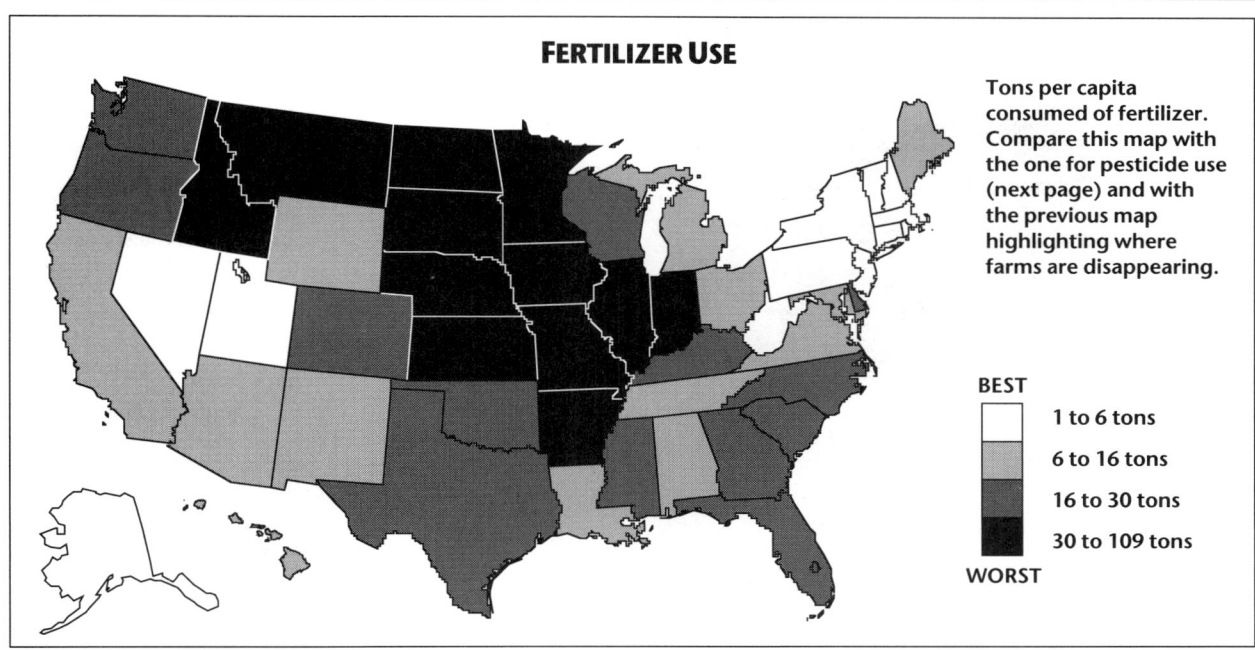

FERTILIZER USE

Tons per capita consumed of fertilizer. Compare this map with the one for pesticide use (next page) and with the previous map highlighting where farms are disappearing.

BEST
- 1 to 6 tons
- 6 to 16 tons
- 16 to 30 tons
- 30 to 109 tons

WORST

ernment. For decades federal policy — through the price-support system, loan programs, and land-grant research colleges — has focused with single-minded determination on creating bigger farms with higher output per acre. The United States has become the agricultural marvel of the world, and consumers have grown accustomed to finding plentiful supplies of flawless, inexpensive food at their corner grocery store.

But the hidden costs of modern agribusiness are mounting, and stirring growing protest. Cancer-sensitized consumers are starting to demand fewer chemicals on their food; the panic over the carcinogenic pesticide Alar on apples, which cost boycotted growers millions of dollars, could repeat itself with dozens of other products. Environmentalists have begun meddling with farm policy, lobbying for conservation measures that threaten the unfettered expansion of agribusiness.

Even the family farmer knows the costs have gotten too steep. Many can no longer keep up the payments on the high-tech equipment that goes with modern agriculture. From the Dakotas to the Deep South, over-leveraged farms went bankrupt by the tens of thousands during the droughts of the early 1980s. The farm loss indicator shows that states with lots of family farms (like Iowa, Illinois, North Carolina, and Minnesota) took the hit much harder than states where corporate agribusiness already prevails (California, Hawaii, Florida, and Arizona).

Farmers are also protesting the way suppliers and buyers are being gobbled up by conglomerates, shrinking their capacity to negotiate a living from the land. ConAgra, Cargill, and IBP (owned by Occidental Petroleum) now control 60 percent of the beef markets; the first two also control half of the nation's grain trade and rank among the top 10 poultry processors.

Ironically, farmers who want to use organic or no-till methods find it difficult to get federal loans because their farms don't fit the standard models. Paralleling the government's support of nuclear over solar energy, policymakers allow corporate agribusiness to define the limits of "reasonable" experiments. In this case, the agenda calls for biotechnology to engineer life itself, so that such chemical companies as DuPont and Monsanto can manufacture plant seeds and animal embryos that depend on their brands of pesticides or antibiotics to survive.

Frustrated by the corporate favoritism of government programs, family farmers are beginning to team up with environmentalists and safe-food consumer advocates to promote resource conservation measures and a radical shift in federal policy away from its mania for "efficient output." The victories have been small, and the follow-through spotty at best. The 1985 Conservation Reserve Program (CRP) pays farmers to remove highly erodible areas from crop cultivation for at least 10 years and to plant them with grasses or trees instead. Eight Southern states lead the nation by enrolling over half of their eligible land in the

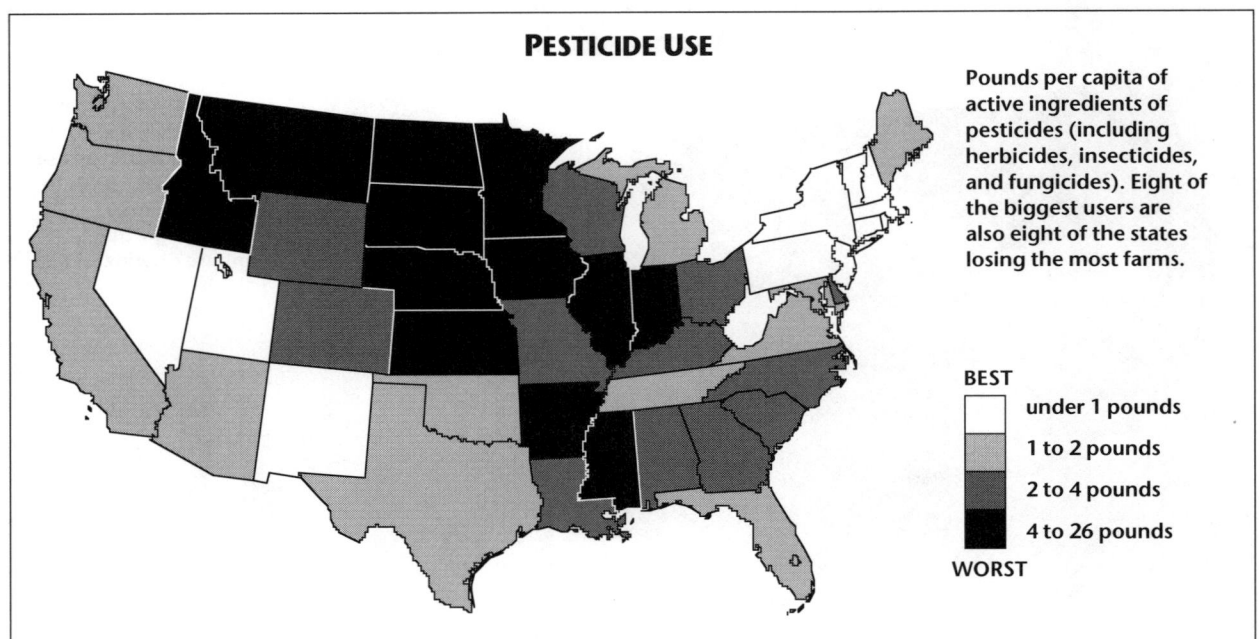

CRP program. By contrast, most Rocky Mountain and Southwestern states have hardly used the program. Montana, Nevada, Colorado, Idaho, Wyoming, New Mexico, Texas, and Oklahoma rank among the worst states for both erosion rates and use of the CRP set-aside. Hawaii and California agribusiness also make little use of either the CRP program or conservation tillage methods that help minimize loss of soil between crops.

The 1990 Farm Bill provides a token $40 million for support of sustainable agriculture, including $15 million for current Low-Input Sustainable Agriculture (LISA) programs. Low-input methods stress crop rotation, reduced chemical use, spot irrigation, and no-till cultivation or tilling that leaves crop residue to anchor the soil. Despite the minimum support from Uncle Sam, more and more farmers in such major grain states as Illinois, Nebraska, Missouri, and Iowa are preaching the no-till gospel; they are now using conservation tillage methods on over a third of their cropland.

Indeed the states, more than the federal government, have taken the lead in adopting measures that promote family farming, safe food, and conservation. Iowa, heartland for the family farmer, has begun addressing the problems of water and food contamination through sustainable agriculture programs, organic labeling laws, and funding for research of new farming methods. Several of these agricultural policies are included on the State Policies Index in Chapter 9.

MANAGING FORESTS

One third of America is covered with trees. Interestingly, the big agriculture states — North and South Dakota, Nebraska, Iowa, and Kansas — are the five states with the smallest proportion of land in forests, less than one acre in 20. In 19 states, more than half the acreage lies in forests. The highest proportions are in New England and along the seaboard to Mississippi. Even in the heavily urbanized states of New York and Pennsylvania, about 60 percent of the land is still covered with trees.

Wooded areas, particularly old-growth forests, prevent erosion, stabilize watersheds, slow global warming by absorbing carbon dioxide, and host the ecosystem for millions of plant and animal species. But trees also feed our appetite for toilet tissue, newsprint, woodframe homes, furniture, and books like this one. Finding a balance between these many uses isn't easy.

The 1960 Multiple-Use Sustained Yield Act said forests should be managed for a variety of purposes, including watershed protection, recreation, and wildlife habitats, but its clear bias favored the paper-pulp and lumber industry. In 1985, the timber industry brought in $54 billion and employed 600,000 people. For a dozen states, the wood-products industry ranks as the first or second largest enterprise, even without counting furniture factories.

The goal of environmentalists is not to eliminate lumber harvesting altogether, but to manage harvesting in the least destructive and disruptive ways possible. Although foresters are experimenting with tree harvesting methods known as New Forestry, which more closely mimic the natural clearing of trees in a forest, the most widely used method of harvesting trees is still clearcutting. With clearcutting, roads are built through to a targeted forest area that is then leveled and replanted with even-aged seedlings. The result is a disturbed ecosystem, increased erosion, and the rise of an artificial monoculture hostile to many formerly indigenous species. Clearcutting also eliminates many recreational opportunities for local people and visitors.

Three-quarters of the nation's timberland is privately owned. Financial incentives encourage owners to preserve or replant forestland, but even the states with the best forest management programs — such as Washington, Idaho, and Massachusetts — lack the personnel and money to enforce their laws. California and Oregon have the best rates of success; in both states, requirements for reforestation are met over 90 percent of the time.

The forestland that is timbered on U.S. Forest Service land is perhaps the most controversial, with environmental groups pushing the Forest Service to practice better management techniques and loosen its ties with timber companies. In the big timber states of the Pacific Northwest, more than half of the industry's harvest comes from national forests, including the old-growth tracts targeted for protection by Earth First!.

Forestland is disappearing fastest precisely in these areas that have depended on it most, which is one reason the old-growth sections are vulnerable to the insatiable chain saw. Oregon, where forests have more economic importance than in any other state, lost nine percent of its forestland between 1982 and 1987, ranking 48th on our indicator of forests lost. Twenty-one percent of the state's forests are owned by timber companies, 58 percent by the federal government.

In Maine, forests cover 90 percent of the land and timber companies own nearly half that acreage — on both counts, the highest share in the nation. Like Oregon, Maine is losing forestland. Meanwhile, timber companies such as Great Northern Nekoosa Corporation, owner of two million acres of Maine timberland, are threatened by buyouts from other companies. Many of the biggest firms, such as Weyerhaeuser and Georgia-Pacific, are diversifying and using their huge landholdings as the base for real-estate development enterprises.

In the past two decades, state legislatures in New England and the Pacific Northwest have placed tougher regulations on everything from logging roads to mill wastewater discharge. Those regulations, in addition to the pine plantation possibilities of the Southeast, have moved the center of the industry's production to Dixie. The region now accounts for nine of the ten states with the most tree farms and for more than half the nation's pulp, paper, and lumber output. Logging in the South's national forests is expected to double by 1995, but a much larger share of the region's trees are held by private landowners and are less subject to shifts in Forest Service policy.

PAPER TIGER

From an environmental standpoint, the most hazardous part of the forestry business is the production of bleached paper. Among all manufacturers, the paper-pulp industry ranks third overall in energy consumption, after chemicals and primary metals. It is first in use of fuel oil, third in electricity and coal purchases, and sixth in natural gas. As a consequence, the industry is also a major producer of sulfur dioxide, the chief cause of acid rain. Inside the plants, exposure to a variety of chemicals — including cancer-causing chloroform and formaldehyde compounds the long-term health risks for workers who suffered 13.1 illnesses or injuries per 100 full-time workers in 1988, a rate 52 percent higher than the average for all private businesses.

More telling, the industry is directly responsible for releasing one million pounds of toxic emissions into the environment every day, ranking it third behind all chemical and primary metal manufacturers. Sixty-two of the 149 plants spewing the most carcinogenic toxins into the air are paper making factories from Maine to Mississippi, Wisconsin to Washington. Significantly, none of these numbers includes the discharge of dioxins, a extremely carcinogenic byproduct of the chloride bleaching process used by about 100 paper mills in the U.S.

The controversy over dioxins is likely to intensify over the next few years as scientists and engineers refine their capacity to measure the impact of a few parts per trillion on fish and people. The fight has already begun as state regulators for the first time are choosing acceptable limits for dioxin discharge. Environmentalists are pressing for zero

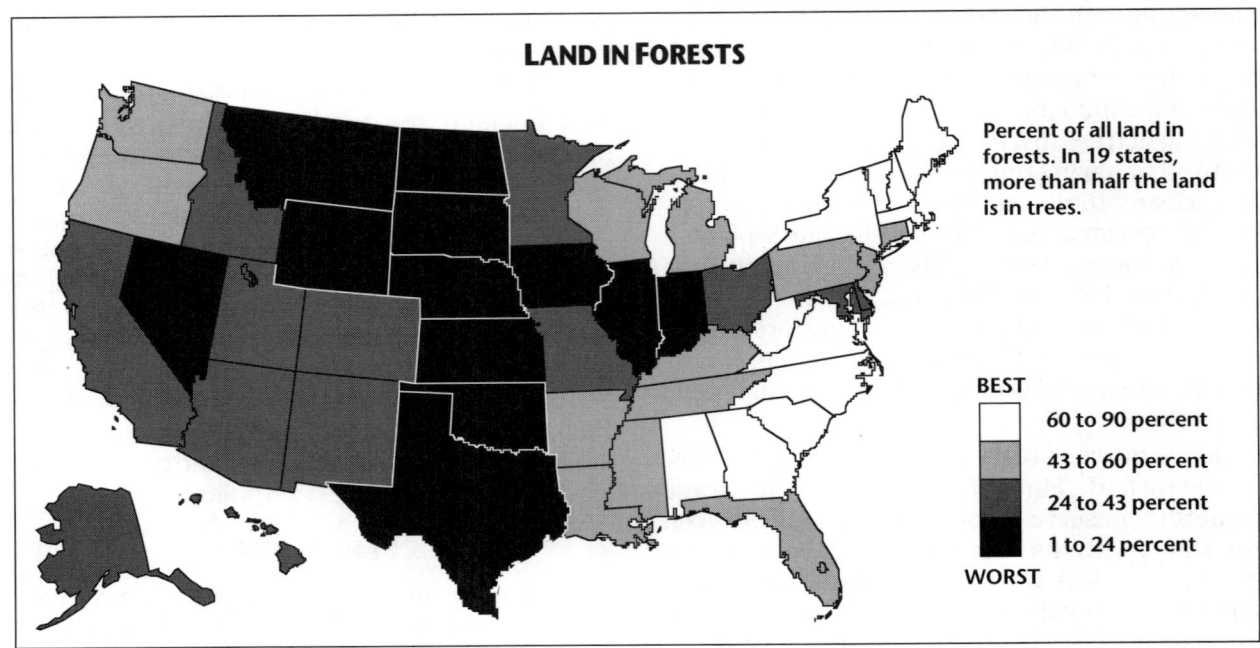

LAND IN FORESTS

Percent of all land in forests. In 19 states, more than half the land is in trees.

BEST
- 60 to 90 percent
- 43 to 60 percent
- 24 to 43 percent
- 1 to 24 percent
WORST

tolerance, emphasizing that alternative technologies exist for making white paper and that less of it is needed anyway. But industry lobbyists are roaming the states, armed with studies that show the Environmental Protection Agency's recommended standards are too tough. So far, most states have gone at least as far as the federal government — with the notable exception of Georgia.

Georgia is the South's leading paper maker, with 21 factories. Almost two-thirds of its land is covered with trees, and forest-product manufacturing ranks second among the state's industries. It is the corporate home for Georgia-Pacific, the nation's second largest timber/paper company with 1990 sales of $12.7 billion. And Georgia's environmental regulators are notorious for their lackluster protection of its resources. Says the *Atlanta Constitution*, "At the request of five Georgia paper mills, state officials have adopted the nation's most permissive limit on cancer-causing dioxin . . . 500 times weaker than the one recommended by the federal Environmental Protection Agency." Four months later, in July 1990, the head of Georgia's Department of Natural Resources resigned to become president of one of the nation's largest consulting companies that helps developers and industry navigate through environmental barriers.

FISH OR FOUL

Forest companies and corporate farms are especially fond of buying up huge tracts of fertile land in or near historic flood plains and marshes. But they are not the only users, or abusers, of this once cheap property. Perhaps no other environment is so stressed by competing demands as the nation's coastal wetlands.

More than half of the people in the U.S. now live within 50 miles of the coast (the Atlantic, Pacific, and Gulf Coast or Great Lakes). Developers have overtaken the shorelines and nearby property — draining, dredging, filling, and constructing roads, sewers, and buildings. Following the premise that "the solution to pollution is dilution," companies have also moved to the water's edge to use rivers and bays as their toilets, pouring five trillion gallons of wastewater into coastal waters each year.

The combined force of agriculture, people, and industry destroys habitats for birds and aquatic life, quickens erosion of beaches, and contaminates water used for swimming and fishing. Coastal wetlands are particularly valuable because they trap many pollutants in their thick soil and regulate the flow of fresh water into the brackish estuaries where fish spawn. Huge tracts of fishing waters are now off-limits, and commercial landings in many states are dramatically lower than their record catches 30 or more years ago — 40 to 60 percent lower in Texas, Massachusetts, and Maryland, 90-plus percent lower in New York, Delaware, and Connecticut.

Louisiana lost 560,000 acres of coastal wetlands from 1956 to 1978, and harvesting shellfish (oys-

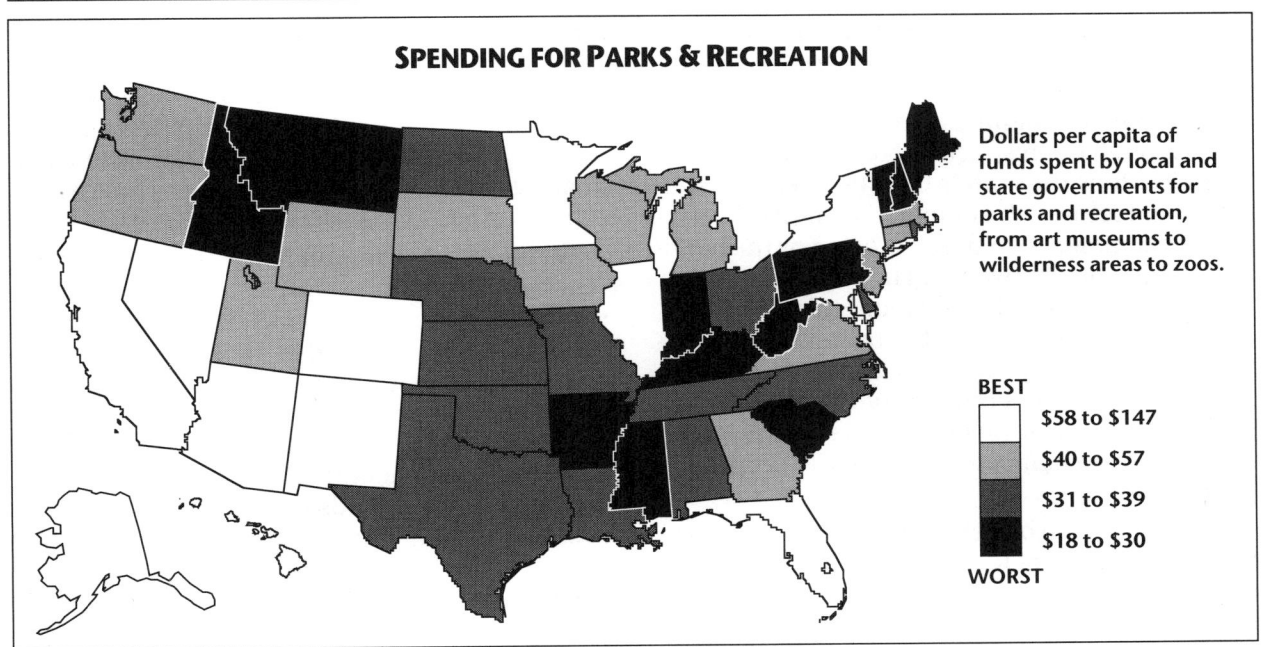

ters, clams, scallops, and mussels) is now severely restricted because the shallow waters they call home are most sensitive to pollution. Chemical companies along the lower Mississippi River, offshore oil rigs, and channel dredging all contribute to the destruction. Nevertheless, Louisiana ranks 2d after Alaska for the nation's biggest commercial fish industry, largely because of its huge off-shore menhaden catch. Before the Valdez disaster, Louisiana also led the nation in oil and hazardous waste spills — with a total of 11.6 million gallons for 1984 through 1986, about equal to the Exxon spill.

In California, where 99 percent of shellfishing waters are restricted because of pollution, discharges of DDT from factories over a 20-year period still contaminate water in Santa Monica Bay. A half century ago, California led the nation in commercial fishing catches with 1.8 million pounds; now the volume is one-third that amount, still enough to rank the state 4th.

In Florida, where the population has jumped 30 percent since 1980, about half of the original coastline and wetlands have been lost to development. More wetlands have disappeared in Florida than in any other state — 9.3 million acres. In March 1989, the Florida Department of Health advised citizens not to eat largemouth bass and warmouth caught in the Everglades because they were contaminated with the highest levels of methyl mercury ever recorded in this country. Pollutants from massive sugar plantations and vegetable farms, combined with mismanaged drainage systems and overuse by south Florida residents, now threaten to turn the Everglades' priceless estuary into a stubby prairie.

ESTUARIES AND WETLANDS

An ongoing "National Estuarine Inventory," conducted by the National Oceanic and Atmospheric Administration, is updating ratings for shellfishing waters and identifying the principle sources of pollution for each estuary. Along the Gulf of Mexico, the nation's fastest growing coastal region, major problems come from overtaxed sewage treatment plants and septic tanks, as well as urban runoff and industrial discharge. Treatment plants are also a major pollution source up the East Coast, along with marinas in the Mid-Atlantic and agricultural runoff in the Southeast. On the West Coast, industrial pollution ranks first; for example, an assortment of 270 paper companies, petroleum refiners, aluminum and steel makers, ship builders, food processors, and lumber mills dump treated effluent, including heavy metals and toxic chemicals, directly into Washington's Puget Sound.

Following passage of the Coastal Zone Management Act in 1972, some states initiated coastal management efforts. For example, North Carolina, with its 3,400 miles of shoreline, has devised a complicated and still evolving set of rules to curb the worst forms of development. But even its program, often heralded as a model for others, hasn't stopped high-rise condominiums from springing up on a barrier island as long as the developer buys enough open space to surround the buildings; nor does the state's Coastal Area Management Act factor in the cumulative impact of several developments on beach erosion or the pollution of fragile fishing waters. The basic approach is to look at each project in isolation and recommend changes that would allow it to be built. Construction rather than conservation is the driving force. And agriculture is completely exempted from regulation; even proposals to mine peat from the state's vast wetlands fell outside the program's jurisdiction.

The protection of wetlands is largely governed by another body of federal law, which the Army Corps of Engineers dominates. Noted for its bridges and efforts to straighten rivers to make navigation easier, the Corps is more in tune with developers than conservationists. In October 1990, it ruled that wetlands converted to farms before 1986 do not need permits to further drain water from fields. "We are pretty easily talking about 40 million acres of wetlands across the country," said Jan Goldman-Carter of the National Wildlife Federation. "They're saying you can do anything with it, pave it over, build a K-mart or whatever you want."

Nationally, 117 million acres of wetlands have already been lost — 53 percent of the original amount in the lower 48 states. While many of these bogs and marshes are along our coasts, millions of acres lie in such inland states as Kentucky and Missouri. In Kansas, the state-owned Cheyenne Bottoms Wildlife Area has lost 80 percent of the water flow through its Walnut Creek because farmers are diverting billions of gallons in new groundwater irrigation systems. The fate of this 20,000-acre wetland refuge for migratory birds, which pits the state's powerful agricultural lobby against conservationists, is yet another example of what happens when renewal resources are subjected to competing, even hostile interests.

FUN AND LIFE QUALITY

Like migratory birds, Americans flock to beaches and national parks each summer to renew themselves and enjoy what nature gives freely. During the year, an amazing 28 percent of all adults hunt or fish, and spend well over $45 billion on supplies, lodging, and travel associated with these two outdoor sports. Recognizing the importance of a state's natural resources for recreation and economic growth, we include 19 indicators under the rubric Fun and Life Quality.

Minnesota, Maine, and Wisconsin, for example, rank best in the number of registered boats per 100 residents, while Hawaii ranks 50th; unlike the top ranking states, Hawaii doesn't benefit from citizens in a neighboring state docking their boats at its summer vacation spots. On the other hand, Hawaii ranks 1st in per-capita visitors to state parks, 2d in tourism spending (behind Nevada), and 2d in local government funds for parks and recreation (behind Alaska). Hawaii also leads the nation in what we call "metro life quality," an indicator based on the grades given each state's major cities by *Places Rated Almanac.*

Population density generally works against people's ability to enjoy their natural surroundings, and 8 of the 12 states with the worst overall Fun and Life Quality scores also are among the nation's most densely populated. The states with the worst overall rankings also include such heavily industrial (and polluted) Great Lakes states as Indiana (rank 50), Ohio (rank 48), and Illinois (rank 46).

The Central and Southern states of Nebraska, Oklahoma, Missouri, Arkansas, and Tennessee turn in a mediocre performance on these 19 indicators, but the others in their regions do even worse. The best overall scores come in the Pacific Northwest and Rocky Mountains, two regions with sizable national parks and other natural attractions. Alaska and South Dakota emerge as 1st and 2d nationally.

Interestingly, there is little correlation between the states with the most per-capita memberships in environmental organizations and those with the best Fun and Life Quality ranking; only Oregon, Vermont, and Alaska rank in the top dozen for both. But an organized constituency for conservation does translate into stronger state policies to protect natural resources. Conversely, 11 of the 17 states with the weakest lobby for the environment also score worst on enacting policies that balance competing demands for renewable resources — the focus of our next two chapters.

FARMS, FORESTS, FISH, AND FUN   105

AGRICULTURE

State	NUMBER OF FARMS Total #	# Per 1,000 Pop.	Rank	# FARMS GAINED OR LOST 1974 TO 87 %	Rank	FARMLAND IN STATE % Land in Farms	Rank	Average Farm in Acres	Rank	FERTILIZER USE PER CAPITA Tons	Rank	HERBICIDES PER ACRE CROPLAND Pounds	Rank	PESTICIDE USE PER CAPITA Pounds	Rank
Alabama	43,318	10.6	21	48.0	19	28.1	34	211	16	15.6	25	1.3	29	2.1	28
Alaska	574	1.1	48	185.6	1	0.3	50	1,789	45	2.0	5	na		na	
Arizona	7,669	2.3	44	77.5	9	50.0	18	4,732	50	12.9	21	2.0	47	1.3	18
Arkansas	48,242	20.2	11	54.3	18	43.1	22	298	26	37.6	41	1.9	46	8.5	45
California	83,217	3.0	42	63.9	15	30.6	29	368	33	12.5	18	1.4	34	1.1	15
Colorado	27,284	8.3	26	29.6	30	51.4	17	1,248	44	16.4	27	0.6	9	2.2	29
Connecticut	3,580	1.1	47	45.5	22	12.8	45	111	4	1.2	2	0.8	12	0.2	3
Delaware	2,966	4.6	36	-0.7	42	49.2	19	205	15	17.2	28	2.3	49	2.9	33
Florida	36,556	3.0	40	74.7	10	32.3	28	306	28	17.2	29	2.3	50	1.3	17
Georgia	43,552	7.0	31	21.5	35	28.9	32	247	23	25.0	35	1.3	30	2.9	32
Hawaii	4,870	4.5	37	132.8	3	41.9	23	353	32	12.1	17	na		na	
Idaho	24,142	24.2	8	23.6	33	26.4	38	577	37	68.3	46	0.9	15	6.4	42
Illinois	88,786	7.7	27	-9.1	48	80.1	6	321	31	31.0	39	1.8	42	5.6	39
Indiana	70,506	12.8	17	-0.6	41	70.3	9	229	20	38.2	42	1.8	44	6.0	41
Iowa	105,180	37.1	4	-10.2	49	88.3	5	301	27	106.7	49	2.1	48	26.2	50
Kansas	68,579	27.7	6	-0.7	43	89.1	4	680	38	56.2	45	0.6	10	5.7	40
Kentucky	92,453	24.8	7	36.7	26	55.2	14	152	6	22.1	33	1.6	40	3.2	35
Louisiana	27,350	6.1	32	47.5	20	28.1	35	293	25	14.1	22	1.9	45	3.3	36
Maine	6,269	5.3	35	37.7	24	6.8	49	214	17	7.1	13	0.3	4	1.2	16
Maryland	14,776	3.3	39	27.5	32	38.1	24	162	9	9.3	15	1.8	43	1.1	14
Massachusetts	6,216	1.1	49	95.2	4	12.3	46	99	3	1.1	1	1.0	18	0.2	2
Michigan	51,172	5.6	34	9.7	39	28.3	33	202	14	12.6	19	1.6	37	1.9	24
Minnesota	85,079	20.0	12	-1.0	44	52.2	16	312	29	45.3	44	1.2	26	10.8	46
Mississippi	34,074	13.0	16	30.8	28	35.5	26	315	30	25.7	36	1.6	41	7.2	44
Missouri	106,105	20.8	10	28.8	31	66.2	10	275	24	33.0	40	1.3	27	3.5	37
Montana	24,568	30.4	5	21.8	34	64.7	11	2,451	46	41.4	43	0.2	2	6.5	43
Nebraska	60,502	38.0	3	-3.3	45	92.4	1	749	41	109.0	50	1.4	33	19.7	48
Nevada	3,027	3.0	41	86.9	6	14.2	44	3,300	48	2.7	7	0.1	1	0.3	5
New Hampshire	2,515	2.4	43	72.5	11	7.4	48	169	10	1.9	4	0.2	3	0.2	4
New Jersey	9,032	1.2	46	64.0	14	18.7	43	99	2	2.5	6	1.5	36	0.3	6
New Mexico	14,249	9.5	22	84.2	7	59.3	12	3,230	47	9.2	14	1.4	32	1.0	12
New York	37,743	2.1	45	17.2	36	27.8	36	223	19	3.1	8	1.3	28	0.5	10
North Carolina	59,284	9.2	23	-5.1	46	30.2	30	159	8	23.1	34	1.3	31	2.8	31
North Dakota	35,289	52.5	1	-13.2	50	90.9	2	1,143	42	92.0	48	0.4	7	19.9	49
Ohio	79,277	7.4	30	12.8	38	57.1	13	189	11	14.5	23	1.6	39	3.0	34
Oklahoma	70,228	21.5	9	46.9	21	71.8	8	449	34	29.6	38	0.4	6	1.4	19
Oregon	32,014	11.8	18	88.1	5	28.9	31	556	36	21.2	32	0.8	13	1.9	23
Pennsylvania	51,549	4.3	38	37.0	25	27.4	37	153	7	4.4	10	1.2	23	0.9	11
Rhode Island	701	0.7	50	67.3	12	8.7	47	84	1	1.5	3	1.1	21	0.1	1
South Carolina	20,517	6.0	33	17.2	37	24.6	39	232	21	15.8	26	1.1	20	2.7	30
South Dakota	36,376	51.3	2	-8.6	47	90.8	3	1,214	43	84.0	47	0.9	16	15.5	47
Tennessee	79,711	16.4	14	65.1	13	44.5	21	147	5	15.2	24	0.9	17	1.8	21
Texas	188,788	11.2	19	78.1	8	77.8	7	691	39	18.1	30	0.9	14	1.6	20
Utah	14,066	8.4	25	60.8	16	19.0	42	710	40	6.0	12	1.0	19	0.5	9
Vermont	5,877	10.7	20	29.7	29	23.7	40	240	22	5.4	11	0.7	11	0.4	7
Virginia	44,799	7.6	28	41.3	23	34.1	27	194	12	10.0	16	1.6	38	1.1	13
Washington	33,559	7.4	29	59.4	17	37.9	25	480	35	18.2	31	0.4	8	1.9	22
West Virginia	17,237	9.1	24	182.6	2	21.9	41	196	13	3.2	9	0.4	5	0.5	8
Wisconsin	75,131	15.6	15	0.4	40	47.7	20	221	18	27.8	37	1.1	22	3.9	38
Wyoming	9,205	18.8	13	33.7	27	54.1	15	3,650	49	12.9	20	1.2	24	2.1	27
U.S. Total	2,087,759	8.6		23.2		42.6		462		18.5		1.2		3.9	

AGRICULTURE

State	PESTICIDE TAINTED GRDWATER %	Rank	UNSAFE NITRATES IN WELLS %	Rank	CROPLAND IRRIGATED %	Rank	CROPLAND EROSION Tons per Acre	Rank	CONSERVATION TILLAGE % Cropland	Rank	ACRES IN CONSERV. RESERVE % Elig.	Rank	AGRICULTURE % OF STATE GROSS PROD. %	Rank	COMPOSITE OF FARMING INDICATORS Score	Rank
Alabama	16.0	35	0.0	1	2.1	16	5.6	24	15.4	38	53.6	9	2.8	22	313	11
Alaska	na		2.4	25	na		na		46.9	6	0.0	44	0.1	50	426	48
Arizona	28.8	42	13.9	48	95.9	50	10.1	46	1.0	49	na		2.6	25	455	50
Arkansas	8.5	27	3.9	31	48.5	41	3.7	11	10.4	42	55.8	7	7.5	7	366	25
California	6.6	21	10.1	45	87.8	48	6.5	31	7.4	45	0.5	33	2.2	31	428	49
Colorado	3.4	13	5.7	36	29.5	37	12.2	47	22.7	25	0.0	47	3.0	21	408	42
Connecticut	0.3	5	2.3	24	7.3	24	3.3	10	15.4	39	100.0	1	0.5	46	294	9
Delaware	35.9	45	9.1	41	11.0	27	2.7	7	51.7	2	17.6	12	1.9	35	389	39
Florida	56.5	49	2.0	20	54.6	43	1.8	4	4.0	47	91.1	3	2.6	26	373	30
Georgia	8.3	26	0.5	4	18.9	34	5.9	28	18.3	30	91.7	2	2.5	28	370	28
Hawaii	na		0.0	1	63.0	46	5.6	24	0.0	50	0.0	41	2.8	23	377	34
Idaho	22.5	39	1.7	19	53.6	42	8.1	38	25.3	20	0.3	35	11.0	5	421	45
Illinois	24.2	41	8.4	40	1.2	10	5.2	20	37.3	9	3.6	21	2.5	29	405	41
Indiana	38.1	47	1.4	15	1.7	11	5.0	18	23.5	23	2.7	22	3.5	17	369	27
Iowa	56.6	50	5.0	35	0.7	8	8.4	40	33.1	14	0.6	32	12.5	4	414	43
Kansas	36.8	46	20.0	49	14.1	32	6.3	29	24.5	21	0.1	38	7.2	8	416	44
Kentucky	6.7	22	4.2	32	0.0	3	8.5	41	55.2	1	0.7	29	4.4	12	290	8
Louisiana	15.3	33	0.6	6	27.7	36	4.3	14	12.2	41	53.8	8	1.7	36	387	38
Maine	4.0	16	2.0	20	0.1	4	1.6	2	36.9	11	6.8	15	2.3	30	266	4
Maryland	6.9	23	6.8	39	4.9	20	5.3	22	51.2	3	8.2	13	1.0	42	337	15
Massachusetts	0.5	7	1.2	13	11.1	28	2.7	7	6.4	46	31.3	11	0.3	48	288	7
Michigan	14.0	31	1.1	12	6.4	22	4.4	15	28.7	17	4.6	19	1.4	38	360	22
Minnesota	33.1	44	9.3	42	1.7	14	7.1	35	18.4	29	2.3	23	6.2	9	424	47
Mississippi	22.7	40	0.2	3	12.9	30	7.3	36	16.5	35	58.9	6	5.6	10	378	36
Missouri	1.9	11	2.1	23	5.8	21	7.8	37	35.7	12	0.7	30	3.5	15	329	12
Montana	3.7	14	3.8	29	11.4	29	9.6	45	29.3	16	0.0	45	8.8	6	367	26
Nebraska	47.8	48	9.3	42	36.8	39	6.6	33	41.5	7	0.2	36	12.7	3	422	46
Nevada	0.0	1	0.9	10	92.6	49	14.9	49	47.3	5	0.0	43	1.0	41	349	20
New Hampshire	0.0	1	1.4	15	1.8	15	1.6	2	10.0	43	na		0.7	44	264	3
New Jersey	16.3	36	1.4	15	15.7	33	6.5	31	23.4	24	0.8	28	0.4	47	370	28
New Mexico	0.5	6	2.9	27	59.7	44	9.0	43	18.2	31	0.0	50	2.7	24	341	16
New York	6.9	24	11.0	46	1.7	12	2.7	7	17.2	32	5.1	18	0.6	45	373	30
North Carolina	4.7	18	0.8	8	7.4	26	6.3	29	15.6	37	59.4	5	3.4	18	348	19
North Dakota	6.2	20	4.6	34	0.7	9	5.8	27	19.0	28	0.0	46	16.7	2	373	30
Ohio	18.7	37	2.6	26	0.2	5	3.8	12	30.2	15	3.6	20	1.5	37	342	18
Oklahoma	4.2	17	11.8	47	7.2	23	6.6	33	27.2	19	0.1	39	3.7	14	329	12
Oregon	0.6	8	1.2	13	40.3	40	4.6	16	27.5	18	0.6	31	3.5	16	295	10
Pennsylvania	10.7	29	5.9	37	0.4	6	5.6	24	37.3	10	2.3	24	1.1	40	332	14
Rhode Island	1.0	10	36.3	50	13.8	31	2.6	5	12.2	40	na		0.3	49	342	17
South Carolina	9.2	28	0.7	7	1.7	13	4.0	13	8.7	44	78.6	4	2.1	32	359	21
South Dakota	15.7	34	6.7	38	3.4	18	4.7	17	23.9	22	0.1	40	18.7	1	376	33
Tennessee	14.9	32	0.9	10	0.7	7	8.8	42	33.9	13	6.3	17	2.6	27	267	6
Texas	5.2	19	9.4	44	30.5	38	14.1	48	21.8	26	0.5	34	2.1	33	377	35
Utah	0.0	1	2.0	20	67.3	47	5.5	23	16.6	34	0.0	49	2.0	34	363	24
Vermont	0.0	1	1.4	15	0.0	1	1.3	1	3.8	48	0.0	42	4.1	13	266	4
Virginia	3.7	15	0.8	8	4.8	19	5.2	20	47.6	4	37.9	10	1.4	39	260	2
Washington	6.9	25	4.3	33	20.9	35	9.0	43	16.3	36	0.1	37	3.2	19	397	40
West Virginia	2.2	12	0.5	4	0.0	1	2.6	5	38.2	8	6.6	16	0.8	43	193	1
Wisconsin	30.1	43	3.6	28	2.8	17	5.1	19	19.4	27	7.3	14	5.0	11	360	22
Wyoming	0.6	9	3.8	29	59.8	45	8.3	39	17.1	33	0.0	48	3.2	20	379	37
U.S. Total	14.9		6.4		15.3		7.1		26.1		6.4		3.9			

FORESTRY

State	FOREST PRODUCTS % Value Added of All Mfg. %	Rank	Industry Rank	FORESTS % OF ALL LAND %	Rank	FORESTS OWNED BY TIMBER FIRMS %	Rank	FORESTS OWNED BY FED. GOVT. %	Rank	CHANGE IN FORESTS 1982 TO 87 %	Rank	PRIVATE TREE FARMS #	Rank	LUMBER AS % STATE GROSS PRODUCT %	Rank
Alabama	19.3	6	1	66.9	5	21	42	4	38	2.4	15	2,615	9	1.73	8
Alaska	19.8	5	2	35.7	30	7	25	55	9	8.4	6	29	46	0.78	18
Arizona	4.3	33	7	26.7	37	0	9	79	2	2.8	12	30	45	0.52	24
Arkansas	16.5	8	1	51.0	17	25	45	16	15	-2.2	44	4,400	3	2.47	7
California	4.0	35	8	39.5	29	12	35	50	10	-1.9	43	713	31	0.60	22
Colorado	2.5	48	10	32.2	33	0	9	69	7	-4.2	47	229	38	0.26	38
Connecticut	3.7	38	8	58.7	14	0	9	1	44	2.2	17	529	33	0.15	48
Delaware	4.1	34	5	33.0	31	8	29	14	17	0.5	27	207	41	0.27	37
Florida	6.5	22	6	48.4	21	33	49	10	21	0.6	25	3,652	4	0.49	25
Georgia	13.4	11	2	64.9	6	21	42	6	33	-1.1	40	4,424	2	1.26	11
Hawaii	2.5	49	5	42.5	26	31	47	1	44	20.1	1	2	50	0.10	49
Idaho	22.1	4	2	41.4	28	6	23	77	3	0.4	28	749	29	5.07	2
Illinois	3.5	42	9	12.0	44	1	13	7	30	18.3	3	935	25	0.21	42
Indiana	4.4	32	10	19.4	40	10	31	8	27	13.1	5	1,002	23	0.82	16
Iowa	3.9	36	7	4.4	46	1	13	3	40	19.9	2	630	32	0.44	28
Kansas	3.7	40	9	2.6	48	0	9	4	38	-0.1	29	328	35	0.31	36
Kentucky	4.7	28	10	48.4	22	2	16	8	27	0.8	22	888	28	0.52	23
Louisiana	12.0	13	3	48.7	20	31	47	6	33	-1.0	39	2,999	7	0.70	20
Maine	36.0	2	1	89.8	1	47	50	1	48	-0.5	34	1,871	13	3.14	4
Maryland	5.6	23	7	41.8	27	5	19	1	44	4.1	10	1,302	21	0.20	43
Massachusetts	3.8	37	7	62.0	10	2	16	1	48	6.2	8	1,359	19	0.19	44
Michigan	2.6	47	9	50.1	19	11	33	14	17	-0.8	36	2,036	12	0.36	33
Minnesota	14.5	10	2	32.8	32	5	19	21	14	-1.5	41	2,459	10	0.76	19
Mississippi	12.4	12	1	55.4	15	20	39	9	26	-0.1	30	5,367	1	2.72	6
Missouri	4.6	30	9	28.4	35	2	16	10	21	-0.9	38	895	27	0.36	34
Montana	33.1	3	1	23.6	39	7	25	73	5	-2.6	45	432	34	2.85	5
Nebraska	2.6	46	12	1.5	49	0	9	6	33	-10.9	49	192	42	0.25	39
Nevada	3.7	39	12	12.7	43	6	23	45	12	16.2	4	3	49	0.16	46
New Hampshire	7.3	19	4	88.1	2	14	37	10	21	0.7	24	1,333	20	1.28	10
New Jersey	4.7	29	7	42.7	25	1	13	2	42	0.6	26	228	39	0.17	45
New Mexico	5.0	26	9	23.9	38	0	9	49	11	2.6	13	109	44	0.40	31
New York	3.2	43	9	62.0	9	11	33	1	44	1.5	19	1,781	15	0.16	47
North Carolina	6.9	21	5	61.0	11	13	36	10	21	-0.9	37	3,175	6	1.17	13
North Dakota	1.3	50	14	1.0	50	0	9	15	16	-11.2	50	302	36	0.07	50
Ohio	5.3	25	14	27.9	36	6	23	2	42	5.2	9	1,851	14	0.32	35
Oklahoma	3.6	41	12	16.6	41	22	43	10	21	6.3	7	292	37	0.25	40
Oregon	44.8	1	1	45.6	23	21	42	58	8	-8.9	48	1,064	22	8.58	1
Pennsylvania	7.1	20	7	59.4	13	6	23	3	40	1.0	21	1,762	16	0.41	30
Rhode Island	2.9	44	10	59.8	12	0	9	0	50	-0.3	31	176	43	0.22	41
South Carolina	10.4	15	4	64.3	7	18	38	7	30	0.7	23	1,646	17	1.19	12
South Dakota	5.5	24	5	3.5	47	4	17	74	4	3.8	11	228	40	0.46	26
Tennessee	7.5	18	6	50.3	18	9	30	6	33	-0.4	33	1,514	18	0.78	17
Texas	4.4	31	8	8.1	45	33	49	6	33	-3.5	46	3,479	5	0.45	27
Utah	2.9	45	13	30.9	34	0	9	69	6	1.0	20	5	48	0.42	29
Vermont	11.4	14	3	75.7	4	8	29	7	30	-0.3	32	899	26	1.51	9
Virginia	8.9	17	5	63.3	8	12	35	11	19	-1.9	42	2,459	11	0.84	15
Washington	17.6	7	2	51.5	16	25	45	39	13	2.2	18	984	24	3.19	3
West Virginia	4.8	27	6	77.5	3	8	29	8	27	2.3	16	715	30	0.62	21
Wisconsin	15.7	9	2	44.1	24	8	29	11	19	2.5	14	2,880	8	0.98	14
Wyoming	9.9	16	6	16.1	42	1	13	86	1	-0.6	35	12	47	0.38	32
U.S. Total	6.7		6	32.4		11				1.8		67,171			

FISHING

State	PAPER, CARDBOARD, PULP MILLS #	Rank	WETLANDS LOST SINCE 1780S %	Rank	SHELLFISH FISHING WATER LIMITED %	Rank	COMMERCIAL FISH LANDINGS Total Pounds 1,000s	Rank	Drop From Peak Year %	Rank	FISHING LICENSES # in 1,000s	# per 100 Pop.	Rank	COMPOSITE OF FORESTRY AND FISH Score	Rank
Alabama	39	45	50	30	80	47	25,444	17	-36	29	579	14.1	28	314	27
Alaska	2	29	<1	1			4,088,780	1	<1	2	314	59.5	1	184	1
Arizona	7	20	36	16							458	12.9	29	261	12
Arkansas	18	42	72	41							733	30.5	6	287	19
California	46	18	91	50	99	49	418,409	4	-76	46	2,164	7.4	39	384	48
Colorado	1	9	50	29							732	22.1	14	304	25
Connecticut	11	26	74	43	21	15	8,588	24	-90	49	223	6.9	42	372	45
Delaware	4	37	54	34	10	3	6,898	25	-98	50	22	3.3	48	384	48
Florida	20	19	46	24	68	42	197,462	7	-18	15	828	6.5	43	301	23
Georgia	41	38	23	5	70	44	15,770	21	-67	44	704	10.9	35	323	28
Hawaii	3	25	12	3			24,397	18	-30	24	9	0.8	50	371	44
Idaho	0	1	56	36							398	39.2	4	203	2
Illinois	13	15	85	45			238	30	na		804	6.9	41	351	39
Indiana	15	24	87	46			1,528	27	na		626	11.2	34	334	36
Iowa	2	11	89	48							408	14.4	26	329	33
Kansas	2	12	48	26							307	12.2	32	356	41
Kentucky	8	21	81	44							646	17.3	21	304	25
Louisiana	32	40	46	25	100	50	1,227,941	2	-36	30	547	12.5	30	346	37
Maine	41	50	20	4	11	5	151,119	11	-58	39	303	24.8	11	271	17
Maryland	6	17	73	42	4	1	84,920	15	-40	32	301	6.4	45	323	28
Massachusetts	43	41	28	9	16	9	268,861	6	-59	40	237	4	47	304	24
Michigan	47	35	50	31			14,215	22	-60	42	1,619	17.5	19	334	35
Minnesota	23	36	42	22			329	29	na		1,531	35.2	5	271	16
Mississippi	20	43	59	37	68	42	298,206	5	-37	31	449	17.1	22	298	22
Missouri	5	13	87	47							1,048	20.3	15	332	34
Montana	2	22	27	7							369	45.7	3	242	7
Nebraska	0	1	35	13							243	15.1	25	354	40
Nevada	0	1	52	32							158	14.2	27	324	30
New Hampshire	16	47	9	2	60	38	11,402	23	na		193	17.4	20	269	15
New Jersey	20	23	39	20	40	33	128,459	12	-76	45	250	3.2	49	379	47
New Mexico	1	10	33	12							275	18	18	254	10
New York	67	28	60	39	19	13	37,080	16	-89	47	1,156	6.4	44	363	42
North Carolina	31	33	49	27	17	11	164,476	9	-62	43	469	7.1	40	292	20
North Dakota	0	1	49	28							152	23	13	347	38
Ohio	43	31	90	49			3,389	26	-89	48	1,148	10.5	36	393	50
Oklahoma	13	30	67	40							598	18.5	17	374	46
Oregon	38	46	38	19	65	40	170,052	8	0	1	769	27.3	9	268	14
Pennsylvania	44	27	56	35			495	28	na		1,173	9.7	37	327	32
Rhode Island	0	1	37	17	25	19	125,041	13	-2	3	41	4.1	46	295	21
South Carolina	23	39	27	8	29	21	20,065	19	-25	23	432	12.3	31	272	18
South Dakota	0	1	35	14							200	27.9	8	225	3
Tennessee	24	34	59	38							760	15.4	24	326	31
Texas	22	16	52	33	21	15	96,421	14	-59	41	1,935	11.4	33	365	43
Utah	0	1	30	10							396	23.2	12	237	5
Vermont	9	48	35	15							154	27.1	10	268	13
Virginia	24	32	42	21	14	7	692,794	3	-8	4	520	8.5	38	240	6
Washington	43	44	31	11	39	31	163,003	10	-17	14	962	20.2	16	247	8
West Virginia	2	14	24	6							287	15.4	23	228	4
Wisconsin	83	49	46	23			17,298	20	na		1,438	29.5	7	247	8
Wyoming	0	1	38	18							238	50.1	2	256	11
U.S. Total	954		30				8,463,080				31,429	13.0			

FUN & LIFE QUALITY

State	ADULTS WHO FISH OR HUNT %	Rank	SPENDING BY SPORTSMEN $ Per Capita	Rank	REGISTERED MOTOR BOATS Per 100 Pop.	Rank	RECREATIONAL WATERS Inland Water as % State	Rank	Coast Line Miles	TOTAL LAND IN MILLION ACRES	% LAND OWNED BY FED. GOV. %	Rank	% LAND OWNED BY FISH & WILD. SERV. %	Rank
Alabama	32.3	23	237	14	5.16	19	1.81	27	607	32.7	1.7	39	0.16	37
Alaska	53.7	1	506	2	5.49	17	3.41	13	31,383	365.5	81.1	1	21.18	1
Arizona	24.5	40	146	33	3.39	35	0.43	49	0	72.7	44.5	7	2.35	5
Arkansas	42.1	7	247	11	6.11	12	2.09	23	0	33.6	7.1	20	0.67	17
California	20.5	44	143	35	2.53	42	1.52	29	3,427	100.2	44.5	8	0.33	28
Colorado	36.3	16	224	16	2.50	43	0.48	47	0	66.5	29.8	10	0.09	42
Connecticut	19.1	48	99	49	2.93	39	2.93	17	618	3.1	0.4	49	0.01	48
Delaware	25.7	39	200	22	6.18	10	5.48	9	381	1.3	2.4	35	2.05	6
Florida	28.1	34	265	7	5.33	18	7.69	2	5,095	34.7	9.4	16	1.50	7
Georgia	31.8	27	251	9	4.11	24	1.45	31	2,344	37.3	4.0	32	1.26	10
Hawaii	20.3	45	102	47	1.28	50	0.71	42	1,052	4.1	6.9	21	6.60	2
Idaho	45.8	4	295	4	6.05	14	1.38	32	0	52.9	60.6	3	0.17	36
Illinois	22.8	42	112	45	2.80	40	1.24	33	0	35.8	1.4	42	0.33	27
Indiana	31.2	28	138	38	3.82	26	0.70	43	0	23.2	2.0	37	0.03	44
Iowa	34.6	18	133	41	6.59	7	0.55	46	0	35.9	0.4	50	0.21	32
Kansas	33.7	20	137	39	3.57	31	0.61	44	0	52.5	1.3	43	0.10	41
Kentucky	33.4	21	141	36	3.07	36	1.83	26	0	25.5	5.5	26	0.01	49
Louisiana	37.3	12	234	15	6.70	6	6.76	5	7,721	28.9	22.6	13	1.37	8
Maine	32.1	25	177	27	10.12	2	6.82	4	3,478	19.8	0.8	47	0.21	31
Maryland	22.8	41	104	46	3.60	29	5.96	6	3,190	6.3	3.1	34	0.45	20
Massachusetts	17.7	49	99	48	3.79	27	5.55	8	1,519	5.0	1.6	40	0.25	30
Michigan	32.2	24	221	18	8.50	4	2.69	19	0	36.5	9.8	15	0.31	29
Minnesota	48.4	3	261	8	15.91	1	5.75	7	0	51.2	4.7	29	0.94	14
Mississippi	40.7	8	250	10	6.08	13	0.96	36	359	30.2	5.5	24	0.45	21
Missouri	37.0	14	293	5	5.13	20	1.08	35	0	44.2	4.6	30	0.13	38
Montana	44.6	6	469	3	4.26	23	1.13	34	0	93.3	29.4	12	1.28	9
Nebraska	33.3	22	155	31	3.45	32	0.92	38	0	49.0	1.1	45	0.34	26
Nevada	27.4	36	245	12	3.45	33	0.60	45	0	70.3	78.9	2	3.38	3
New Hampshire	26.4	38	126	43	1.32	49	3.08	15	131	5.8	13.0	14	0.03	46
New Jersey	19.3	46	132	42	2.24	46	4.10	10	1,792	4.8	3.4	33	0.99	12
New Mexico	27.8	35	170	28	2.26	45	0.21	50	0	77.8	33.1	9	0.49	19
New York	16.9	50	79	50	2.14	48	3.52	12	1,850	30.7	0.8	46	0.08	43
North Carolina	30.1	30	188	24	3.90	25	7.26	3	3,375	31.4	7.1	19	0.90	16
North Dakota	44.6	5	284	6	6.14	11	1.98	24	0	44.5	4.4	31	2.95	4
Ohio	27.1	37	119	44	3.44	34	0.79	41	0	26.2	1.3	44	0.03	47
Oklahoma	37.2	13	213	19	5.62	16	1.86	25	0	44.1	2.0	38	0.34	25
Oregon	37.0	15	244	13	5.67	15	0.92	39	1,410	61.6	52.3	5	0.91	15
Pennsylvania	22.6	43	151	32	2.21	47	0.93	37	89	28.8	2.3	36	0.03	45
Rhode Island	19.1	47	143	34	2.99	38	13.03	1	384	0.7	0.7	48	0.20	34
South Carolina	28.5	33	224	17	8.05	5	2.92	18	2,876	19.4	6.1	22	0.97	13
South Dakota	39.7	9	165	29	6.41	8	1.51	30	0	48.9	5.5	25	1.19	11
Tennessee	28.5	32	188	25	4.55	22	2.35	22	0	26.7	5.1	28	0.39	24
Texas	30.7	29	208	21	3.57	30	1.80	28	3,359	168.2	1.6	41	0.21	33
Utah	35.9	17	199	23	2.65	41	3.33	14	0	52.7	60.0	4	0.19	35
Vermont	37.8	10	134	40	6.39	9	3.55	11	384	5.9	6.0	23	0.10	40
Virginia	29.4	31	162	30	3.06	37	2.61	20	3,315	25.5	7.5	18	0.44	23
Washington	34.1	19	182	26	3.76	28	2.39	21	3,026	42.7	29.6	11	0.44	22
West Virginia	32.0	26	139	37	2.44	44	0.46	48	0	15.4	9.1	17	0.00	50
Wisconsin	37.6	11	210	20	9.88	3	3.08	16	0	35.0	5.4	27	0.64	18
Wyoming	50.9	2	609	1	4.62	21	0.84	40	0	62.3	46.5	6	0.12	39
U.S. Total	27.8		174		4.17		2.20		83,165	2,271.3	30.3		4.02	

FUN & LIFE QUALITY

State	VISITS TO NATL. PARKS Per 100 Pop.	Rank	% LAND IN STATE PARKS & REC. AREAS %	Rank	VISITORS TO STATE PARKS Per 100 Pop.	Rank	% STATE BUDGET FOR PARKS %	Rank	LOCAL FUNDS FOR PARKS & RECREATION $ p/c	Rank	TOURISM & TRAVEL SPENDING $ p/c	Rank	NATL. RESOURCES AS % STATE GROSS PRODUCT Pop.	Rank
Alabama	28	34	0.15	40	140	43	0.46	9	32.88	36	500	50	7.3	20
Alaska	201	12	0.89	11	1,047	3	0.20	35	147.01	1	1,631	10	31.3	2
Arizona	317	9	0.05	49	57	49	0.20	34	60.09	11	1,664	8	5.5	26
Arkansas	108	20	0.14	43	277	23	0.44	11	18.92	50	799	42	12.4	14
California	134	17	1.29	4	266	26	0.88	4	73.12	5	1,294	13	4.3	32
Colorado	172	13	0.35	25	239	31	0.21	31	79.48	4	1,655	9	6.8	22
Connecticut	0	48	1.02	8	266	27	0.12	46	41.95	23	968	27	0.8	47
Delaware	0	48	0.96	9	259	28	0.47	7	39.43	26	1,125	20	2.2	43
Florida	57	29	1.21	5	120	47	0.19	39	63.37	9	2,024	4	4.2	33
Georgia	77	25	0.17	37	223	33	0.35	15	40.72	24	917	33	4.3	31
Hawaii	385	8	0.60	17	1,559	1	0.21	32	102.29	2	3,048	2	2.9	40
Idaho	42	31	0.09	45	210	34	0.19	38	22.66	47	1,063	21	17.7	9
Illinois	5	44	1.08	7	304	19	0.12	47	67.46	8	916	34	3.6	36
Indiana	38	32	0.25	29	168	40	0.15	43	24.65	44	595	47	5.1	28
Iowa	14	40	0.15	42	379	15	0.25	24	39.83	25	704	44	13.2	13
Kansas	5	45	0.06	47	203	35	0.28	21	32.72	37	875	39	11.4	18
Kentucky	85	22	0.16	38	703	6	0.72	5	26.44	39	651	46	11.5	17
Louisiana	23	36	0.13	44	23	50	0.11	49	37.42	31	862	40	24.7	4
Maine	445	6	0.35	24	181	37	0.27	22	26.07	40	1,815	6	5.5	27
Maryland	80	24	1.53	2	190	36	0.20	36	69.18	7	1,174	17	1.4	45
Massachusetts	165	14	1.19	6	239	29	0.16	42	51.32	17	1,148	19	0.6	50
Michigan	20	37	0.72	16	266	25	0.14	44	46.08	18	937	31	2.5	42
Minnesota	15	39	0.39	23	177	38	0.25	25	71.32	6	1,307	12	8.2	19
Mississippi	395	7	0.08	46	167	41	0.18	41	20.10	49	507	49	12.0	16
Missouri	88	21	0.25	28	279	22	0.23	27	38.52	28	1,037	23	4.4	30
Montana	461	5	0.06	48	520	12	0.23	26	23.57	45	900	36	20.1	7
Nebraska	13	41	0.30	26	542	9	0.43	13	36.34	34	853	41	13.4	12
Nevada	580	2	0.20	34	268	24	0.26	23	88.95	3	8,189	1	3.4	38
New Hampshire	4	46	0.57	18	401	14	0.57	6	25.00	42	1,894	5	2.1	44
New Jersey	49	30	1.92	1	137	44	0.19	40	55.47	14	1,732	7	0.7	48
New Mexico	142	16	0.15	39	316	17	0.30	19	59.13	12	1,279	14	21.6	5
New York	76	26	0.85	12	312	18	0.96	3	60.50	10	965	28	0.9	46
North Carolina	259	11	0.41	21	121	46	0.11	48	37.05	32	1,051	22	4.8	29
North Dakota	82	23	0.04	50	152	42	0.13	45	31.24	38	963	29	25.2	3
Ohio	13	42	0.79	14	601	8	0.22	29	32.93	35	699	45	2.9	41
Oklahoma	61	28	0.22	31	522	11	1.00	2	36.35	33	895	37	18.0	8
Oregon	31	33	0.15	41	1,384	2	0.30	20	43.77	22	1,026	24	12.3	15
Pennsylvania	108	19	0.96	10	302	20	0.36	14	23.17	46	978	26	2.9	39
Rhode Island	2	47	1.37	3	618	7	0.34	16	39.07	27	579	48	0.6	49
South Carolina	19	38	0.41	22	239	30	0.20	33	25.56	41	1,254	16	3.5	37
South Dakota	499	3	0.19	36	765	5	0.47	8	45.06	19	883	38	20.4	6
Tennessee	159	15	0.51	20	528	10	0.45	10	38.23	29	940	30	4.1	34
Texas	27	35	0.26	27	123	45	0.20	37	38.04	30	936	32	15.6	11
Utah	494	4	0.22	30	287	21	0.44	12	44.20	21	1,278	15	7.3	21
Vermont	0	48	0.79	15	173	39	0.32	17	22.54	48	2,876	3	6.0	25
Virginia	305	10	0.20	32	64	48	0.08	50	44.79	20	1,161	18	3.7	35
Washington	130	18	0.54	19	854	4	0.31	18	56.78	13	985	25	6.6	23
West Virginia	62	27	0.82	13	472	13	1.20	1	24.96	43	755	43	16.4	10
Wisconsin	8	43	0.20	33	238	32	0.22	28	51.36	16	912	35	6.1	24
Wyoming	932	1	0.19	35	379	16	0.22	30	55.13	15	1,551	11	36.5	1
U.S. Total	98		0.44		294		0.30		49.10		1,127			

FARMS, FORESTS, FISH, AND FUN   111

FUN & LIFE QUALITY

State	1990 POPULATION 1,000s	PEOPLE PER SQUARE MILE Population Density 1990 #	Rank	1970 #	Rank	POPULATION CHANGE 1970-1990 %	Rank	PEOPLE IN RURAL AREAS %	Rank	METRO LIFE QUALITY Rate	Rank	CONSERVATION MEMBERS Per 1,000 Pop.	Rank	COMPOSITE FUN & LIFE QUALITY Score	Rank
Alabama	4,041	79.6	26	67.8	24	17.3	24	40.0	15	248	49	3.4	49	578	43
Alaska	550	1.0	1	0.5	1	81.5	47	35.7	22	157	27	12.3	8	215	1
Arizona	3,665	32.3	14	15.6	10	106.5	49	16.2	42	39	2	8.0	28	500	27
Arkansas	2,351	45.1	16	36.9	16	22.2	27	48.4	9	222	46	3.9	47	454	16
California	29,760	190.4	39	127.8	38	49.0	42	8.7	50	129	15	13.1	4	475	22
Colorado	3,294	31.8	13	21.3	12	49.1	43	19.4	39	176	34	12.7	5	455	17
Connecticut	3,287	674.7	47	622.3	47	8.4	15	21.2	36	152	24	14.2	3	648	49
Delaware	666	344.8	44	283.6	44	21.6	25	29.4	31	89	5	11.5	10	461	19
Florida	12,938	238.9	41	125.4	37	90.5	48	15.7	43	188	39	7.5	31	489	24
Georgia	6,478	111.6	30	79.0	27	41.2	38	37.6	17	208	43	5.3	38	524	36
Hawaii	1,108	172.5	38	119.8	36	43.9	40	13.5	47	32	1	9.6	20	491	25
Idaho	1,007	12.2	7	8.7	6	41.2	37	46.0	12	111	11	7.9	29	420	13
Illinois	11,431	205.4	40	199.7	41	2.9	6	16.7	40	167	30	8.6	25	606	46
Indiana	5,544	154.3	35	144.6	39	6.7	13	35.8	21	175	33	6.6	35	655	50
Iowa	2,777	49.6	18	50.5	22	(1.7)	1	41.4	14	190	40	8.3	26	518	33
Kansas	2,478	30.3	12	27.5	14	10.2	17	33.3	24	173	32	7.2	32	591	44
Kentucky	3,685	92.9	28	81.2	29	14.4	19	49.1	8	125	14	4.2	46	511	30
Louisiana	4,220	94.8	29	81.9	30	15.8	22	31.4	29	238	47	3.5	48	518	34
Maine	1,228	39.6	15	32.1	15	23.5	29	52.5	5	155	26	12.6	6	394	7
Maryland	4,781	486.1	46	398.9	46	21.9	26	19.7	38	109	10	11.2	12	521	35
Massachusetts	6,016	769.0	48	727.1	48	5.8	11	16.2	41	165	29	12.3	7	563	41
Michigan	9,295	163.2	37	156.0	40	4.7	9	29.3	32	210	45	8.1	27	512	31
Minnesota	4,375	55.0	20	47.8	20	15.0	20	33.1	25	117	13	10.6	14	336	3
Mississippi	2,573	54.5	19	46.9	19	16.1	23	52.7	4	198	41	2.5	50	517	32
Missouri	5,117	74.2	24	67.9	25	9.4	16	31.9	28	134	19	6.9	34	467	21
Montana	799	5.5	3	4.8	4	15.1	21	47.1	11	210	44	9.7	18	367	6
Nebraska	1,578	20.6	9	19.4	11	6.3	12	37.1	19	112	12	7.1	33	466	20
Nevada	1,202	10.9	6	4.4	3	145.8	50	14.7	46	132	17	8.6	24	402	9
New Hampshire	1,109	123.3	33	82.1	31	50.3	44	47.8	10	169	31	15.3	2	531	38
New Jersey	7,730	1,035.1	50	960.2	50	7.8	14	11.0	49	99	9	11.4	11	556	40
New Mexico	1,515	12.5	8	8.4	5	49.0	41	27.9	33	133	18	8.9	23	436	14
New York	17,990	379.7	45	385.0	45	(1.4)	2	15.4	45	99	7	10.6	15	551	39
North Carolina	6,629	135.7	34	104.1	34	30.4	32	52.0	6	176	35	6.2	36	503	28
North Dakota	639	9.2	5	8.9	8	3.4	7	51.2	7	164	28	4.9	40	406	10
Ohio	10,847	264.5	42	259.9	42	1.8	4	26.7	34	143	21	7.8	30	634	48
Oklahoma	3,146	45.8	17	37.3	17	22.9	28	32.7	26	201	42	4.3	45	461	18
Oregon	2,842	29.6	11	21.7	13	35.9	35	32.1	27	77	4	11.9	9	358	5
Pennsylvania	11,882	264.7	43	262.9	43	0.7	3	30.7	30	155	25	9.7	19	577	42
Rhode Island	1,003	951.2	49	900.5	49	5.6	10	13.0	48	135	20	10.2	17	592	45
South Carolina	3,486	115.4	31	85.8	32	34.5	34	45.9	13	148	23	4.6	41	499	26
South Dakota	696	9.2	4	8.8	7	4.5	8	53.6	3	185	38	5.7	37	324	2
Tennessee	4,877	118.5	32	95.4	33	24.2	30	39.6	16	144	22	4.5	43	477	23
Texas	16,987	64.8	22	42.7	18	51.7	45	20.4	37	242	48	4.5	42	611	47
Utah	1,723	21.0	10	12.9	9	62.7	46	15.6	44	50	3	5.2	39	409	11
Vermont	563	60.7	21	48.0	21	26.5	31	66.2	1	99	8	20.2	1	411	12
Virginia	6,187	155.8	36	117.1	35	33.0	33	34.0	23	92	6	9.0	22	527	37
Washington	4,867	73.2	23	51.3	23	42.6	39	26.5	35	131	16	10.5	16	399	8
West Virginia	1,793	74.4	25	72.3	26	2.8	5	63.8	2	177	36	4.4	44	510	29
Wisconsin	4,892	89.9	27	81.2	28	10.7	18	35.8	20	182	37	10.7	13	449	15
Wyoming	454	4.7	2	3.4	2	36.6	36	37.3	18	294	50	9.3	21	347	4
U.S. Total	248,101	70.1		57.2		22.5									

SOURCES FOR FARMS, FORESTS, FISH, & FUN INDICATORS

Number of farms
Total farms in 1987 with sales of at least $1,000. Numbers presented in thousands and per 1,000 residents; ranked on a per-capita basis.
Source: 1987 Census of Agriculture, Bureau of the Census, U.S. Department of Commerce, Washington.

Farms lost or gained
Percent change in number of farms with annual sales of at least $1,000, between 1974 and 1987.
Source: Census of Agriculture, 1974 and 1987, Bureau of the Census, U.S. Department of Commerce, Washington.

Farmland in state
Percent of state's land in farms and average size of farm in acres.
Source: 1987 Census of Agriculture, Bureau of the Census, U.S. Department of Commerce, Washington.

Fertilizer use
Tons per capita of commercial fertilizer consumed, 1989.
Source: "Commercial Fertilizers," December 1989. Published by National Fertilizer Development Center, Tennessee Valley Authority, Muscle Shoals, AL 35660; telephone (205) 386-3551.

Herbicide use
Pounds of active ingredient per acre of cropland of herbicide applied. Corn and soybean acreage accounts for two-thirds of the 500 million pound total.
Source: Leonard P. Gianessi and Cynthia Puffer, "Herbicide Use in the United States," December, 1990. Published by Resources for the Future, 1616 P Street, NW, Washington, DC 20036; telephone (202) 328-5000.

Pesticide use
Pounds per capita of active ingredient of pesticides (herbicide, fungicide, insecticide, etc.) applied.
Source: Leonard P. Gianessi, "A National Pesticide Usage Data Base," 1986. Published by Resources for the Future, Washington.

Pesticide-tainted groundwater
Percent of state's population in counties served by public water supplies from groundwater potentially contaminated by pesticides.
Source: Elizabeth G. Nielsen and Linda K. Lee, "The Magnitude and Costs of Groundwater Contamination from Agricultural Chemicals." Agricultural Economic Research Report No. 576, October 1987. Published by Economic Research Service, U.S. Department of Agriculture.

Unsafe nitrates in wells
Percent of wells tested that had 10 or more milligrams per liter of nitrogen or nitrates, which exceeds the Safe Drinking Water standard set by U.S. Environmental Protection Agency. Data comes from wells tested over a 25-year period.
Source: Table 8, "National Water Summary, 1984," U.S. Geological Survey, U.S. Department of Interior, Washington.

Cropland irrigated
> Percent of cultivated and noncultivated cropland artificially irrigated, 1987.
> *Source:* "Summary Report, 1987 National Resources Inventory," December 1989. Published by Soil Conservation Service, U.S. Department of Agriculture, Washington.

Cropland erosion
> Rate of erosion from wind and water, tons per year of cropland lost (not to be confused with erosion rate for all rural land).
> *Source:* "Summary Report, 1987 National Resources Inventory," December 1989. Published by Soil Conservation Service, U.S. Department of Agriculture, Washington.

Conservation tillage
> Percent of planted acres using no-till, ridge-till, or mulch-till conservation methods, which minimize erosion between harvest and planting of next crop.
> *Source:* "1990 National Survey of Conservation Tillage Practices," November 1990. Published by Conservation Technology Information Center, 1220 Potter Drive, West Lafayette, IN 47906; telephone (317) 494-9555.

Acres in Conservation Reserve Program (CRP)
> Percent of eligible acres enrolled by landowners in program to protect wetlands, highly erodible, or other lands. Rather than being farmed, land is planted in trees or grasses for at least 10 years.
> *Source:* Conservation Reserve Program status report, September 1990, from U.S. Forest Service, Cooperative Forestry, Atlanta, and January 13, 1986 press release on CRP from U.S. Department of Agriculture, Office of Information, Washington.

Agriculture as percent of state gross product
> Average contribution of agriculture to state's total goods and services during period 1963-1986.
> *Source:* Ronald H. Schmidt, "Natural Resources and Regional Growth," *Economic Review*, Fall 1989. Published by the Federal Reserve Bank of San Francisco. Updated tables were provided by the author.

Composite score for farming
> Rankings of 14 agriculture indicators were totaled to produce a composite score. Lowest score receives best composite rank.

Forest products, economic significance
> Value added by forest-products industry as percent of total value added by 21 manufacturing industries monitored by U.S. Department of Commerce. Also, relative significance of forest products among those 21 industries, ranked on value added. Data for 1986. Forest products include lumber and paper-pulp (SIC 24 and 26), but not wood furniture.
> *Source:* March 1990 computer printout from National Forest Products Association, 1250 Connecticut Avenue, NW, Washington; telephone (202) 463-2700.

Forest land and its ownership
> Percent of state's land in forests, 1987. Also percent of forest acreage owned by paper/pulp and wood products companies; percent owned by federal agencies; and percent of forest acreage gained or lost between 1982 and 1987.
> *Source:* "Analysis of the Timber Situation in the U.S., 1989-2040" and "Forest Statistics of the U.S., 1987," September 1989. Published by U.S. Forest Service, U.S. Department of Agriculture, Washington.

Private tree farms
> Number of privately owned tree farms.
> *Source:* "Ranking of States by Number of Tree Farms." January 1, 1990 fact sheet from American Forest Council, 1250 Connecticut Avenue, NW, Washington, DC 20036; telephone (202) 463-2455.

Lumber products as percent of state gross product
> Average contribution of forest products to state's total goods and services during period 1963-1986.
> *Source:* Ronald H. Schmidt, "Natural Resources and Regional Growth," *Economic Review*, Fall 1989. Published by the Federal Reserve Bank of San Francisco. Updated tables were provided by the author.

Paper, paperboard (cardboard), and pulp mills
> Number of mills in 1989, including some at multi-plant sites, ranked on per-capita basis.
> *Source: Lockwood-Post's Pulp and Paper 1990 Directory*. Published by Miller Freeman Publications, 500 Howard Street, San Francisco, CA 94105.

Wetlands lost
> Percent of inland and coastal wetlands lost in past 200 years.
> *Source:* "Wetland Losses in the U.S., 1780s to 1980s," December 1990. Published by U.S. Department of Interior, Washington.

Shellfish waters limited for fishing
> Percent of shellfish-productive waters capable of commercial harvesting which are restricted from fishing due to high levels of pollution.
> *Source:* "1985 National Shellfish Register of Classified Estuarine Waters," National Oceanic and Atmospheric Administration, U.S. Department of Commerce, Washington.

Commercial fish landings
> Pounds of fish (excluding shells) brought to state's shore for sale in 1989.
> *Source:* "Fisheries of the United States, 1989," May 1990. Published by Fisheries Statistics Division, National Oceanic and Atmospheric Administration, U.S. Department of Commerce, Washington.

Drop in fish landings
> Percent decrease of fish landed from state's peak year of harvest, which ranged from 1880 in New York and 1889 in Rhode Island to 1989 for Oregon.
> *Source:* "Fisheries of the United States, 1989," May 1990. Published by Fisheries Statistics Division, National Oceanic and Atmospheric Administration, U.S. Department of Commerce, Washington.

Fishing licenses
> Number of fishing licenses issued during fiscal 1989, in thousands and ranked as licenses per 100 residents.
> *Source:* News release dated July 3, 1990 from Fish and Wildlife Service, U.S. Department of Interior, Washington.

Composite score for forestry and fishing
> Rankings of 13 forestry and fishing indicators were totaled to produce a composite score. Lowest score receives best composite rank.

Adults who fish or hunt
>Percent of population 16 years or older who fish and/or hunt, 1985.
>*Source:* "1985 National Survey of Fishing, Hunting, and Wildlife-Associated Recreation," March 1989. Published by U.S. Fish and Wildlife Service, U.S. Department of Interior, Washington.

Spending by sportsmen and sportswomen
>Dollars per capita spent by fishers and hunters for supplies, lodging, etc.
>*Source:* "1985 National Survey of Fishing, Hunting, and Wildlife-Associated Recreation," March 1989. Published by U.S. Fish and Wildlife Service, U.S. Department of Interior, Washington.

Registered motor boats
>Number of motorized boats owned per 100 people, 1989.
>*Source: Boating Industry* magazine, January 1990. Published by Communications Channels, Atlanta, GA.

Recreational waters
>Inland water as percent of state's total area. Also, miles of coastal shoreline.
>*Source: Boating Industry* magazine, January 1990. Published by Communications Channels, Atlanta, GA.

Total land in million acres
>Size of state (excluding inland water) in acres.
>*Source:* "Public Lands Statistics, 1989," Bureau of Land Management, U.S. Department of Interior, Washington.

Land owned by federal government
>Percent of land owned by federal agencies. Total is 30 percent, or 21 percent if Alaska is excluded.
>*Source:* "Public Lands Statistics, 1989," Bureau of Land Management, U.S. Department of Interior, Washington.

Land owned by Fish & Wildlife Service
>Percent of land owned by U.S. Fish & Wildlife Service, 1989.
>*Source:* "Annual Report of Lands Under the Control of the U.S. Fish and Wildlife Service as of September 30, 1989," U.S. Department of Interior, Washington.

Visits to National Parks
>Recreational visits per 100 residents to National Park Service areas, 1989.
>*Source:* "National Park Service Statistical Abstract, 1989," National Park Service, U.S. Department of Interior, Denver, CO.

State park lands, visitors, and budget
>Percent of land owned by state park agencies (which in some states also have jurisdiction over historic, wildlife, or other sites). Also, visitors per 100 residents to these sites and percent of state budget allocated for park agency, with rankings, for 1989.
>*Source:* "Annual Information Exchange," April 1990. Published by National Association of State Park Directors, care of Jim Riggs, Texas Parks & Wildlife Commission, 4200 Smith School Road, Austin, TX 78744; telephone (512) 389-4904.

Funds for parks and recreation
> Per-capita spending by state and local governments for parks, cultural, and recreational activities, from art galleries to zoos.
> *Source:* "Government Finances in 1987-88," Bureau of Census, U.S. Department of Commerce, Washington.

Tourism and travel spending
> Per-capita spending on tourism, overnight travel, and related lodging, food service, and other activities, including spending for travel 100 miles or more away from home.
> *Source:* "Impact of Travel on State Economies, 1987," May 1989. Published by U.S. Travel Data Center, 1133 21st Street, NW, Washington, DC 20036; telephone (202) 293-1040.

Natural resources as percent of state gross product
> Average total contribution from agriculture, mining, timber, and energy industries to state's total goods and services during period 1963-1986.
> *Source:* Ronald H. Schmidt, "Natural Resources and Regional Growth," *Economic Review*, Fall 1989. Published by the Federal Reserve Bank of San Francisco. Updated tables were provided by the author.

Population, population density, and population change
> Number of people in thousands from 1990 Census, with number of people per mile, and change since 1970.
> *Source:* "Statistical Abstract of the United States, 1990," Bureau of Census, U.S. Department of Commerce, Washington; 1990 data from Census Bureau.

People in rural areas
> Percent of the population in 1980 living in rural areas or towns of fewer than 2,500 people.
> *Source:* "1980 Census of Population, Volume 1," Bureau of Census, U.S. Department of Commerce, Washington.

Metro life quality
> Average rating of the cities evaluated in each state for recreation, climate, education, the arts, crime, job outlook, living costs, transportation, and health care. A total of 333 metro areas were evaluated.
> *Source:* Richard Boyer and David Savageau, *Places Rated Almanac*, 1989. Published by Prentice Hall, New York.

Conservation members
> Members per 1,000 residents of three conservation organizations: Sierra Club, Greenpeace, and National Wildlife Federation. An indicator of both the lobbying strength of conservationists and participation in environmental activities.
> *Source:* State data from Names in the News, 1 Bush Street, San Francisco, CA 94104.

Composite score for fun and quality of life.
> Rankings of 19 previous indicators were totaled to produce a composite score. Lowest score receives best composite rank.

CHAPTER 8

Congressional Leadership

INDICATORS

Score for voting record of state's Congressional delegation
Composite scores for 1970-1990, 1970-84, 1985-1990
Score for voting record on nuclear issues
Score for each Senator's and Representative's voting record
Contributions received from energy-related PACs

Earth Day 1990 pushed environmental issues into the spotlight and inspired Americans to evaluate their personal contribution to the planet's pollution. Lost in this emphasis on individual accountability, however, was a political analysis that identified the voting booth as the best place to begin cleaning up our environmental mess. As a result, while millions planted trees and rallied for recycling, members of Congress sanctioned another decade of poisoning through passage of flawed amendments to the Clean Air Act.

Pollution persists because politicians approve permissive policies. Who will hold *these* individuals accountable? They are the ones who make the laws and allocate the money that determines how much the environment is valued, how tough regulators will be, how long the cleanup will take, how many lives will be sacrificed before a product or process is banned.

In this chapter, we focus on the environmental records of the states' policymakers in Congress; in the next, we examine the performance of the 50 state legislatures. Whether at the federal or local level, these elected officials define, then balance, public priorities — jobs, clean water, taxes, health care, on and on. They set the standards for the public's welfare. It's a difficult chore, full of risks that can jeopardize reelection. As a consequence, most politicians — especially those in Congress — follow the leadership of others, primarily those who give them money or those who give them votes.

CLEAN VOTES, DIRTY VOTES

Although some laws protecting air and water passed in the 1950s and 1960s, it wasn't until the 1970s that Congress answered the groundswell of public (i.e., voter) concern with far-reaching environmental legislation — the 1970 Clean Air Act, 1970 Occupational Safety and Health Act, 1972 Clean Water Act, 1972 Coastal Zone Management Act, 1973 Endangered Species Act, 1974 Safe Drinking Water Act, 1976 Resource Conservation and Recovery Act. In the 1980s, President Ronald Reagan followed the advice of his big-money backers by putting anti-regulators in charge of EPA and

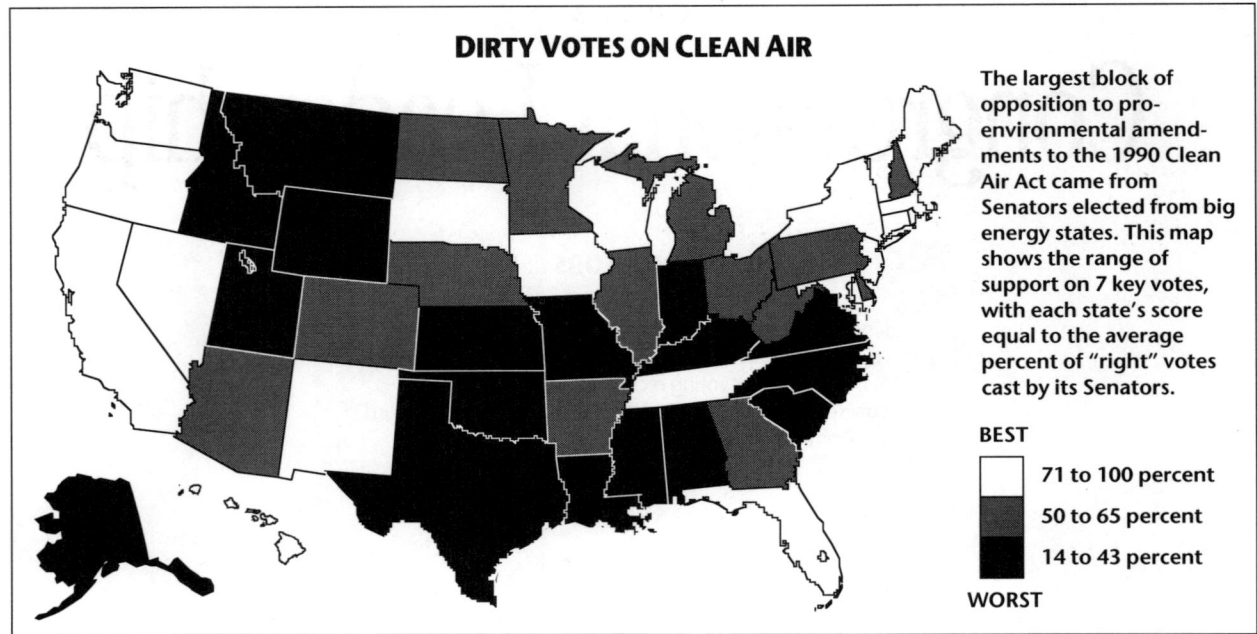

DIRTY VOTES ON CLEAN AIR

The largest block of opposition to pro-environmental amendments to the 1990 Clean Air Act came from Senators elected from big energy states. This map shows the range of support on 7 key votes, with each state's score equal to the average percent of "right" votes cast by its Senators.

BEST
- 71 to 100 percent
- 50 to 65 percent
- 14 to 43 percent

WORST

other agencies. Pollution standards were degraded, put on hold, or not enforced; funding for everything from sewage treatment plants to solar energy was slashed.

Many members of Congress went along with the heavy hand of deregulation, while others maintained the federal government should set high standards for the public's health and welfare. The stalemate resulted in little real progress during most of the 1980s: Congress barely managed to reauthorize or amend key legislation from the '70s, often over President Reagan's veto, but 535 bickering Senators and Representatives were unable to appropriate the funds needed to enforce what they approved on paper.

To keep score of friends and foes inside Congress, environmental organizations created the League of Conservation Voters (LCV) to monitor voting behavior and endorse candidates. Each year since 1970, LCV has chosen about a dozen roll-call votes that separate the sheep from the goats on environmental issues — curbing nuclear power, cutting pork-barrel water projects, strengthening pollution standards, protecting wetlands and national forests, promoting alternative energy, stopping toxic wastes.

A review of these votes illustrates the truth of former House Speaker Tip O'Neill's maxim that "all politics is local." For example, the impasse between two powerful legislators representing vastly different local constituencies stymied renewal of the Clean Air Act throughout the 1980s. On the one side, John D. Dingell, chair of the House Energy and Commerce Committee, has Ford Motor's Detroit headquarters in his district; he believed car manufacturers had done their share in cutting emissions. On the other side, Henry A. Waxman, chair of the House Subcommittee on Health and the Environment, represents a liberal district in smog-laden Los Angeles; he kept pushing for tougher automobile pollution standards.

Even after these two powerbrokers finally began crafting a compromise Clean Air package, other lawmakers weighed in to protect their local interests. Senate Appropriations Chair Robert Byrd wanted coal miners back home in West Virginia to receive compensation if they lost their jobs to clean-fuel requirements. Similarly, lawmakers from Midwest states won a system of pollution credits for their acid rain-making electric utilities. The final bill "is riddled with exemptions and extensions for the steel, oil, chemical, and other industries," says Richard L. Grossman, former director of Greenpeace. "It substitutes industry's 'almost best' technology for public health standards mandated in earlier laws."

GOATS AND SHEEP

An analysis of voting patterns for entire delegations reveals the strong correlation between what drives the economy in a politician's home district and how he or she votes in Washington. Overall,

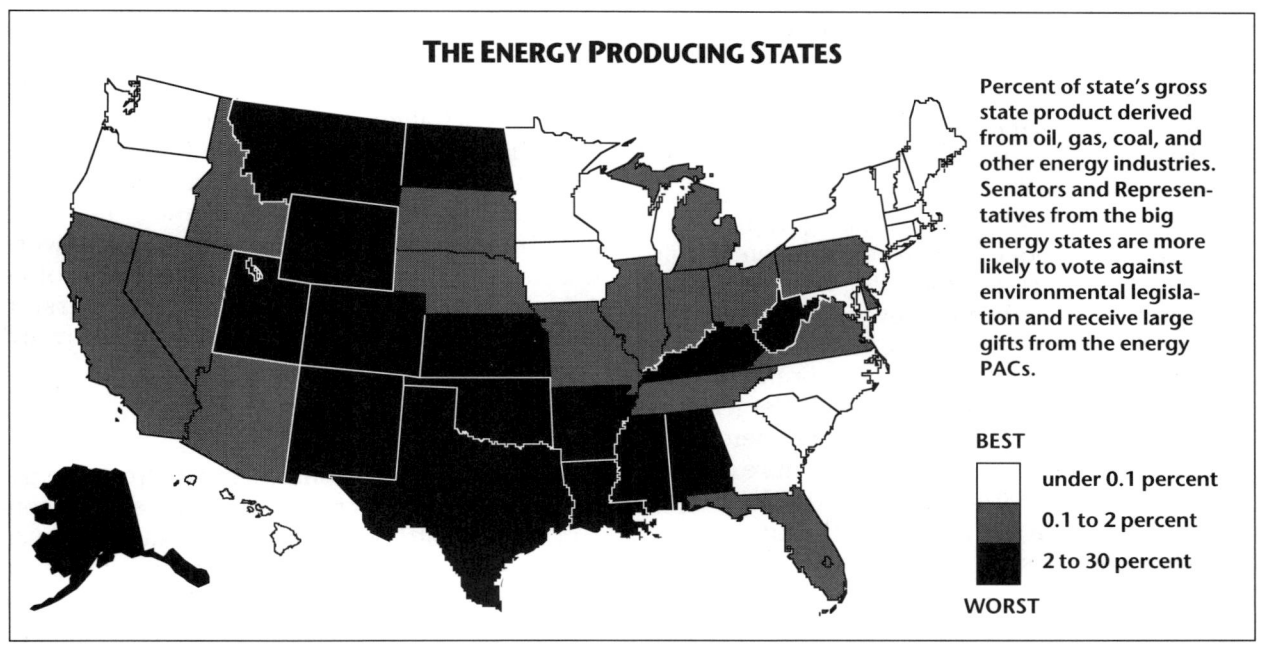

the staunchest foes of environmental legislation come from the Rocky Mountain and Southern states where energy production, agriculture, and small business mindsets prevail. Public officials from the two regions champion an anti-government philosophy that supports the freewheeling exploitation of natural resources by mining companies, utilities, oil corporations, agribusiness, and timber interests. They favor nuclear power and water subsidies for farmers, while voting against the development of renewable energy and sustainable agriculture.

A review of seven key floor votes on the 1990 Clean Air Act shows that the strongest opposition came from 11 of the 15 states which get the highest proportion of their gross state product from oil, gas, coal, and other energy industries (see maps). Here are other highlights based on an analysis of League of Conservation Voters scorecards over the past 21 years.

• The delegations (House and Senate members) with the 10 worst average scores for 1985-1990 come from energy-producing states — Wyoming (rank 50), Utah, Alaska, Arizona, Kentucky, Mississippi, Louisiana, and Alabama — or from the farming states of Idaho and Nebraska.

• The delegations with the best records in the same period are elected from many of the states least dependent on energy resources, including Vermont (rank 1), Massachusetts, Rhode Island, Maine, Connecticut, Wisconsin, and Washington. The other delegations in the top 10 are from Delaware, New Jersey, and New York, liberal states with serious pollution problems that need government intervention.

• Looking at individuals, Florida's Ileana Ros-Lehtinen (who replaced Claude Pepper) is the only Southerner among the 50 Representatives with the best environmental voting records. In the Senate, Florida lawmaker Bob Graham is the only Southerner in the top 25, while 11 of the worst 25 Senators are from the South. None of the best-scoring House or Senate members comes from the Rocky Mountain region.

• Democrats in Congress vote for environmental measures almost twice as often as Republicans. During 1985-90, House Democrats voted right 68 percent of the time, compared to an average score of 36 percent for Republicans. In the Senate, the gap narrowed to 63 for Democrats versus 36 for Republicans. The 27 women in the House in 1990 and two in the Senate had an average score of 67, compared to 55 for the men.

• Black members of the House (there are none in the Senate) generally favor an activist federal government and are strong supporters of environmental regulation. Overall, they voted right 76 percent of the time and posted the best records in Missouri, Georgia, and Maryland. The nine Hispanics in the 1990 House, including four members from Texas, favor the environment less often, 62 percent of the time.

- The 25 Senators with the worst environmental records include *both* Senators from 8 states, all of whose economies depend heavily on natural resources — Idaho, Wyoming, Utah, Oklahoma, and Alaska in the West, plus Mississippi, Alabama, and Louisiana in the South.

- California has the largest delegation — and one of the most polarized on environmental policies. For the period 1985-1990, Senators Alan Cranston and Pete Wilson (now governor) ranked 8th and 43d, respectively. The state's 45-member House delegation ranged from top-ranked Tom Campbell, with a score of 100, to Wally Herger, who came in dead last by voting right only 3 percent of the time. The average score for the entire delegation makes it the 18th best for the 1985-1990 period, a drop from 15th place on the cumulative 1970-1990 rankings.

- Several other states have decidedly polarized delegations. In the case of both Colorado and North Carolina, the splits follow the ideological gulf between one Democratic and one right-wing Republican Senator and a similar division among House members. Nebraska has the same split among its three-member House delegation, but its sharply divided Senators are both Democrats. In populist Iowa, Republicans span the extremes, from Jim Leach's perfect 100 in 1989-90 to Jim Ross Lightfoot's 11.

- Seven states — Mississippi, Utah, Alaska, Idaho, Arizona, Louisiana, and Alabama — stayed among the worst 10 from 1970 through 1990. Among other states, the most dramatic changes were downward. Wyoming dropped from 29th place during 1970-1984 to 50th for 1985-1990, largely because a Democratic Senator and Representative were replaced by conservative Republicans. Montana dropped from 15th to 33d between the same periods, Iowa went from 8th to 24th, and Kentucky sank from 30th to 43d.

- Eight states have remained in the top 10 since 1970 — Connecticut, Maine, Massachusetts, New Jersey, Rhode Island, Vermont, Wisconsin, and New York. New Hampshire improved its ranking between periods, from 22d to 12th, thanks to the modest greening of its Republican leadership; before his 1990 retirement, Senator Gordon Humphrey voted with Jesse Helms on most matters, but often departed from the far right on environmental issues. North Dakota also advanced 10 positions, from 32d to 22d, and Washington climbed from 21st to 10th, reflecting a growing preoccupation with quality-of-life issues.

- During 1989-90, Massachusetts' John Kerry had the Senate's only perfect score. Nine members of the House also scored 100: Tom Campbell and Jim Bates of California; Christopher Shays of Connecticut; Jim Leach of Iowa; Peter Hoagland of Nebraska; Ted Weiss, Benjamin Gilman and Sherwood Boehlert of New York; and Peter Smith of Vermont. House members scoring zero were California's Charles Pashayan, Jr., Minnesota's Arlan Strangeland, Missouri's Bill Emerson, Nebraska's Virginia Smith, and Utah's Howard Nielson — all Republicans.

FOCUSED ENERGY

While most Congressional members from energy-dependent states act as if energy workers and consumers need little protection, these same lawmakers work hard for mining interests, oil companies, and utilities — and they are richly rewarded for their efforts. Senator Orrin Hatch of Utah received $114,335 from energy-related political action committees (PACs) in 1988. The same year, he voted against holding nuclear contractors liable for negligence or misconduct, even though his state is a major route for radioactive waste transported for storage in Nevada. The next year, he voted for delaying strict protection of groundwater and against holding oil companies fully liable for their spills. Then, in 1990, he sided with mining and utility interests against stronger regulations for radioactive emissions; he agreed with oil firms and automakers against improving fuel efficiency; and he stood with timber interests against protecting national forests.

As a consequence, Hatch ranks 89th out of 100 Senators on the 1985-1990 scorecard. The other Senator from Utah, Jake Garn, ranks even lower. Across the country, Mississippi's freshman Senator Trent Lott received major help from energy-related PACs and followed the oil industry's lead in opposing double-hulled tankers and limiting liability for off-shore spills. Lott and fellow Mississippian Thad Cochran were the only Senators to vote wrong on every environmental issue rated by LCV in 1990. According to a study by Common Cause, the two Senators took in $305,633 from energy PACs between 1983 and 1988, more than any other state's pair except Big Oil's traditional champions from Texas and Louisiana.

Two more Senators from big energy states — Don Nickles of Oklahoma and Malcolm Wallop of Wyoming — are aggressive opponents of environmental regulations, favoring only 1 of 22 measures studied in the 1989-90 Congress and none in the 1987-88 Congress. Nickles was a principle sponsor of measures to gut the 1990 Clean Air amendments; when he ran for reelection in 1986, Nickles got $65,000 from nuclear and petrochemical PACs, the fourth largest amount that election cycle. Wallop co-sponsored legislation to open Alaska's Arctic National Wildlife Refuge to oil drilling, opposed forcing oil companies to bear the full costs of their spills — and received 13 percent of his campaign treasury in 1988 from oil PACs. On the House side, Wyoming's lone Representative Craig Thomas ranks 425th out of 435 members on environmental votes.

As Senate Minority Whip and a member of the Environment and Public Works Committee, Wyoming's other Senator, Alan Simpson, exerts considerable influence over environmental issues. In 1990, Simpson proposed an amendment to weaken EPA's regulation of radioactive air emissions at facilities licensed by the Nuclear Regulatory Commission (NRC). "The Simpson Amendment would have reversed a recently issued EPA standard and returned us to a far weaker standard set by the NRC in the 1960s," said Environmental Action lobbyist Leon Lowery. The amendment lost, but one Hill staffer commented, "Simpson has clout. He's listened to."

In his 1990 reelection campaign, Simpson attracted $800,674 in PAC contributions, largely from energy, agribusiness, and chemical interests. In response to criticism that most of the money came from outside his district, Simpson explained, "Some of the PACs that contribute are 'out of state' but they are not 'out of touch' with Wyoming." Overall, energy PACs have kept in touch with Congress by giving $18.8 million in contributions between 1983 and 1988.

NUCLEAR PROTECTION

The pro-nuclear lobby is among the most active parts of the energy industry in Congress, despite its loss of public support. Idaho's 4-member delegation, which ranks worst on all environmental legislation, also ranks last for caving in to nuclear energy advocates. Mississippi, Nebraska, Kentucky, Georgia, Alabama, Wyoming, Virginia, New Mexico, and Alaska all score 8 or less (out of a possible 100) on nuclear votes evaluated by Public Citizen's Critical Mass Energy Project. Alabama, Nebraska, and Virginia each get over 20 percent of their electricity from nuclear plants. With its uranium mines, bomb-making plants, research labs, waste sites, and related facilities, New Mexico's economy is the most nuclear dependent in the nation, and its two Senators are among the biggest recipients of energy PAC dollars.

Despite the free-enterprise rhetoric against government meddling, a majority of lawmakers from these states voted to continue subsidizing nuclear energy research and to protect the nuclear industry from the full financial liability of a meltdown. They are joined by other self-styled conservatives who don't mind using taxpayer money to bail out industry. Republican William Dannemeyer of southern California is a perfect example. As a member of the House Energy and Commerce Committee, Dannemeyer has repeatedly proposed a one-step nuclear plant licensing system that would squeeze out citizen participation in regulatory reviews. He tried to cut $80 million earmarked for state conservation efforts, while allowing Department of Energy contractors to pass on their environmental fines and legal defense costs to the federal government. Dannemeyer has an average score of 17 percent, putting him 398th among the 435 House members.

Overall, Rhode Island scored best on nuclear votes, followed by Massachusetts and Maine, reflecting New England's nervous reliance on nuclear power. While these legislators want tighter controls, their colleagues from Connecticut diverge from their normal pro-environment record to defend the local industry. Connecticut gets more electricity from nuclear power than any other state in the country — over 45 percent. As an illustration of the nuclear lobby's clout, Connecticut's Representative Barbara Kennelly and Senator Joseph Leiberman both broke an otherwise perfect record on LCV's 1990 scorecard by respectively voting to continue subsidies for plutonium production and to weaken regulation of radioactive emissions.

Interestingly, the fourth best score on nuclear issues came from West Virginia's delegation, which opposes federal help for nuclear power at the expense of the state's chief local interest — coal. By contrast, legislators from the big oil states generally side with nuclear interests. After picking up $16,000 in speakers' fees from the nuclear industry in 1986, Senator J. Bennett Johnston of Louisiana pushed through siting of a high-level radioactive waste site in Nevada.

As the chair of the Senate's Energy and Natural Resources Committee, Johnston is in a position to get what he wants. Unfortunately, he opposes envi-

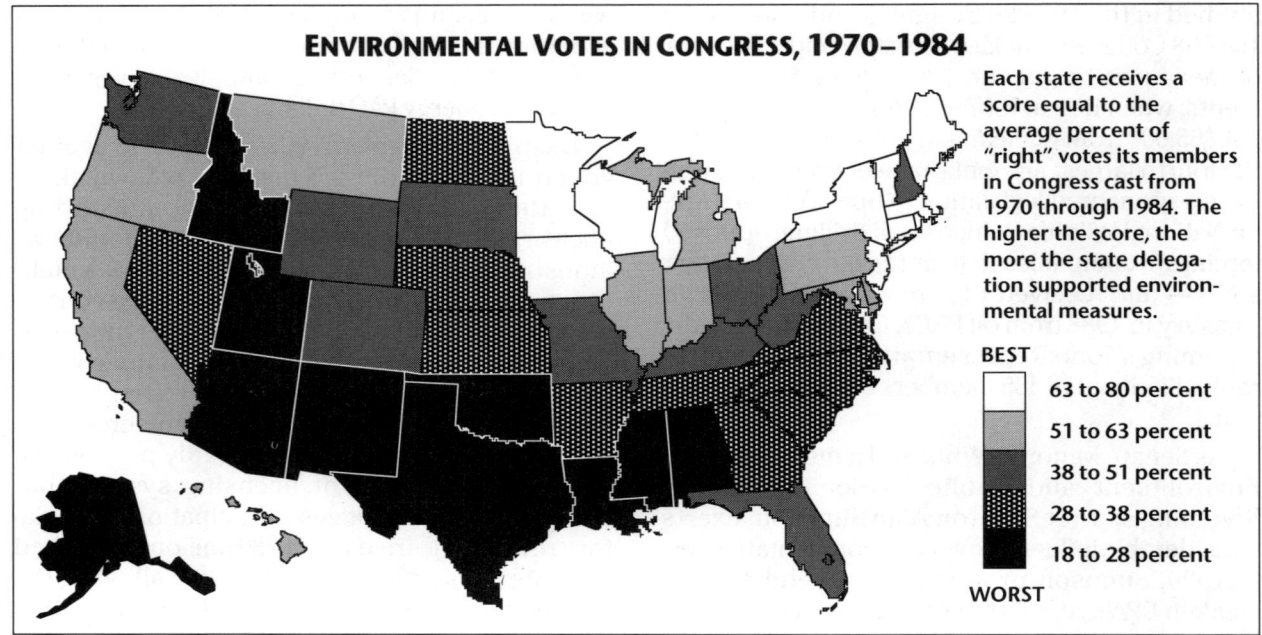

ronmentalists on four out of five measures that reach the Senate floor and prevents even more from getting that far. He blocked unlimited liability for nuclear power accidents and single-handedly saved his oil friends millions by having their drilling waste classified as "non-hazardous" for regulatory purposes. Until the *Exxon Valdez* spill, he successfully held back demands for double-hulled oil tankers.

NEARSIGHTED INTERESTS

In 1991 Johnston teamed up with Wyoming's Malcolm Wallop to sponsor a bill that would open Alaska's Arctic National Wildlife Refuge for oil exploration, expand offshore drilling, and undercut attempts to set higher fuel efficiency goals for automobiles. In 1990, it took a Republican filibuster to kill a popular bill pushed by Nevada Senator Richard Bryan that would have raised the current 27.5 miles-per-gallon standard 40 percent by the year 2001. That measure could have saved 2.5 million barrels of oil a day by 2005, more than Alaska's current output. Johnston's alternative directs the Secretary of Transportation to study the feasibility of new goals — and do nothing if he or she so chooses.

Like Johnston, other oil-state lawmakers are quick to support the auto industry's commitment to gas-guzzling vehicles. In early sparring over the Clean Air Act in the House, Texans Ralph M. Hall and Jack Fields successfully knocked out a mandate found even in Bush's version that would require auto firms to build up to a million cars that run on clean, alternative fuels. Hall and Fields took their cues from a formidable lobby of oil, auto, and chemical firms called the Clean Air Working Group. The two Texans' past loyalty has earned them the second and third largest slices of energy PAC contributions for House members. Number one on the list is fellow Texan and another member of the Energy and Commerce Committee, Joe Barton; in 1984, he won Phil Gramm's vacated seat in a hotly contested race and his overall anti-green voting record ranks him 390th out of 435.

Even Louisiana liberal Lindy Boggs sided with big oil on such issues as requiring double hulls for tankers. Before retiring in 1990, her voting record on energy was not much better than Billy Tauzin, her conservative colleague from Louisiana's Cajun and oil heartland. Tauzin uses his position on the House Energy and Commerce Committee to weaken proposals for tougher federal standards promoted by members from non-oil states, such as Minnesota's Gerry Sikorski, Ed Markey of Massachusetts, and Cardiss Collins from Chicago, Illinois.

The call of local interests is remarkably persuasive, especially when backed with lots of money. Florida's Senator Bob Graham passed up a perfect LCV score in 1990 by favoring price supports for his state's sugar industry, even though the plantations are wreaking havoc on the Everglades. Philip

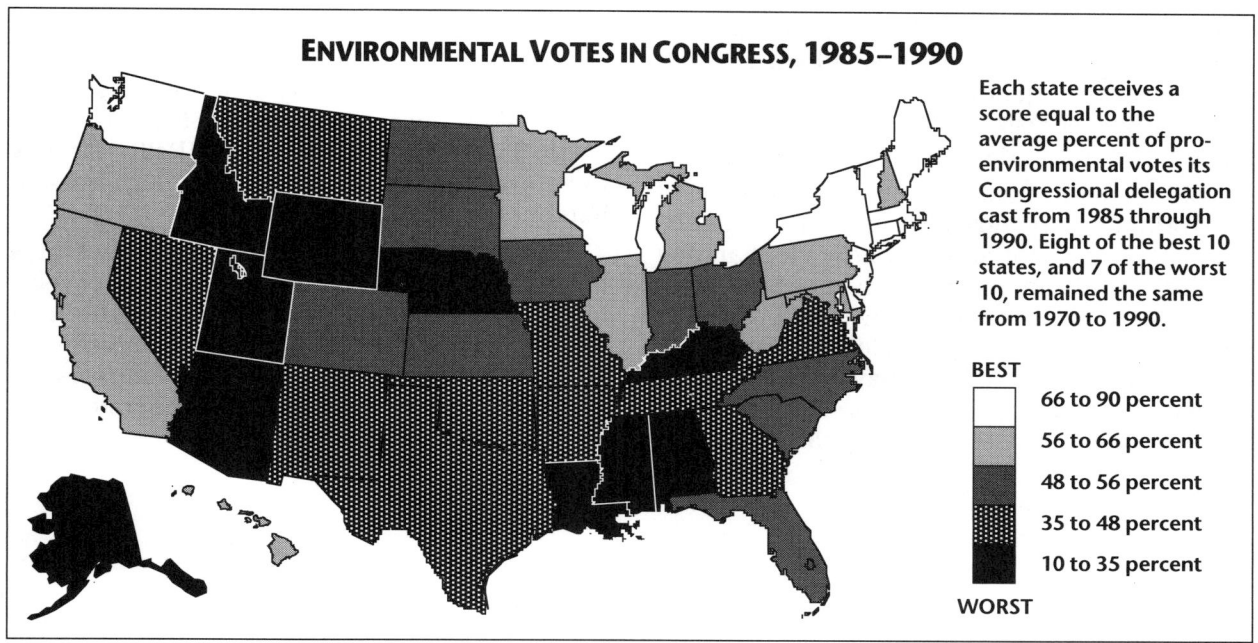

ENVIRONMENTAL VOTES IN CONGRESS, 1985–1990

Each state receives a score equal to the average percent of pro-environmental votes its Congressional delegation cast from 1985 through 1990. Eight of the best 10 states, and 7 of the worst 10, remained the same from 1970 to 1990.

BEST
- 66 to 90 percent
- 56 to 66 percent
- 48 to 56 percent
- 35 to 48 percent
- 10 to 35 percent

WORST

R. Sharp, one of several Indiana Democrats who increasingly favors environmental regulation, still gets plenty of energy PAC money and uses his position as chair of the House Subcommittee on Energy and Power to protect his state's coal-burning utilities from tough restrictions designed to curb acid rain.

Idaho's conservative delegation routinely lambasts government spending, but huge federal subsidies for Western water projects win consistent favor; thanks to that cheap supply, Idaho leads in per-capita water consumption and its economy is the fifth most dependent on agriculture. And after two tries, timber interests finally got Slade Gorton reelected as Senator from Washington, making him the largest recipient of their PAC funds and a militant ally in their fight to push aside the spotted owl and pursue cutting the Pacific Northwest's ancient forests. Timber's point man in the fight is their second largest PAC recipient, Senator Mark Hatfield of Oregon, who votes with environmentalists on most other issues — except a few that hit closest to home.

DISMAL LEADERSHIP

The list of politicians whose principles get shaped or squeezed by money goes on and on. Environmentalists have gained rhetorical support in Congress, and won important victories. But when the issue gets framed as jobs (or local economic interests) versus the environment, success becomes illusive, mired in compromise and loopholes and delays.

Even when environmentalists win passage of a federal law, its implementation depends on leadership, funding, and commitment from the executive branch. In most cases, that means the Environmental Protection Agency — which is woefully understaffed, underfunded, and overloaded with duties. Worse, the agency's chief executives since the days of Anne Gorsuch Burford and James Watt have worried more about pleasing industry and campaign contributors than about protecting natural habitats and public health. William Ruckleshaus followed Burford by installing a program of risk assessment that quantified "acceptable" death rates in setting pollution standards. As a logical next step, his successor, Lee Thomas, proposed an extraordinarily weak standard for benzene, a known human carcinogen and common ingredient in gasoline, solvents, and varnishes. Natural Resources Defense Council attorney David Doniger called the proposal "the most shocking public health decision to come from the EPA during the Reagan era."

Observers see a modest improvement under George Bush's administration. "Since the darker era in the early years of the Reagan administration, the new leadership at EPA has built a better relationship with Congress and calmed some of the more egregious abuses at the agency," says Bill Roberts, legislative aid to the primary author of the Superfund program, former Representative (now Governor) Jim Florio of New Jersey. "But if you look at the agency's environmental report card, as opposed to its ethical and legal abuses . . . the results are fairly dismal."

William Reilly, Bush's EPA chief, formerly led the World Wildlife Fund and Conservation Foundation, but his credentials carry little clout among the President's inner circle. Chief of Staff John Sununu is an ardent nuclear power advocate, and he forcefully blocked Reilly's global-warming initiatives. Vice President Dan Quayle was named to Environmental Action's "Dirty Dozen" in 1986, and Secretary of Defense Dick Cheney earned an LCV score of zero as a Wyoming congressman in 1987-88. "The best thing an EPA administrator can do is enforce the law harshly against polluters," says Dave Baker, political director of Friends of the Earth. "I've seen no indication that [Reilly] is ready to enforce the law with the speed, fairness, and harshness necessary."

Frustrated by federal inaction, many states have accepted or taken over leadership for regulating environmental protection. As the next chapter's indicators show, the gap between the best and worst is huge, and it largely mirrors the performance of the public officials the states send to Washington.

CONGRESSIONAL LEADERSHIP

AVERAGE LCV SCORE FOR EACH CONGRESSIONAL DELEGATION, BY HOUSE AND YEAR

State	HOUSE 89-90 Score	SENATE 89-90 Score	HOUSE 87-88 Score	SENATE 87-88 Score	HOUSE 85-86 Score	SENATE 85-86 Score	BOTH HOUSES, MULTI-YEAR PERIODS 1985-1990 Score	Rank	1970-1984 Score	Rank	1970-1990 Score	Rank	DELEGATION SCORE ON NUCLEAR ISSUES Score	Rank
Alabama	48	25	31	15	26	18	31.4	44	24.5	46	26.4	44	7	45
Alaska	17	20	25	35	16	8	20.4	47	23.2	48	22.4	48	8	41
Arizona	27	39	29	50	30	32	31.9	42	23.8	47	26.1	46	23	35
Arkansas	34	68	35	35	46	52	42.7	35	34.9	31	37.1	30	21	38
California	57	75	56	70	56	70	57.1	18	55.4	16	55.9	15	52	18
Colorado	54	52	51	45	43	49	49.1	28	46.6	24	47.3	24	32	26
Connecticut	82	89	76	60	74	60	75.5	5	67.2	6	69.5	6	38	22
Delaware	61	71	88	75	84	77	75.3	6	62.6	11	66.3	8	59	13
Florida	60	59	49	55	48	70	53.3	23	41.2	28	44.7	28	34	24
Georgia	51	66	48	40	42	40	47.1	31	31.0	34	35.6	34	6	46
Hawaii	71	45	56	65	57	51	57.5	16	58.1	14	57.9	14	43	21
Idaho	28	8	22	0	33	0	15.2	49	25.7	43	22.7	47	0	50
Illinois	65	73	54	30	53	67	57.4	17	50.9	19	52.8	20	30	27
Indiana	70	34	59	30	46	38	54.3	21	50.5	20	51.6	22	29	30
Iowa	51	48	52	50	55	62	52.7	24	65.1	8	61.5	11	21	37
Kansas	60	29	59	30	49	22	47.7	30	29.6	37	34.8	36	30	28
Kentucky	41	18	33	30	25	34	31.6	43	37.7	30	35.9	32	5	47
Louisiana	24	18	26	25	40	13	27.8	45	25.6	44	26.3	45	9	40
Maine	89	78	82	80	68	88	80.8	4	68.1	5	71.7	4	82	3
Maryland	68	82	65	75	55	76	65.6	11	58.5	12	60.5	12	60	10
Massachusetts	87	93	83	85	83	85	84.9	2	79.6	1	81.1	1	84	2
Michigan	63	55	60	65	59	86	61.5	14	58.2	13	59.1	13	70	6
Minnesota	61	46	71	65	65	71	64.6	13	64.7	9	64.7	9	59	11
Mississippi	38	4	31	15	22	17	25.1	46	18.0	50	20.0	50	3	49
Missouri	49	23	43	30	43	71	44.2	34	46.5	25	45.9	27	32	25
Montana	37	23	47	50	40	72	44.7	33	55.9	15	52.7	21	59	11
Nebraska	37	60	25	24	25	46	34.7	41	27.9	40	29.8	40	4	48
Nevada	34	89	41	35	35	13	41.0	36	28.1	39	31.8	37	38	23
New Hampshire	75	48	60	65	65	79	65.3	12	48.7	22	53.5	19	53	16
New Jersey	71	95	70	80	67	95	71.9	7	70.9	2	71.2	5	49	20
New Mexico	41	48	27	40	34	40	37.3	37	25.4	45	28.8	43	8	42
New York	73	64	70	65	61	59	67.8	9	63.4	10	64.6	10	49	19
North Carolina	67	36	52	40	35	29	48.7	29	30.1	35	35.4	35	25	34
North Dakota	67	43	69	60	58	42	53.8	22	34.6	32	40.1	29	71	5
Ohio	53	73	52	60	48	67	52.5	25	48.1	23	49.4	23	55	14
Oklahoma	41	13	42	10	41	22	34.7	39	26.7	42	29.0	42	22	36
Oregon	55	66	64	65	53	54	58.7	15	53.8	17	55.2	17	64	9
Pennsylvania	57	64	55	40	54	83	55.8	19	53.7	18	54.3	18	29	29
Rhode Island	94	71	81	90	82	79	82.8	3	68.5	4	72.6	3	93	1
South Carolina	62	43	61	35	42	38	50.9	27	29.9	36	35.9	33	26	32
South Dakota	83	57	75	40	71	21	51.7	26	45.2	26	47.0	25	64	8
Tennessee	51	82	41	50	37	59	46.8	32	31.8	33	36.1	31	25	33
Texas	36	27	33	30	42	34	36.5	38	26.8	41	29.6	41	27	31
Utah	32	11	35	15	12	9	20.3	48	21.2	49	21.0	49	13	39
Vermont	100	84	94	85	82	100	90.4	1	65.5	7	72.6	2	70	7
Virginia	33	39	42	30	28	42	34.7	40	29.6	38	31.0	38	7	43
Washington	69	68	68	65	62	67	66.4	10	49.8	21	55.3	16	53	17
West Virginia	57	64	52	65	53	50	55.8	20	42.5	27	46.3	26	78	4
Wisconsin	64	73	69	65	67	84	68.1	8	69.3	3	68.9	7	54	15
Wyoming	11	4	0	10	16	17	9.9	50	39.3	29	30.9	39	7	44
U.S. Total	57	51	47	51	52	51	53.0		47.2		48.9		39	

CONGRESSIONAL LEADERSHIP

U.S. HOUSE MEMBER	LEAGUE OF CON. VOTERS SCORES			CONTRIBUTIONS FROM ENERGY PACS			U.S. HOUSE MEMBER	LEAGUE OF CON. VOTERS SCORES			CONTRIBUTIONS FROM ENERGY PACS		
	1989-90	Average 85-90	Rank	$ in 1983-88	Rank	% All PACs		1989-90	Average 85-90	Rank	$ in 1983-88	Rank	% All PACs
Alabama							**California (cont.)**						
CALLAHAN	17	15.7	402	67,450	393	12.2	DYMALLY	72	69.0	168	14,600	195	3.9
DICKINSON	17	13.3	413	29,050	298	5.3	ANDERSON	50	60.3	214	50,850	366	7.3
BROWDER	72	72.0	149	na			DREIER	50	43.7	281	13,500	182	4.0
BEVILL	39	29.0	348	75,675	403	25.4	TORRES	89	79.3	92	6,600	102	2.1
FLIPPO	50	42.7	286	85,850	418	9.1	LEWIS, J.	22	21.0	375	29,700	300	8.4
ERDREICH	78	60.3	214	20,950	253	3.0	BROWN, G.	61	73.7	142	10,700	148	1.5
HARRIS	61	55.5	233	19,410	240	4.5	McCANDLESS	11	15.3	405	12,300	169	6.3
Alaska							DORNAN	6	11.7	420	42,660	342	10.7
YOUNG	11	17.3	395	146,550	432	20.8	DANNEMEYER	17	17.0	398	63,350	388	16.7
Arizona							COX	61	61.0	212	12,600	171	6.6
RHODES	11	12.0	418	25,575	277	10.8	LOWERY	33	24.3	367	33,710	313	6.8
UDALL	72	74.0	139	45,700	351	15.3	ROHRABACHER	28	28.0	151	13,150	178	7.5
STUMP	6	5.7	434	28,850	297	8.8	PACKARD	6	11.7	420	23,875	273	7.1
KYL	17	18.0	392	33,000	310	8.1	BATES	100	92.0	19	15,550	207	2.9
KOLBE	28	32.3	332	79,450	408	13.9	HUNTER	6	13.3	413	17,720	226	4.2
Arkansas							**Colorado**						
ALEXANDER	50	49.7	254	23,575	270	3.1	SCHROEDER	89	90.0	30	2,800	55	0.9
ROBINSON	17	39.3	299	30,350	301	5.6	SKAGGS	89	82.0	77	1,750	42	0.3
HAMMERSCHMIDT	17	17.0	398	18,100	232	5.6	CAMPBELL, B.	28	48.5	262	13,650	185	2.7
ANTHONY	50	37.3	308	56,050	373	6.9	BROWN, H.	61	41.3	290	26,376	283	8.6
California							HEFLEY	33	32.0	335	18,970	238	8.4
BOSCO	67	66.7	180	15,800	211	4.8	SCHAEFER	22	19.0	386	78,169	406	12.5
HERGER	6	3.0	435	38,100	325	8.6	**Connecticut**						
MATSUI	78	80.3	85	72,759	398	7.5	KENNELLY	83	82.3	76	15,050	200	2.2
FAZIO	72	62.7	205	65,075	390	6.6	GEJDENSON	94	88.0	39	4,058	66	0.7
PELOSI	89	84.0	61	17,750	227	3.5	MORRISON	78	88.7	34	2,550	53	0.3
BOXER	89	92.3	15	5,660	91	1.1	SHAYS	100	94.5	8	1,250	36	1.0
MILLER, G.	89	87.3	40	35,885	318	8.3	ROWLAND, J.	72	62.7	205	21,250	256	5.3
DELLUMS	89	92.7	14	1,650	40	0.6	JOHNSON, N.	67	62.0	210	22,330	264	4.5
STARK	89	91.7	21	8,750	125	1.0	**Delaware**						
EDWARDS, D.	83	88.7	34	5,100	82	1.6	CARPER	61	77.7	112	6,500	99	1.2
LANTOS	78	82.0	77	2,250	49	0.9	**Florida**						
CAMPBELL, T.	100	100.0	1	10,600	147	4.7	HUTTO	33	36.7	309	17,250	220	7.6
MINETA	78	75.7	125	11,950	165	1.8	GRANT	44	47.0	268	34,900	316	15.2
SHUMWAY	6	9.3	428	21,450	258	5.0	BENNETT	83	73.7	142	5,750	92	3.5
CONDIT	60	60.0	217	na			JAMES	78	78.0	104	1,000	34	12.9
PANETTA	83	84.3	60	7,950	118	2.4	McCOLLUM	39	35.3	318	5,800	93	2.1
PASHAYAN	0	13.3	413	39,000	331	11.7	STEARNS	50	65.7	187	1,750	42	3.3
LEHMAN, R.	72	70.0	160	10,155	142	2.3	GIBBONS	89	72.7	146	87,138	419	8.2
LAGOMARSINO	44	36.0	315	68,478	395	14.1	YOUNG, B.	39	32.0	335	15,750	209	5.8
THOMAS, W.	22	26.7	356	64,650	389	11.8	BILIRAKIS	61	44.0	276	55,620	370	13.1
GALLEGLY	33	32.0	335	32,000	306	10.5	IRELAND	44	34.7	321	45,650	350	8.7
MOORHEAD	17	17.3	395	74,235	401	16.2	NELSON	44	59.7	219	20,925	252	4.4
BEILENSON	94	92.0	19	0	1	0.0	LEWIS, T.	22	26.7	356	15,800	211	6.9
WAXMAN	89	92.3	15	11,250	157	2.2	GOSS	61	61.0	212	7,250	110	5.3
ROYBAL	72	75.3	129	4,750	76	2.9	JOHNSTON, H.	83	83.0	67	4,900	80	1.6
BERMAN	78	84.0	61	7,800	115	1.9	SHAW	44	34.0	324	26,500	285	7.5
LEVINE	78	85.0	56	11,515	159	3.2	SMITH, L.	83	80.0	89	16,300	215	1.8
DIXON	78	75.0	134	7,700	113	3.0	LEHMAN, W.	78	70.0	160	6,650	103	2.1
HAWKINS	67	68.3	170	5,600	88	2.3	ROS-LEHTINEN	87	87.0	42	na		
MARTINEZ	72	68.3	170	6,650	103	1.4	FASCELL	83	79.0	94	16,500	217	3.4

CONGRESSIONAL LEADERSHIP

U.S. HOUSE MEMBER	LEAGUE OF CON. VOTERS SCORES			CONTRIBUTIONS FROM ENERGY PACs			U.S. HOUSE MEMBER	LEAGUE OF CON. VOTERS SCORES			CONTRIBUTIONS FROM ENERGY PACs		
	1989 -90	Average 85-90	Rank	$ in 1983-88	Rank	% All PACs		1989 -90	Average 85-90	Rank	$ in 1983-88	Rank	% All PACs
Georgia							**Iowa**						
THOMAS, R.	50	51.0	247	24,120	275	6.1	LEACH	100	86.0	47	0	1	0.0
HATCHER	39	35.3	318	22,150	262	5.6	TAUKE	61	52.7	243	38,250	329	6.3
RAY	44	41.7	288	26,350	282	6.6	NAGLE	78	76.5	121	3,350	62	0.6
JONES, B.	72	72.0	149	5,400	86	1.8	SMITH, N.	33	43.3	285	10,950	152	2.8
LEWIS, J.	89	82.0	77	11,100	155	2.9	LIGHTFOOT	11	21.0	375	56,150	374	9.9
GINGRICH	11	31.3	340	32,300	307	5.3	GRANDY	22	30.0	345	41,500	336	8.1
DARDEN	56	49.3	259	50,325	364	6.9	**Kansas**						
ROWLAND, R.	61	49.0	260	13,350	181	4.7	ROBERTS	22	24.7	363	10,856	151	4.2
JENKINS	44	47.0	268	34,100	314	4.9	SLATTERY	89	72.3	147	56,550	375	8.3
BARNARD	39	40.7	293	16,200	213	3.5	MEYERS	78	67.7	176	20,650	249	4.9
Hawaii							GLICKMAN	94	85.3	53	13,100	177	2.5
SAIKI	56	56.0	230	22,550	265	5.6	WHITTAKER	17	29.0	348	47,700	358	12.0
AKAKA	86	67.3	177	na			**Kentucky**						
Idaho							HUBBARD	39	32.7	328	51,050	368	7.1
CRAIG	6	7.7	433	61,025	384	14.6	NATCHER	61	47.0	268	0	1	0.0
STALLINGS	50	47.7	265	17,750	227	2.4	MAZZOLI	78	55.3	236	6,500	99	1.9
Illinois							BUNNING	17	18.0	392	45,600	349	9.4
HAYES	89	82.7	72	1,750	42	0.5	ROGERS	11	13.7	410	26,700	287	12.5
SAVAGE	83	83.3	64	0	1	0.0	HOPKINS	17	19.0	386	30,685	302	7.7
RUSSO	83	70.7	159	23,900	274	3.0	PERKINS	61	47.3	267	12,600	171	2.7
SANGMEISTER	78	78.0	104	0	1	0.0	**Louisiana**						
LIPINSKI	67	65.0	189	3,250	61	1.5	LIVINGSTON	11	15.7	402	50,465	365	17.6
HYDE	17	21.0	375	13,035	175	4.4	BOGGS	50	47.7	265	72,000	397	12.2
COLLINS	78	80.3	85	14,650	196	2.4	TAUZIN	39	32.3	332	140,848	431	22.3
ROSTENKOWSKI	72	51.0	247	66,400	392	6.8	McCRERY	11	18.0	392	42,635	341	16.2
YATES	89	90.7	26	4,550	72	6.3	HUCKABY	39	39.0	300	50,200	363	15.8
PORTER	61	54.3	239	8,750	125	3.2	BAKER	6	12.5	416	27,250	291	13.0
ANNUNZIO	67	59.7	219	2,850	56	0.7	HAYES	33	35.5	317	26,750	288	10.5
CRANE	39	25.0	362	0	1	0.0	HOLLOWAY	6	12.5	416	44,050	343	11.8
FAWELL	78	65.3	188	11,375	158	4.9	**Maine**						
HASTERT	22	20.5	378	21,650	259	7.5	BRENNAN	89	88.5	36	3,450	63	0.8
MADIGAN	22	26.7	356	59,845	382	8.5	SNOWE	89	77.3	117	2,950	58	1.3
MARTIN, L.	67	43.7	281	22,150	262	5.1	**Maryland**						
EVANS, L.	94	96.3	5	6,900	106	0.8	DYSON	61	50.7	250	34,622	315	4.2
MICHEL	17	9.3	428	106,585	426	7.6	BENTLEY	28	26.7	356	94,350	422	11.4
BRUCE	83	75.3	129	41,554	337	6.1	CARDIN	78	79.5	91	12,913	174	3.5
DURBIN	78	74.7	136	14,550	194	2.3	McMILLEN	67	68.0	174	9,700	139	1.4
COSTELLO	78	78.0	104	4,800	77	1.5	HOYER	83	68.0	174	13,650	185	2.5
POSHARD	78	78.0	104	2,500	51	1.1	BYRON	50	43.7	281	45,350	347	12.0
Indiana							MFUME	83	91.5	22	1,550	39	1.2
VISCLOSKY	72	66.0	186	9,125	134	3.0	MORELLA	94	91.0	24	46,150	353	10.1
SHARP	89	82.7	72	128,676	430	15.9	**Massachusetts**						
HILER	39	36.3	313	49,039	361	7.3	CONTE	89	82.7	72	8,550	124	2.8
LONG	94	94.0	10	0	1	0.0	NEAL, R.	94	94.0	10	2,500	51	2.9
JONTZ	94	97.0	4	4,550	72	0.6	EARLY	83	76.3	122	6,000	96	2.9
BURTON	22	19.0	386	20,625	248	5.4	FRANK	83	92.3	15	1,325	37	0.4
MYERS	17	19.3	383	26,107	281	10.3	ATKINS	89	85.3	53	0	1	0.0
McCLOSKEY	89	73.7	142	14,900	199	1.6	MAVROULES	78	79.0	94	12,150	168	3.9
HAMILTON	94	74.3	138	18,075	231	4.8	MARKEY	89	92.3	15	250	26	0.7
JACOBS	89	85.7	50	0	1	0.0	KENNEDY	94	91.0	24	5,600	88	1.6

CONGRESSIONAL LEADERSHIP

U.S. HOUSE MEMBER	LEAGUE OF CON. VOTERS SCORES			CONTRIBUTIONS FROM ENERGY PACS			U.S. HOUSE MEMBER	LEAGUE OF CON. VOTERS SCORES			CONTRIBUTIONS FROM ENERGY PACS		
	1989 -90	Average 85-90	Rank	$ in 1983-88	Rank	% All PACs		1989 -90	Average 85-90	Rank	$ in 1983-88	Rank	% All PACs
Massachusetts (cont.)							**Nebraska**						
MOAKLEY	78	83.7	63	19,925	241	4.5	BEREUTER	11	27.0	354	13,525	183	5.0
STUDDS	94	96.0	6	500	27	0.2	HOAGLAND	100	100.0	1	3,000	59	1.0
DONNELLY	89	78.3	99	14,850	198	4.2	SMITH, V.	0	11.7	420	31,750	305	10.0
Michigan							**Nevada**						
CONYERS	72	85.7	50	4,835	79	2.2	BILBRAY	61	65.0	189	10,450	144	2.3
PURSELL	61	45.0	274	39,715	332	10.7	VUCANOVICH	6	9.7	427	77,425	405	16.2
WOLPE	94	90.3	29	16,650	219	2.2	**New Hampshire**						
UPTON	39	38.5	302	11,175	156	6.4	SMITH, R.	78	66.3	183	23,800	271	6.0
HENRY	83	69.7	165	41,915	338	12.3	DOUGLAS	72	72.0	149	7,750	114	4.9
CARR	61	51.0	247	56,019	372	5.3	**New Jersey**						
KILDEE	89	87.0	42	5,300	84	2.2	FLORIO	20	66.3	183	na		
TRAXLER	50	52.0	244	15,535	206	4.9	HUGHES	78	77.7	112	5,840	95	1.9
VANDER JAGT	22	22.3	373	50,895	367	7.4	PALLONE	89	89.0	32	2,600	54	0.6
SCHUETTE	33	32.7	328	84,675	416	10.6	SMITH, C.	78	69.3	166	16,600	218	4.6
DAVIS	44	40.0	295	62,410	386	11.5	ROUKEMA	78	72.3	147	16,400	216	3.6
BONIOR	83	78.3	99	18,180	233	2.9	DWYER	83	75.3	129	3,200	60	1.0
CROCKETT	72	72.0	149	4,650	75	3.5	RINALDO	83	75.3	129	25,700	278	3.5
HERTEL	94	86.3	46	4,300	70	1.2	ROE	56	58.3	225	23,200	267	3.6
FORD, W.	72	72.0	149	11,935	164	1.8	TORRICELLI	89	79.0	94	12,413	170	2.1
DINGELL	56	61.7	211	113,360	428	10.6	PAYNE	67	67.0	178	8,380	122	4.8
LEVIN, S.	78	77.3	117	11,750	162	3.1	GALLO	72	64.3	195	42,395	340	8.0
BROOMFIELD	33	34.0	324	4,550	72	3.3	COURTER	33	43.7	281	20,097	243	5.4
Minnesota							SAXTON	78	62.3	208	47,550	357	9.6
PENNY	72	71.7	155	6,900	106	1.4	GUARINI	89	81.3	83	17,450	222	2.2
WEBER	44	57.7	229	31,300	304	4.6	**New Mexico**						
FRENZEL	39	45.3	273	37,250	321	4.5	SCHIFF	33	33.0	327	26,800	289	15.2
VENTO	83	90.0	30	6,475	98	1.5	SKEEN	6	10.0	426	55,900	371	18.5
SABO	83	77.3	117	11,950	165	2.6	RICHARDSON	83	71.7	155	81,650	412	10.3
SIKORSKI	94	90.7	26	20,150	244	1.9	**New York**						
STRANGELAND	0	15.3	405	44,850	345	5.4	HOCHBRUECKNER	83	85.5	52	1,350	38	0.2
OBERSTAR	72	78.0	104	13,090	176	2.0	DOWNEY	89	85.0	56	8,900	132	1.1
Mississippi							MRAZEK	83	79.3	92	3,550	64	0.5
WHITTEN	50	36.7	309	26,400	284	6.0	LENT	28	33.3	326	92,650	421	11.6
ESPY	28	39.0	300	14,500	192	1.9	McGRATH	78	63.7	199	29,650	299	5.0
MONTGOMERY	28	24.7	363	12,850	173	8.9	FLAKE	67	77.5	116	2,000	46	0.9
PARKER	17	17.0	398	9,450	138	4.1	ACKERMAN	89	90.7	26	2,100	48	0.5
TAYLOR	67	67.0	178	1,000	34	1.4	SCHEUER	83	77.3	117	1,700	41	1.3
Missouri							MANTON	50	51.7	245	23,550	269	3.3
CLAY	78	83.3	64	1,999	45	0.5	SCHUMER	89	88.3	38	0	1	0.0
BUECHNER	56	53.0	242	32,850	309	8.8	TOWNS	78	70.0	160	7,450	112	1.8
GEPHARDT	83	58.7	223	37,746	324	3.7	OWENS, M.	83	80.3	85	2,400	50	0.7
SKELTON	44	40.0	295	15,425	204	3.1	SOLARZ	89	86.0	47	500	27	0.4
WHEAT	89	83.0	67	10,200	143	1.5	MOLINARI	63	63.0	202	na		
COLEMAN	28	23.3	371	8,454	123	2.1	GREEN	78	82.7	72	28,150	295	6.3
HANCOCK	17	17.0	398	4,900	80	5.7	RANGEL	67	78.3	99	20,325	245	2.4
EMERSON	0	8.0	432	80,950	410	9.0	WEISS	100	95.7	7	985	33	0.5
VOLKMER	44	45.7	271	12,150	167	1.9	SERRANO	75	75.0	134	na		
Montana							ENGEL	83	83.0	67	500	27	0.4
WILLIAMS, P.	67	68.3	170	4,200	69	1.0	LOWEY	89	89.0	32	500	27	0.3
MARLENEE	6	13.7	410	80,825	409	18.5	FISH	72	75.7	125	17,710	225	4.2

CONGRESSIONAL LEADERSHIP

U.S. HOUSE MEMBER	LEAGUE OF CON. VOTERS SCORES			CONTRIBUTIONS FROM ENERGY PACS			U.S. HOUSE MEMBER	LEAGUE OF CON. VOTERS SCORES			CONTRIBUTIONS FROM ENERGY PACS		
	1989-90	Average 85-90	Rank	$ in 1983-88	Rank	% All PACs		1989-90	Average 85-90	Rank	$ in 1983-88	Rank	% All PACs
New York (cont.)							SYNAR	78	75.3	129	4,825	78	22.4
GILMAN	100	87.3	40	15,576	208	3.9	WATKINS	28	31.0	342	27,850	294	13.1
McNULTY	78	78.0	104	500	27	0.4	McCURDY	78	60.3	214	32,750	308	8.9
SOLOMON	39	35.7	316	9,000	133	4.2	EDWARDS, M.	11	15.7	402	44,718	344	17.2
BOEHLERT	100	86.7	45	11,550	160	3.8	ENGLISH	39	38.3	304	36,500	319	8.7
MARTIN, D.	33	34.7	321	13,700	187	6.5	**Oregon**						
WALSH	50	50.0	252	17,800	229	9.4	AuCOIN	72	81.0	84	15,500	205	1.3
McHUGH	78	77.7	112	5,230	83	1.5	SMITH, R.	11	15.3	405	27,500	293	7.4
HORTON	67	63.7	199	10,970	153	3.6	WYDEN	94	84.7	59	25,173	276	4.0
SLAUGHTER, L.	89	88.5	36	4,050	65	0.6	DeFAZIO	89	91.5	22	5,400	86	1.3
PAXON	44	44.0	276	18,325	234	7.3	SMITH, D.	11	17.3	395	82,829	413	13.2
LaFALCE	78	71.3	157	7,900	117	2.7	**Pennsylvania**						
NOWAK	83	75.7	125	5,800	93	2.5	FOGLIETTA	89	82.0	77	9,300	136	1.6
HOUGHTON	39	38.5	302	20,850	251	8.4	GRAY	78	75.7	125	21,075	254	2.2
North Carolina							BORSKI	72	72.0	149	15,325	203	2.4
JONES, W.	56	49.7	254	56,750	378	16.7	KOLTER	61	49.7	254	19,060	239	3.6
VALENTINE	94	64.7	192	46,400	355	14.3	SCHULZE	28	31.3	340	61,600	385	9.6
LANCASTER	83	76.0	124	10,800	149	4.0	YATRON	78	64.0	197	4,450	71	1.8
PRICE	89	79.0	94	10,000	141	1.4	WELDON	61	58.5	224	73,660	399	13.9
NEAL, S.	83	78.3	99	15,300	202	1.7	KOSTMAYER	94	94.0	10	13,800	188	1.3
COBLE	44	32.0	335	58,550	379	8.7	SHUSTER	11	13.7	410	20,600	247	4.3
ROSE	83	58.3	225	13,240	180	2.5	McDADE	39	40.0	295	40,700	334	6.4
HEFNER	61	41.0	292	26,600	286	3.9	KANJORSKI	83	66.3	183	8,800	129	1.1
McMILLAN, A.	28	29.0	348	52,700	369	7.2	MURTHA	61	44.0	276	48,250	360	6.7
BALLENGER	22	23.5	370	18,900	237	7.2	COUGHLIN	61	71.3	157	20,682	250	3.9
CLARKE	89	82.0	77	8,800	129	1.5	COYNE	83	76.3	122	6,750	105	2.4
North Dakota							RITTER	33	37.7	307	83,891	414	11.4
DORGAN	67	64.7	192	36,700	320	3.7	WALKER	28	38.3	304	4,150	68	3.7
Ohio							GEKAS	22	31.0	342	8,091	120	5.2
LUKEN	56	51.3	246	62,524	387	6.7	WALGREN	78	79.7	90	38,226	327	5.0
GRADISON	56	44.0	276	0	1	0.0	GOODLING	22	34.3	323	0	1	0.0
HALL, T.	83	69.0	168	18,436	235	5.4	GAYDOS	67	54.7	238	14,425	191	4.1
OXLEY	22	18.7	390	78,962	407	16.7	RIDGE	50	59.3	222	39,825	333	6.9
GILLMOR	44	44.0	276	18,695	236	6.8	MURPHY	78	55.7	232	28,771	296	9.5
McEWEN	28	24.7	363	37,256	322	10.0	CLINGER	28	32.7	328	100,347	423	16.2
DeWINE	56	48.0	263	17,522	223	6.0	**Rhode Island**						
LUKENS	11	12.0	418	15,075	201	6.6	MACHTLEY	94	94.0	10	5,300	84	7.5
KAPTUR	78	74.0	139	2,875	57	0.5	SCHNEIDER	94	87.0	42	6,435	97	1.3
MILLER, C.	11	19.3	383	25,800	279	10.8	**South Carolina**						
ECKART	72	78.0	104	56,635	376	7.5	RAVENEL	72	64.0	197	11,550	160	5.6
KASICH	44	30.0	345	41,930	339	9.3	SPENCE	33	32.7	328	31,050	303	6.7
PEASE	72	73.7	142	23,495	268	4.5	DERRICK	61	68.3	170	41,250	335	6.0
SAWYER	78	86.0	47	8,750	125	1.6	PATTERSON	61	55.5	233	22,650	266	4.2
WYLIE	33	24.7	363	16,214	214	3.5	SPRATT	89	78.3	99	13,550	184	5.0
REGULA	33	36.3	313	0	1	0.0	TALLON	56	58.0	227	23,821	272	3.7
TRAFICANT	61	64.3	195	750	32	0.4	**South Dakota**						
APPLEGATE	56	49.7	254	11,870	163	6.5	JOHNSON	83	79.0	94	7,250	110	1.3
FEIGHAN	78	82.0	77	6,500	99	0.8	**Tennessee**						
OAKAR	72	74.7	136	9,445	137	1.3	QUILLEN	6	11.7	420	67,800	394	6.8
STOKES	78	77.7	112	7,050	108	2.3	DUNCAN	28	23.3	371	5,600	88	5.7
Oklahoma							LLOYD	50	32.3	332	56,650	377	7.3
INHOFE	11	15.0	409	46,300	354	13.1	COOPER	78	74.0	139	27,400	292	5.6

CONGRESSIONAL LEADERSHIP

U.S. HOUSE MEMBER	LEAGUE OF CON. VOTERS SCORES			CONTRIBUTIONS FROM ENERGY PACS			U.S. HOUSE MEMBER	LEAGUE OF CON. VOTERS SCORES			CONTRIBUTIONS FROM ENERGY PACS		
	1989-90	Average 85-90	Rank	$ in 1983-88	Rank	% All PACs		1989-90	Average 85-90	Rank	$ in 1983-88	Rank	% All PACs
Tennessee (cont.)							**Vermont**						
CLEMENT	61	55.5	233	10,550	146	2.9	SMITH, P.	100	100.0	1	8,050	119	5.2
GORDON	83	63.0	202	14,500	192	2.2	**Virginia**						
SUNDQUIST	28	24.3	367	38,250	328	7.2	BATEMAN	11	21.7	374	77,350	404	13.0
TANNER	56	56.0	230	10,850	150	3.9	PICKETT	39	44.5	275	13,950	189	3.7
FORD, H.	72	64.7	192	8,750	125	1.5	BLILEY	17	19.7	381	90,900	420	13.1
Texas							SISISKY	44	45.7	271	21,900	261	6.5
CHAPMAN	39	41.3	290	49,257	362	9.8	PAYNE, L.	50	50.0	252	14,350	190	6.4
WILSON, C.	44	38.3	304	84,100	415	10.6	OLIN	50	50.7	250	20,500	246	4.2
BARTLETT	33	29.7	347	59,449	381	10.7	SLAUGHTER, F.	11	15.3	405	33,400	312	11.2
HALL, R.	6	19.7	381	165,602	433	30.0	PARRIS	6	20.0	380	71,900	396	11.4
BRYANT	50	63.3	201	103,500	425	11.2	BOUCHER	72	62.7	205	47,100	356	5.9
BARTON	11	18.7	390	214,000	435	27.4	WOLF	28	36.7	309	115,000	429	14.9
ARCHER	28	30.3	344	0	1	0.0	**Washington**						
FIELDS	11	19.3	383	203,071	434	23.5	MILLER, J.	89	80.3	85	38,770	330	6.4
BROOKS	44	41.7	288	45,462	348	6.0	SWIFT	67	66.7	180	47,700	359	7.2
PICKLE	67	62.3	208	59,363	380	11.9	UNSOELD	83	83.0	67	0	1	0.0
LEATH	28	25.3	361	17,550	224	7.9	MORRISON, S.	28	36.7	309	13,200	179	5.8
GEREN	27	27.0	354	2,000	46	2.8	FOLEY		54.0	241	75,547	402	5.9
SARPALIUS	28	28.0	351	9,250	135	4.5	DICKS	83	70.0	160	26,950	290	4.9
LAUGHLIN	28	28.0	351	11,050	154	3.9	McDERMOTT	83	83.0	67	7,100	109	3.2
DE LA GARZA	33	40.0	295	7,805	116	2.2	CHANDLER	50	49.0	260	21,695	260	5.0
COLEMAN, R.	67	59.7	219	45,902	352	7.0	**West Virginia**						
STENHOLM	28	26.7	356	37,700	323	12.7	MOLLOHAN	33	32.0	335	33,200	311	6.8
WASHINGTON	63	63.0	202	na			STAGGERS	50	58.0	227	8,350	121	1.8
COMBEST	6	19.0	386	85,740	417	21.0	WISE	72	65.0	189	17,250	220	4.5
GONZALEZ	72	78.0	104	0	1	0.0	RAHALL	72	60.0	217	45,250	346	11.4
SMITH, L.	22	20.5	378	38,213	326	15.7	**Wisconsin**						
DeLAY	17	9.3	428	111,100	427	20.7	ASPIN	56	66.7	180	20,050	242	2.9
BUSTAMANTE	39	48.0	263	26,100	280	7.2	KASTENMEIER	89	94.3	9	4,100	67	1.1
FROST	56	49.7	254	81,096	411	9.2	GUNDERSON	33	42.0	287	18,057	230	5.0
ANDREWS	72	54.3	239	101,725	424	15.1	KLECZKA	67	70.0	160	8,850	131	2.1
ARMEY	17	24.3	367	73,700	400	16.5	MOODY	89	83.3	64	21,200	255	2.7
ORTIZ	33	40.7	293	35,700	317	11.4	PETRI	78	69.3	166	14,820	197	4.9
Utah							OBEY	78	85.3	53	9,800	140	1.5
HANSEN	6	9.3	428	66,040	391	12.2	ROTH	33	35.3	318	21,320	257	4.8
OWENS, W.	89	85.0	56	10,548	145	1.3	SENSENBRENNER	56	55.0	237	15,750	209	5.8
NIELSON	0	11.7	420	60,500	383	17.8	**Wyoming**						
							THOMAS, C.	11	11.0	425	na		
							Total U.S. House		55.6		11.8 million		6.1

CONGRESSIONAL LEADERSHIP

U.S. SENATE MEMBER	LEAGUE OF CON. VOTERS SCORES			CONTRIBUTIONS FROM ENERGY PACS			U.S. SENATE MEMBER	LEAGUE OF CON. VOTERS SCORES			CONTRIBUTIONS FROM ENERGY PACS		
	1989-90	Average 85-90	Rank	$ in 1983-88	Rank	% All PACs		1989-90	Average 85-90	Rank	$ in 1983-88	Rank	% All PACs
Alabama							**Louisiana**						
HEFLIN	27	15	89	99,150	77	9.7	BREAUX	18	24	77	195,691	96	14.2
SHELBY	22	21	82	150,349	91	11.2	JOHNSTON	18	18.3	84	180,461	93	30.4
Alaska							**Maine**						
MURKOWSKI	22	20	83	129,521	85	19.1	COHEN	91	84.7	12	17,000	21	4
STEVENS	18	22	80	87,604	68	11.4	MITCHELL	64	78.7	18	19,000	24	2.3
Arizona							**Maryland**						
DeCONCINI	50	54.3	50	48,550	50	4.5	MIKULSKI	77	73.5	25	21,050	26	2.3
McCAIN	27	38.5	67	132,450	86	13.7	SARBANES	86	86	9	6,000	10	1
Arkansas							**Massachusetts**						
BUMPERS	68	54	51	30,075	30	5.8	KENNEDY	86	78	19	6,000	10	1.7
PRYOR	68	49.3	56	40,250	44	5.1	KERRY	100	97.3	2	0	1	0
California							**Michigan**						
CRANSTON	91	86.3	8	51,650	52	3.3	LEVIN	46	59	40	15,870	19	2.2
WILSON	59	57	43	128,806	84	5.5	RIEGLE	64	78	19	42,225	47	2.8
Colorado							**Minnesota**						
ARMSTRONG	13	16.7	86	93,099	73	11.6	BOSCHWITZ	36	45.3	60	81,882	65	8.1
WIRTH	91	80.5	16	66,993	59	4.7	DURENBERGER	55	75.7	22	87,245	67	4.9
Connecticut							**Mississippi**						
DODD	82	71.3	29	4,750	9	0.6	COCHRAN	4	15.7	88	125,183	83	12.7
LIEBERMAN	95	95	3	1,500	6	0.7	LOTT	4	4	98	180,450	92	11.7
Delaware							**Missouri**						
BIDEN	86	80.7	15	4,000	8	0.9	BOND	13	11.5	93	136,950	87	9.5
ROTH	55	67.7	33	67,950	60	8.1	DANFORTH	32	48.3	57	90,840	70	6.4
Florida							**Montana**						
GRAHAM	95	82.5	13	52,750	53	5.5	BAUCUS	32	57.7	42	22,550	27	2.4
MACK	22	22	80	150,000	90	11.9	BURNS	13	13	92	34,400	36	9.3
Georgia							**Nebraska**						
FOWLER	73	66.5	35	57,150	56	4.6	EXON	46	35.3	68	16,200	20	3.1
NUNN	59	39	66	31,550	33	7.9	KERREY	73	73	26	19,650	25	2.4
Hawaii							**Nevada**						
INOUYE	46	44.7	62	18,800	23	2.8	BRYAN	95	95	3	8,400	13	1.1
MATSUNAGA	44	62.3	38				REID	82	66	36	30,775	31	2.5
Idaho							**New Hampshire**						
McCLURE	8	2.7	100	120,875	81	21.1	HUMPHREY	59	74	23	37,150	41	4.9
SYMMS	8	2.7	100	182,372	94	12.6	RUDMAN	36	53.7	52	450	5	3.9
Illinois							**New Jersey**						
DIXON	59	43	63	61,950	57	5	BRADLEY	95	85	9	43,087	48	4.3
SIMON	86	69.7	31	11,200	14	0.9	LAUTENBERG	95	94.7	6	15,750	18	1
Indiana							**New Mexico**						
COATS	32	32	71	55,945	55	13.2	BINGAMAN	73	62	39	140,873	88	10.2
LUGAR	36	42	64	62,180	58	7.4	DOMENICI	22	23	78	145,813	89	16.3
Iowa							**New York**						
GRASSLEY	22	28.3	72	72,350	62	6.4	D'AMATO	41	45	61	71,100	61	5.4
HARKIN	73	77.7	21	13,650	17	1.3	MOYNIHAN	86	80	17	40,850	45	3.3
Kansas							**North Carolina**						
DOLE	22	25.7	75	102,750	80	7.2	HELMS	8	8.3	94	97,975	76	9.8
KASSEBAUM	36	28	74	13,500	16	5.9	SANFORD	64	72	28	37,500	42	3
Kentucky							**North Dakota**						
FORD	13	28.3	72	89,783	69	10.6	BURDICK	50	56	47	97,103	75	8.2
McCONNELL	22	25.7	75	76,753	64	15.7	CONRAD	36	48	58	31,000	32	4.9

CONGRESSIONAL LEADERSHIP

U.S. SENATE MEMBER	LEAGUE OF CON. VOTERS SCORES 1989-90	Average 85-90	Rank	CONTRIBUTIONS FROM ENERGY PACS $ in 1983-88	Rank	% All PACs
Ohio						
GLENN	55	51.7	56	29,636	28	4.3
METZENBAUM	91	81.3	15	11,405	14	1
Oklahoma						
BOREN	22	22.7	80	0	1	0
NICKLES	4	7	97	197,392	96	19.8
Oregon						
HATFIELD	73	56.3	46	41,066	45	8.6
PACKWOOD	59	66.7	35	50,915	50	4.9
Pennsylvania						
HEINZ	64	68	33	101,752	77	7.2
SPECTER	64	56.3	46	122,850	81	8.2
Rhode Island						
CHAFEE	46	73.7	25	45,760	48	3.9
PELL	95	86	10	1,575	6	0.7
South Carolina						
HOLLINGS	59	58.7	42	33,884	34	3
THURMOND	27	18.3	85	34,950	36	5.8
South Dakota						
DASCHLE	64	57	44	36,000	39	2.2
PRESSLER	50	35	70	35,975	38	5.7
Tennessee						
GORE	95	70.7	31	35,500	37	3.3
SASSER	68	56	48	38,000	42	2.3
Texas						
BENTSEN	50	46.7	60	327,717	98	12.8
GRAMM	4	13.7	92	382,103	99	18.9
Utah						
GARN	13	7.7	96	55,340	53	8.9
HATCH	8	15	90	92,935	71	7.1
Vermont						
JEFFORDS	73	73	27	28,504	27	3.2
LEAHY	95	98.3	1	18,750	21	2.1
Virginia						
ROBB	55	55	50	91,147	70	9.9
WARNER	22	32.3	71	94,310	73	13
Washington						
ADAMS	95	87.5	8	7,500	11	0.9
GORTON	41	41	66	216,019	97	9.7
West Virginia						
BYRD	50	53.3	54	102,650	78	10.2
ROCKEFELLER	77	63.7	38	31,850	33	5
Wisconsin						
KASTEN	50	52.3	55	82,487	65	6.8
KOHL	95	95	4	0	1	0
Wyoming						
SIMPSON	4	16.3	88	74,290	62	14.5
WALLOP	4	4	99	188,261	94	19.2
Total U.S. Senate		50.9		7.0 million		7.3

BEST AND WORST MEMBERS OF CONGRESS

State Member	LCV Score 85-90	Rank	Energy % All PACs	State Member	LCV Score 85-90	Rank	Energy % All PACs
SENATE BEST				**WORST**			
VT LEAHY	98.3	1	2.1	ID McCLURE	2.7	100	21.1
MA KERRY	97.3	2	0	ID SYMMS	2.7	100	12.6
NV BRYAN	95	3	1.1	MY WALLOP	4	98	19.2
CT LIEBERMN	95	3	0.7	MS LOTT	4	98	11.7
WI KOHL	95	3	0	OK NICKLES	7	96	19.8
NJ LAUTNBRG	94.7	6	1	UT GARN	7.7	95	8.9
WA ADAMS	87.5	7	0.9	NC HELMS	8.3	94	9.8
CA CRANSTN	86.3	8	3.3	MO BOND	11.5	93	9.5
NJ BRADLEY	85	9	4.3	MT BURNS	13	92	9.3
RI PELL	86	9	0.7	TX GRAMM	13.7	91	18.9
MD SARBANES	86	9	1	AL HEFLIN	15	89	9.7
ME COHEN	84.7	12	4	UT HATCH	15	89	7.1
HOUSE BEST				**WORST**			
NE HOAGLND	100	1	1	CA HERGER	3	435	8.6
VT SMITH, P.	100	1	5.2	AZ STUMP	5.7	434	8.8
CA CAMPBLL	100	1	4.7	ID CRAIG	7.7	433	14.6
IN JONTZ	97	4	0.6	MO EMERSN	8	432	9
IL EVANS, L.	96.3	5	0.8	CA SHUMWY	9.3	428	5
MA STUDDS	96	6	0.2	TX DeLAY	9.3	428	20.7
NY WEISS	95.7	7	0.5	IL MICHEL	9.3	428	7.6
CT SHAYS	94.5	8	1	UT HANSEN	9.3	428	12.2
WI K'MEIER	94.3	9	1.1	NV VUCNVCH	9.7	427	16.2
IN LONG	94	10	0	NM SKEEN	10	426	18.5
MA NEAL, R.	94	10	2.9	WY THOMAS	11	425	na
RI MACHTLY	94	10	7.5	CA DORNAN	11.7	420	10.7
PA K'MAYER	94	10	1.3	CA PACKRD	11.7	420	7.1
CA DELLUMS	92.7	14	0.6	UT NIELSON	11.7	420	17.8
MA MARKEY	92.3	15	0.7	TN QUILLEN	11.7	420	6.8
MA FRANK	92.3	15	0.4	NE SMITH, V.	11.7	420	10
CA BOXER	92.3	15	1.1	AZ RHODES	12	418	10.8
CA WAXMAN	92.3	15	2.2	OH LUKENS	12	418	6.6
CA BEILNSN	92	19	0	LA BAKER	12.5	416	13
CA BATES	92	19	2.9	LA HOLLWY	12.5	416	11.8
CA STARK	91.7	21	1	CA PASHAYN	13.3	413	11.7
MD MFUME	91.5	22	1.2	CA HUNTER	13.3	413	4.2
OR DeFAZIO	91.5	22	1.3	AL DICKNSN	13.3	413	5.3
MA KENNEDY	91	24	1.6	KY ROGERS	13.7	410	12.5
MD MORELLA	91	24	10.1	PA SHUSTER	13.7	410	4.3
NY ACKRMN	90.7	26	0.5	MT MARLENE	13.7	410	18.5
IL YATES	90.7	26	6.3	OK INHOFE	15	409	13.1
MN SIKORSKI	90.7	26	1.9	VA SLAUGHTR	15.3	405	11.2
MI WOLPE	90.3	29	2.2	CA McCNDLSS	15.3	405	6.3
CO SCHROEDR	90	30	0.9	MN STRNGLND	15.3	405	5.4
MN VENTO	90	30	1.5	OR SMITH, R.	15.3	405	7.4
NY LOWEY	89	32	0.3	OK EDWARDS	15.7	402	17.2
NJ PALLONE	89	32	0.6	AL CALLAHN	15.7	402	12.2
				LA LIVNGSTN	15.7	402	17.6

SOURCES FOR CONGRESSIONAL LEADERSHIP INDICATORS

Average LCV Score
   Percent of pro-environment votes cast by members of House, Senate, or total delegation averaged together for designated years. Key votes were chosen and evaluated by League of Conservation Voters (LCV). For the House, 19 votes on key issues were selected for 1985-86, 16 were chosen for 1987-88, and 18 for 1989-90. For the Senate, 12 were chosen for 1985-86, 10 for 1987-88, and 22 for 1989-90. Not voting counts as an anti-environmental position and lowers the member's score.
   Source: "National Environmental Scorecard," annual editions, 1970-1990. Published by League of Conservation Voters, 1150 Connecticut Avenue, NW, Washington, DC 20036; telephone (202) 785-8683.

Delegation Score on Nuclear Issues
   Percent of "right" votes cast by state's delegation on selected nuclear power and nuclear safety issues during 1986, 1987, and 1988.
   Source: "The Nuclear Congress: How Congress Voted, 1986-1988," July 1988. Published by Public Citizen's Critical Mass Energy Project, 215 Pennsylvania Avenue, SE, Washington, DC 20003; telephone (202) 546-4996.

LCV Score for Members of Congress
   Percent of pro-environment votes cast by each member of House and Senate in office at end of 1990. Scores are for votes cast in 1989-90 sessions and for average percent of right votes cast during 1985-90 (or as long as person served during that period). See comments above for votes selected. Ranking is based on average scores for 1985-90. There are 435 Representatives and 100 Senators, so worst score is 435 in House and 100 in Senate.
   Source: "National Environmental Scorecard," annual editions, 1985-1990. Published by League of Conservation Voters, Washington.

Contributions from Energy PACs
   Campaign contributions received by members of Congress from energy-related political action committees (PACs) from 1983 through 1988, and the percent these gifts represent of all PAC donations received during the period. Ranking is based on dollar amount, with most money getting worst rank (435 for House, 100 for Senate). Energy PACs include oil, gas, and coal companies, electric and gas utilities, and nuclear power contractors.
   Source: Press releases and supplementary printouts furnished by Common Cause, 2030 M Street, NW, Washington, DC 20036; telephone (202) 833-1200.

CHAPTER 9

State Policy Initiatives

INDICATORS

Status of 50 environmental regulations
Scores on 17 policy areas
Spending for environmental programs

Sixty years ago, U.S. Supreme Court justice Louis Brandeis observed, "It is one of the happy incidents of the federal system that a single courageous state may serve as a laboratory and try novel social and economic experiments." Today, after a decade of Reagan-Bush deregulation and deficits, states are taking a wide range of initiatives less out of courage than desperation. As the federal government abdicates its leadership role, states must fill the gap if they value public health and the environment.

"States are leading the way in solid waste reduction, groundwater protection, right-to-know legislation, global warming, you name it," says Jeff Tryens, associate director of the Center for Policy Alternatives. "That's where Washington gets its models for environmental regulation — from the state capitals." In fact, the plethora of state laws has led some polluters to seek help from the federal government to standardize (and weaken) the mishmash of rules they face. For example, merchandisers of so-called "biodegradable" or "earth friendly" products are so troubled by the assortment of rules emerging from state capitals that they are lobbying the Federal Trade Commission to set national guidelines for what the labels mean.

The growing political clout of conservationists in big-market states like California and New Jersey is spurring other corporations to abandon their former passion for state's rights and federal deregulation. As more polluters look to Washington for protection, the fate of such "novel experiments" as Maine's ban on CFCs in auto air conditioners or Massachusetts' limits on toxic emissions may wind up in the hands of Congress or, just as likely, with Brandeis' less-liberal successors at the U.S. Supreme Court.

MISSING MONEY

One of the main reasons states have taken over leadership on environmental issues is the stinginess of the federal government — or, more accurately, the diversion of tax money to the Pentagon and other interests. In 1979, federal grants for state environmental programs addressing air, water, and waste problems totaled $479 million; by 1989, the total had dropped to $303 million in constant dollars. Meanwhile, the scope and the cost of state regulatory programs have skyrocketed. To keep up, many states have vastly increased their environmental budgets. According to the National Governors' Association, state budgets for air, water, and waste programs increased from $512 million to $721 million between 1982 and 1986.

A more detailed survey conducted by the Council of State Governments includes all funds that pass through the state budget for natural resource programs (fish and wildlife, forestry, land reclamation, etc.) as well as for environmental protection (air quality, waste management, drinking water, etc.) The Council found that state spending for all these programs leaped 38 percent in just two years, from $5.3 billion in 1986 to $7.3 billion in 1988.

There are huge disparities between states, however, and sometimes the states with the worst pollution spend the least to correct their problems. Texas, for example, ranks among the worst states for toxic chemical releases, energy inefficiency, high-risk jobs, and cropland erosion, yet it spends the least per capita on environment and natural resource protection. Texas also ranks 49th on environmental spending as a percent of the total state budget. Other states in the bottom 10 for per-capita environmental spending are Indiana (rank 49), Ohio, Oklahoma, New York, Arizona, Georgia, North Carolina, Alabama, and Tennessee. Seven of these are also among the worst 15 states for their composite scores on the Green Index's 179 pollution condition indicators.

The list of states devoting the most money per resident to the environment presents a more complicated picture. The bulk of the funds spent by four of the top six states — Wyoming, Alaska, Montana, and Idaho — goes for reclamation of mining sites and for fish and wildlife programs, mostly on federal property. The federal government owns an amazing 67 percent of these four states, compared to 18 for the other 46 states; and while local politicians and many citizens rail against Big Government intrusion, a large chunk of the budget for these four states is federal money. Meanwhile, these states' commitment to such basics as solid waste recycling and groundwater protection lags well behind the national norm.

The other four states among the leading eight for per-capita environmental spending — New Jersey, Oregon, Washington, and California — face enormous pollution problems from industrial growth and population density, and their elected officials have responded with relatively bold programs and state dollars. In fact, California, New Jersey, and Oregon rank 1st, 2d, and 5th as the states with the best environmental policies in place.

To supplement funds available from general revenues, states have pioneered a variety of alternative funding methods, including permit and emissions fees, environmental taxes, bonds, and revolving loan funds. These sources now contribute $3.2 billion annually for conservation programs, including land purchases, with bonds alone raising $1.3 billion. State officials told the National Governors' Association they believe alternative financing methods will never equal the funds contributed by general tax revenues, but they agree there's still lots of room for innovation and growth. The potential just from fees levied against different kinds of waste generators boggles the mind.

Sticking polluters with the bill through emission fees avoids politically unpopular tax hikes while also discouraging unhealthy, inefficient waste. California, for example, adopted a program which imposes fees on emissions of sulfur dioxide and nitrogen oxides. The program raised $800,000 for acid rain research and monitoring in 1987-88. The fees also provide an economic incentive to cut emissions, but this approach is not always appreciated by the champions of free enterprise. Maine's paper industry bitterly fought a proposed state law that would replace permit fees with an annual charge of $8 for every ton of industrial air pollutant released. Regulators welcomed the change, with its promised 14-fold increase in revenue, as a way to get money to implement air quality rules. "The legislature ordered that a toxic pollution program be inaugurated seven years ago, but the funds to carry it out have never been provided," says Ronald Keisman, staff attorney for the Natural Resources Defense Council.

Passing a law and then withholding the money to make it work is standard practice for legislatures throughout the nation, perhaps especially in states with progressive leanings. Minnesota, which has innovative policies on the books regarding everything from ozone-depleting chemicals to contract farming, is a case in point. "The laws look good, but they lack teeth," points out Judy Bellairs of Minneapolis' North Star Sierra Club. "Lawmakers cave in to agricultural interests and won't put the money that's needed into enforcement." Minnesota ranks 7th for overall state policy, but 31st in the percent of its budget devoted to environmental protection.

Connecticut, number 6 on state policy, ranks 46th on state budget spending. North Carolina passes more environmental laws than any Southern state except Florida, but inside the region only

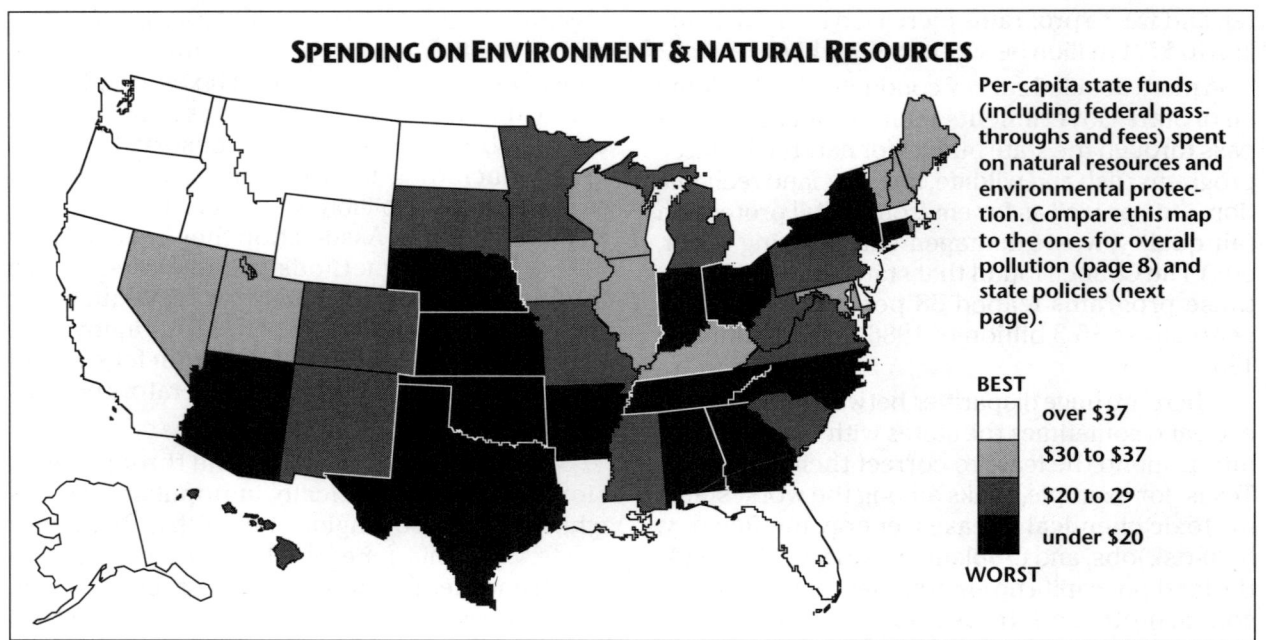

SPENDING ON ENVIRONMENT & NATURAL RESOURCES

Per-capita state funds (including federal pass-throughs and fees) spent on natural resources and environmental protection. Compare this map to the ones for overall pollution (page 8) and state policies (next page).

BEST
- over $37
- $30 to $37
- $20 to 29
- under $20

WORST

Texas spends a smaller share of its budget on enforcement and implementation. The Tarheel state gets points for policies that provide grants to assist local recycling and toxic reduction — but those programs have hardly any money to spend. Similarly, New York ranks 4th in policies on the books and 50th, dead last, in spending priorities for the environment.

New Hampshire, ranking about average for policies and spending, illustrates another problem. Supposedly to save money, its legislature sliced more than $100,000 from the environmental enforcement staff's 1991 budget, a move that jeopardizes the regulators' capacity to repeat their record of collecting $4 million in fines and cost recovery during fiscal 1990. In a more typical move to cripple regulation, Arizona's Agriculture Commission has simply refused to set guidelines for implementing a new law that requires farmers to minimize water pollution through best-management plans for fertilizer use. In dozens of ways, what one government body gives, another can take away.

THE INNOVATORS

The difficulty in measuring follow-through or enforcement, beyond presenting spending figures, is an important caveat to the discussion of state policy below. As with many indicators in this book, the policy tables should be used as a starting point for further investigation. It is also important to recognize that the tables present a series of snapshots of policies in place at a certain moment. "State environmental laws are constantly changing," notes Tina Hobson of Renew America, the sponsor of numerous studies used in this chapter. "Each study records how the states compare at a given point in time; while some improve the next month or next year, the innovators also take new steps and generally remain the leaders."

The states with the best overall records on 67 policy indicators — from recycling and seat belt laws to Superfund programs and pesticide regulations — are Maine, Connecticut, Massachusetts, New Jersey, New York, Rhode Island, and Florida along the East Coast; Wisconsin, Minnesota, and Michigan in the Midwest; and California and Oregon on the West Coast. For years, these have been the states that initiate programs others later imitate. Florida, for instance, passed an energy conservation act in 1987 which set home appliance energy efficiency standards tougher than those of the federal government; the law saved consumers and Mother Nature the high cost of a new coal-fired power plant, and is now policy in several other states.

In 1990, many of these same states pioneered policies that gained national exposure through the Center for Policy Alternative's database and "Best Bets" profiles. Here's a sample:

• *Ozone Protection.* Cars with CFC-based air conditioners, the nation's largest source of ozone-

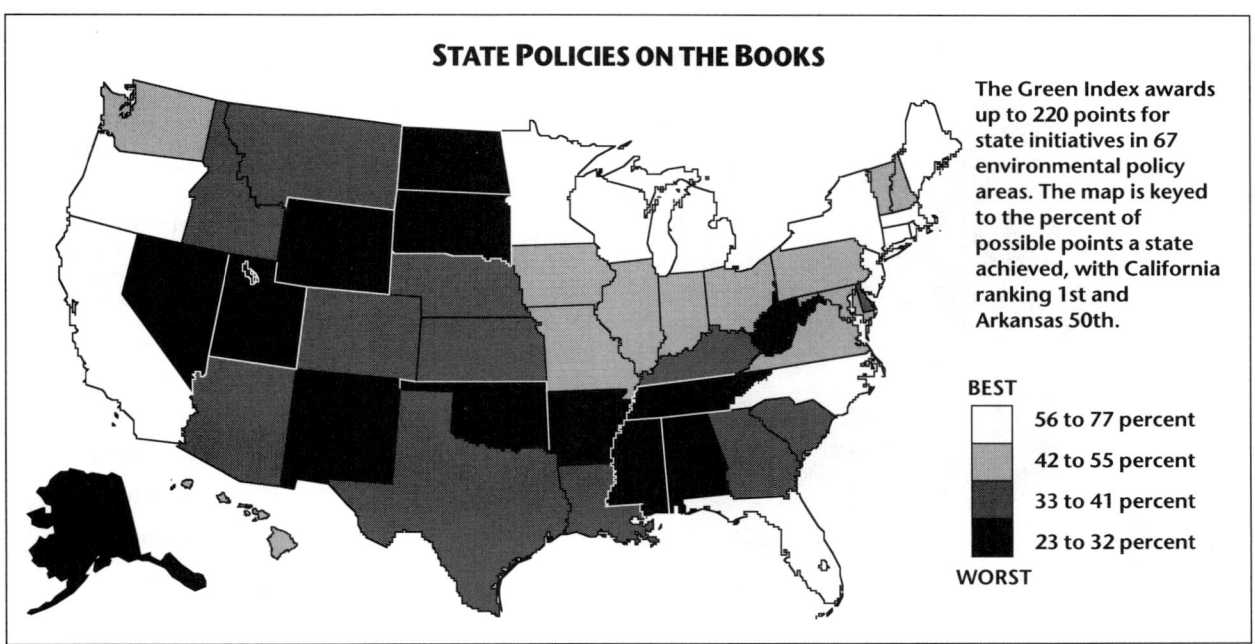

STATE POLICIES ON THE BOOKS

The Green Index awards up to 220 points for state initiatives in 67 environmental policy areas. The map is keyed to the percent of possible points a state achieved, with California ranking 1st and Arkansas 50th.

BEST
- 56 to 77 percent
- 42 to 55 percent
- 33 to 41 percent
- 23 to 32 percent

WORST

depleting CFCs, will be banned from Vermont after 1993. The same law restricts the sale of halon-using fire extinguishers, spray cleaners, and noise horns; it also sets up procedures for recycling CFCs from building air conditioners and large refrigeration units.

• *Solid Waste Reduction.* In addition to imposing a ban on CFCs by 1998, Iowa's new pollution prevention law requires a 25 percent drop in solid waste output by 1994 and a 50 percent cut by 2000. Yard waste, used oil, and lead acid batteries cannot go to landfills; tires must be shredded, and the state offers money for processing or developing markets for tires and other waste.

• *Global Warming.* In one of his last executive orders, retiring Governor Thomas Kean of New Jersey created the nation's first state climate protection program. It directs all state agencies to reduce emissions of carbon dioxide, CFCs, and other global-warming gases by increasing energy efficiency, particularly in buildings, promoting tree planting to absorb carbon dioxide, and recycling CFCs.

• *Groundwater Protection.* After years of study, Minnesota finally enacted a policy of nondegradation for groundwater. It sets fees on chemical use, well construction, and other activities that endanger groundwater. And it authorizes funds to reimburse farmers who initiate cleanup of spills from agricultural chemicals.

• *Bottle Bill.* While most states are still debating bottle bills, Maine expanded its law to encompass liquor, juice, and bottled water containers. It also bans juice boxes (a recycling headache because of their mixed materials) and sets a recycling goal of 50 percent by 1994.

• *Toxic Waste.* Massachusetts passed the first comprehensive toxic use reduction law, with a goal of slashing chemical waste generation in half by 1997. The 2,400 largest users of over 1,000 chemicals must file annual compliance reports; fees support a research center on reduction methods; and citizens have a right-to-know and right-to-sue without first proving direct economic loss.

DROP THE BALL

While even the best states lag behind in some areas and need to improve their follow-through, they at least demonstrate a willingness to pick up the regulatory ball dropped by the federal government. Unfortunately, the diminished federal role means an uneven playing field exists. Polluters can play one state against another, in search of the best bargain or weakest regulation. The pressure on politicians seeking to reconcile economic growth with quality of life issues is real: do they keep up with the innovators by setting high standards that promise long-term security, or do they match the weaker rules of competing states to entice, or keep, an industry?

Not surprisingly, the poorer states — at least those that perceive themselves as economically desperate — tend to give the least weight to envi-

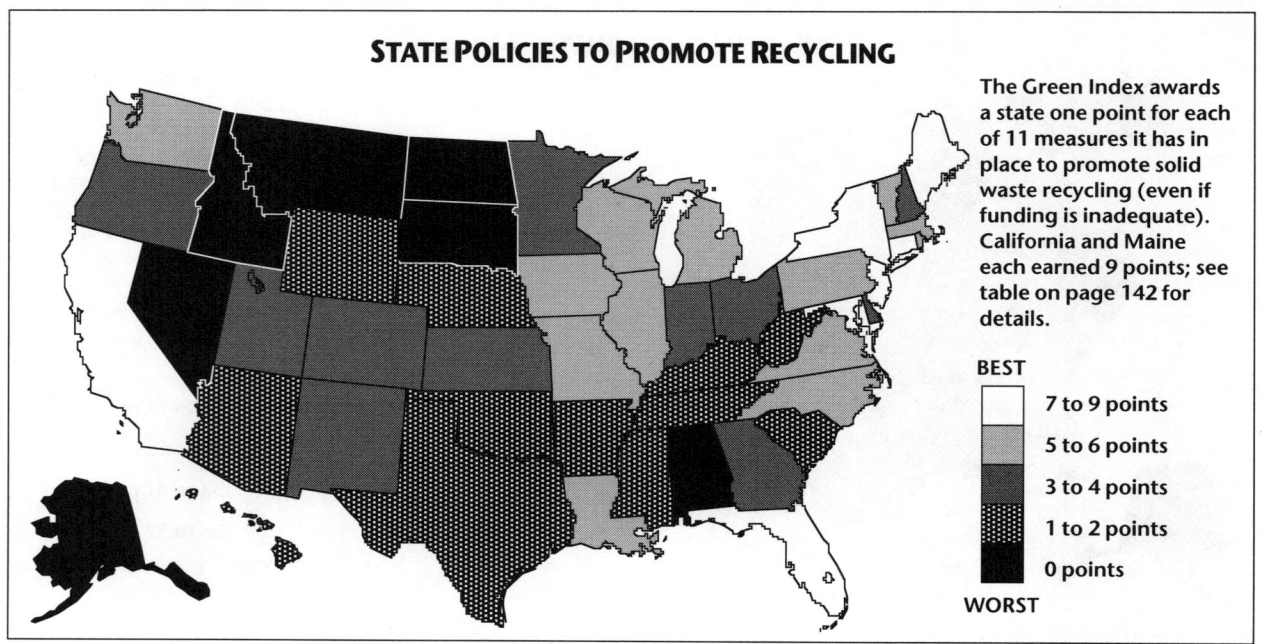

ronmental factors. Lacking both capital and a well educated workforce, these states bargain away their natural heritage for the promise of better jobs. Ironically, the casualties in this high-stakes game now include family farmers, ranchers, fishermen, steelworkers, oil well roughnecks, woodcutters, underground miners, and other resource harvesters considered expendable by agribusiness, coastal developers, and multinational corporations.

The true cost of forgetting the environment has not yet come home to lawmakers in these states. As in the case of federal policy, the states with legislators who most consistently vote against environmental protection are the natural resource-dependent states in the South, Rocky Mountains, and Farm Belt. The 12 states ranking worst on state policy are Arkansas, Alabama, Mississippi, West Virginia, and Tennessee in the South, and Alaska, Nevada, Utah, South Dakota, North Dakota, Wyoming, and Oklahoma to the West. With the exception of Nevada and Tennessee, all of these states are among those whose economies depend the most on natural resources, with Alaska and Wyoming leading the nation in this respect.

Arkansas, for example, depends heavily on farming, lumbering, and fossil-fuel extraction, and it ranks 50th overall on state policy, with few recycling measures, poor implementation of Superfund and right-to-know laws, and lackluster control of pesticide use or groundwater contamination. Another anti-regulatory agricultural state, such as South Dakota or Idaho, might survive such a laggard approach to environmental protection. But Arkansas already faces profound pollution problems, ranking among the worst 10 states for toxics released to air and water, oil spills, carbon emissions, reliance on pesticides, and fertilizer use.

Mississippi and Alabama rank 45th and 48th on overall state policy and have taken no progressive steps to make industry pay for its pollution or allow citizens access to information about emissions. Yet both states host large chemical, paper, and energy industries whose abnormal levels of toxic discharge produce health problems, ruined rivers, and dozens of contaminated waste sites. State legislators juggle protection of the environment with protection of industry — and they drop the green ball nearly every time. They vote in favor of the oil, nuclear power, pesticide manufacturers, paper makers, and agribusiness which fuel their economies — and foul their air, water, and land.

Even in the best-ranking states, laws challenging industry to reduce production of poisons are among the last to make it through the legislature. By contrast, recycling programs that cost industry little and elicit broad public support become law first. Forty-three states have passed some sort of recycling legislation compared to 16 with toxic reduction laws.

RECYCLING

Solid waste recycling does not stop waste at its source by eliminating packaging, for example, or reducing chemical emissions; however, it does decrease the need for virgin materials. And since it is relatively inexpensive and enjoys widespread support, recycling is the focus of many state policies. The effectiveness of these programs varies widely. Programs that require participation, source separation, or other mandatory provisions, and those that provide practical economic incentives, like bottle bills, tend to be the most effective, especially compared to voluntary efforts. Legislation that diverts nonbiodegradable goods from landfills — tires, diapers, appliances, batteries or that channels recyclables to a market, such as for newsprint, is also especially beneficial.

The legislatures in California, Connecticut, Maine, and New York have enacted some of the broadest recycling laws. All four states receive points for enacting bottle bills, establishing mandatory recycling goals, offering financial assistance to communities for recycling programs, and directing state agencies to give preference to goods made with recycled materials, even if the cost is slightly higher.

The California law allows the state to pay up to 5 percent extra to procure everything from office paper to paving material made from recycled material. It also extends tax credits to businesses that use recycled goods, creating new markets for old materials. The lack of markets has been one of the greatest obstacles to promoting recycling; without an end use, the mounting piles of recyclables lose their value and revert to waste. In Connecticut, newspaper companies were told in 1989 that they would be required to use 90 percent recycled fiber by 1998. In 1990 the law was amended to require 50 percent by 1999, a substantial cut, but the measure still provides a large market for recycled paper. Arizona, California, Florida, Maryland, Missouri, and Wisconsin have also passed laws imposing minimum standards for the recycled content of daily newspapers.

Bottle bills mandating fees on beverage containers are among the most controversial recycling measures. Proponents see them as a way to reduce waste at no government expense, while opponents say they single out a small part of the wastestream at the expense of selected industries and can deter more expansive recycling efforts. After analyzing various programs, Jeff Tryens of the Center for Policy Alternatives concludes that not even mandatory recycling programs are "as effective as a good bottle bill." The added bonus — or penalty of cash deposits captures consumer attention like nothing else.

Only 10 states have bottle bills levying a deposit on certain glass, aluminum, or plastic containers. These states — California, Connecticut, Delaware, Iowa, Maine, Massachusetts, Michigan, New York, Oregon, and Vermont generally rank well on other recycling indicators, although Delaware has no curbside recycling programs.

Diapers are another controversial subject in today's waste reduction/recycling debate. Disposable diapers comprise 2 to 3 percent of all municipal solid waste; they also use six times more energy and generate three times more manufacturing waste in their production than reusable diapers. On the other hand, reusables consume more water in cleaning and send more sewage to waste treatment systems. On balance, disposables still produce seven times more waste. In 1990, 24 states introduced legislation to add a surcharge on disposable diapers or otherwise promote the use of reusables, but only Wisconsin, Maine, Virginia, and Nebraska have passed diaper laws. California's bill to stop disposable diaper use in daycare centers passed both houses of the legislature but was vetoed by the governor. Interestingly, legislators in Nebraska agreed to ban non-biodegradables from the Cornhusker state not because of a concern for landfill space, but because the bill promoted the use of biodegradable plastics made from corn starch.

The states with the worst recycling records, receiving no credit for any of our 11 recycling indicators, are the rural states of Alaska, Idaho, Montana, Nevada, North Dakota, and South Dakota, plus Alabama. All these states, except Alabama, also rank 37th or worse on the per-capita number of municipal landfills and open dumps in their states, indicating they need to get serious about recycling and waste reduction.

AIR AND WATER PROTECTION

Another popular area for state laws is the monitoring of air and water pollution, but only a few states have pursued strategies that will lead to reducing contamination, especially by toxic chemicals. The best-ranking states for clean air legislation, New Hampshire and New York, have both instituted air toxic control programs, acid rain monitoring, programs to encourage least-cost energy production, and fees charged to air-polluting industries. Louisiana, a state not known for its pro-environmental legislation, passed an air toxics law in 1990 that requires a 50 percent cut of emissions from 100 air pollutants by 1994. In all three states, however, low funding or administrative delays have slowed progress.

States providing little monitoring or management of air pollution include West Virginia, Utah, South Dakota, Wyoming, New Mexico, and Nevada. Several of these states have intense energy and chemical production centers that pollute their surroundings and endanger their neighbors. Utah has none of the air pollution control programs on our policy indicators, despite its poor ranking on several indicators of actual conditions — 37th on air with ozone and carbon monoxide violations, 37th on state spending for air pollution, and 50th on per-capita industrial toxic releases, thanks to its AMAX Magnesium plant, the single largest source of air toxics in the nation. The state is 42d in the overall policy ranking.

Surface water is regulated by the federal Clean Water Act, but groundwater remains largely untouched by federal legislation. Surface and groundwater provide all of our drinking water, yet they are often contaminated by pesticides, other chemicals, and acid rain. New York, which has experienced each of these problems in its most acute form, now has some of the best water protection programs, with provisions to control acid rain, restrict pesticides and phosphates, detect underground storage tank leaks, and monitor groundwater. The state has also launched a Self-Help Support System, a public-private partnership that helps rural communities get the technical assistance and finances needed to complete their own water treatment systems.

Connecticut, Florida, Illinois, Maryland, Minnesota, New Jersey, North Carolina, Oregon, Virginia, and Wisconsin also have extensive water protection programs — but the quality of their water hasn't always improved because the programs are not adequately funded, staffed, or enforced. Some states do not even make a pretense of protecting water quality. Alaska and Texas, the nation's two biggest oil producers, had no groundwater monitoring policy and only the most minimal policies to control runoff, according to a 1989 survey by the U.S. General Accounting Office. Alaska ranks 50th on water systems violating Safe Drinking Water standards; Texas ranks 50th in per-capita underground injections, 37th in water systems in noncompliance, and 50th in per-capita spending on water quality.

SOLUTIONS TO POLLUTION

Monitoring air and water quality measures pollution but does not stop it. Recycling laws focus on individual responsibility at the end of the wastestream, not reducing how much is created at the beginning. Every state is affected by hazardous and toxic chemicals, but only a handful devote substantial resources and laws to blocking poisons at their source; most still worry about finding the funds to clean up the mess after it happens.

New Jersey has one of the best records for non-Superfund cleanup. The state's program places liens on property to force responsible parties to pay for cleanups and gives the state Department of Environmental Protection authority to take over when responsible parties cannot be found. Along with California, Connecticut, and Massachusetts, New Jersey also has relatively strong right-to-know laws, which enable citizens to obtain information about the chemicals being used and discharged in their communities.

Even in the most aggressive states, cleanup efforts remain a frustrating game of catch-up. Progressive public officials and principled fiscal conservatives now recognize that source reduction — changing industrial methods and materials to reduce toxic waste production — is the best way to prevent pollution before it begins. Toxic reduction laws, however, have only worked their way through 16 legislatures. Lawmakers fear that the cost of new equipment and manufacturing processes required to reduce waste will overwhelm the industries in their districts. But a true accounting would show the long-term benefits of such changes, as well as count the current costs of chronic illness, cancer, birth defects, and other toxic health problems.

"Consumers, workers, and the environment all suffer from hazards caused by our society's ever-increasing use of toxic chemicals," says Richard Schrader, a former Center for Policy Alternatives researcher. "Reducing toxic chemical use is a common-sense solution to all of those problems." Economic incentives, including high fees or taxes for waste disposal and grants or loans for waste reduction, have proven most effective in pushing industry to reduce hazardous and toxic waste. Many states also provide waste exchange referrals and

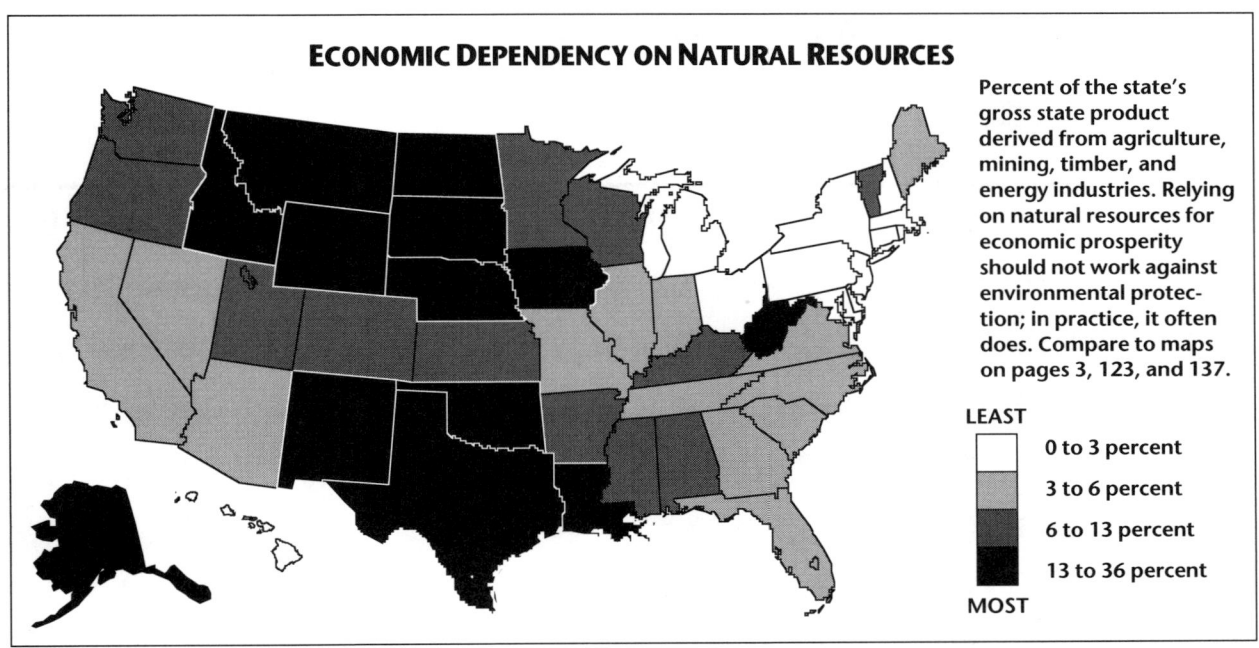

ECONOMIC DEPENDENCY ON NATURAL RESOURCES

Percent of the state's gross state product derived from agriculture, mining, timber, and energy industries. Relying on natural resources for economic prosperity should not work against environmental protection; in practice, it often does. Compare to maps on pages 3, 123, and 137.

LEAST
- 0 to 3 percent
- 3 to 6 percent
- 6 to 13 percent
- 13 to 36 percent

MOST

other technical assistance to encourage pollution prevention.

Some of the most progressive states are phasing in complex toxic use reduction laws. According to a report on pollution prevention laws published by the National Environmental Law Center (NELC), U.S. PIRG, and the Center for Policy Alternatives, Massachusetts far surpasses other states in its source reduction measures. "Massachusetts citizens will have safer air, water, workplaces, and products, and Massachusetts businesses will save money through prevention," writes William Ryan, NELC policy director and report co-author. Oregon, Indiana, Washington, Illinois, Maine, Minnesota, and California had "fair" prevention laws according to the report, but Massachusetts goes beyond those states in promoting toxic reduction, requiring companies to report on their efforts, and providing technical assistance.

Georgia and Tennessee received the lowest rating of the 10 states studied. Once again, legislators in the South and Rocky Mountains demonstrate the weakest will to force industry to meet its social obligations. The states with the worst hazardous waste cleanup programs and provisions for liability of toxic producers include Alabama, Mississippi, North Carolina, Virginia, West Virginia, Colorado, and Nevada.

Ironically, lawmakers excuse themselves by claiming they lack resources for waste prevention programs. In reality, source reduction measures save money in the long run. The average cost of a state hazardous waste minimization program is $150,000, a tiny figure compared to the $25 million required to clean up the average Superfund site. Even a modest effort like Minnesota's Technical Assistance Program (MnTAP), which uses University of Minnesota engineering interns to review industry processes, can pay off handsomely. A simple waste reduction program developed for one company cost $2,900 and now saves that business $7,000 each year.

In the spirit of Justice Brandeis' "novel experiments," state solutions to toxic waste problems may eventually influence federal legislation. As we write, Congress is debating reauthorization of the Resource Conservation and Recovery Act (RCRA). "A key part of the debate over RCRA will be how to detoxify hazardous wastes and municipal trash," explains attorney Carolyn Hartman of U.S. PIRG, a sponsor of the 10-state waste reduction survey. "Toxic use reduction should be the preferred prevention solution, and this report highlights states which are setting good examples for Congress to follow."

We likewise hope the *1991-92 Green Index* will encourage lawmakers, conservationists, and concerned citizens to take the lessons from other states and use them in their own.

STATUS OF 50 STATE POLICIES

State	Statewide law 1	Grants or Loans 2	Sets Specific Goals 3	Mandatory Action 4	Source Separation 5	Buy Recycled Goods 6	Goals for Buying 7	Offer Tax Aid 8	Bottle Return Law 9	Limit One-Time Diapers 10	Newsprint Reuse 11	Test Groundwater 12	Cleanup Standards 13
Alabama												■	
Alaska													
Arizona											■		
Arkansas	■	■											
California	■	■	■	■		■	■	■	■			■	■
Colorado		■				■	■	■				■	
Connecticut	■	■	■		■	■			■			■	■
Delaware		■	■						■			■	
Florida	■	■	■	■								■	
Georgia	■	■		■									
Hawaii	■											■	
Idaho												■	
Illinois	■	■	■				■	■					
Indiana	■	■	■					■				■	■
Iowa	■	■	■				■		■			■	
Kansas		■				■	■					■	
Kentucky		■						■				■	■
Louisiana	■	■	■			■						■	
Maine	■	■	■		■	■	■	■	■	■		■	
Maryland	■	■	■	■							■	■	■
Massachusetts	■	■	■						■		■	■	
Michigan	■	■	■			■	■		■			■	■
Minnesota	■	■	■									■	
Mississippi		■	■									■	
Missouri	■		■			■	■					■	
Montana												■	
Nebraska		■									■	■	■
Nevada													
New Hampshire		■				■	■					■	
New Jersey	■	■	■	■	■	■	■	■				■	
New Mexico	■	■				■						■	
New York	■	■	■		■	■			■		■	■	
North Carolina	■	■	■			■		■				■	■
North Dakota												■	
Ohio	■	■	■	■								■	■
Oklahoma	■	■										■	
Oregon						■		■	■			■	■
Pennsylvania	■	■	■		■	■						■	
Rhode Island	■	■	■									■	■
South Carolina		■										■	
South Dakota													
Tennessee	■						■					■	
Texas								■				■	■
Utah						■	■	■					
Vermont	■	■	■				■		■		■	■	
Virginia	■		■	■		■		■		■			
Washington	■	■	■			■		■				■	
West Virginia	■		■										
Wisconsin								■		■	■	■	
Wyoming		■										■	
# States	30	34	28	7	7	20	15	17	10	4	10	37	12

STATUS OF 50 STATE POLICIES

State	TOXIC WASTE									AIR POLLUTION			
	Superfund Plan 14	Right to Sue 15	Strict Liability 16	Right to Know 17	Aid For R-T-K Access 18	Worker Protection 19	Toxic Cuts Law 20	Plan & Report Cuts 21	Focus: Reduce Toxics 22	Stop Acid Rain 23	Control Air Toxics 24	Emission Fees 25	Ozone Protection 26
Alabama						■	■				■	■	
Alaska			■		■	■						■	
Arizona	■	■	■			■					■	■	
Arkansas											■	■	
California	■	■	■	■	■	■	■	■			■	■	■
Colorado						■						■	
Connecticut	■		■	■		■					■	■	■
Delaware				■		■						■	
Florida	■					■					■	■	
Georgia							■	■				■	
Hawaii		■	■			■							■
Idaho		■		■		■				■		■	
Illinois	■		■	■		■	■				■	■	■
Indiana	■		■	■		■	■					■	
Iowa		■	■			■					■	■	■
Kansas	■			■	■	■					■	■	
Kentucky		■	■			■					■	■	
Louisiana		■	■	■	■	■		■			■	■	
Maine	■	■	■	■		■					■	■	■
Maryland			■	■		■					■	■	
Massachusetts	■	■	■	■		■	■	■	■	■	■	■	■
Michigan	■			■	■					■	■		
Minnesota	■	■	■	■	■	■	■	■		■	■	■	■
Mississippi						■	■	■			■	■	
Missouri	■		■								■	■	■
Montana			■								■	■	
Nebraska		■	■								■	■	
Nevada						■					■	■	
New Hampshire	■			■						■	■	■	
New Jersey	■		■	■		■					■	■	
New Mexico					■	■					■		
New York	■						■	■		■	■	■	■
North Carolina						■	■	■			■		
North Dakota		■				■					■	■	
Ohio	■	■	■	■		■					■	■	
Oklahoma						■						■	
Oregon	■	■	■	■	■	■	■	■	■		■	■	
Pennsylvania	■		■	■		■					■		
Rhode Island	■	■	■	■		■					■	■	■
South Carolina	■		■	■		■					■	■	
South Dakota			■										
Tennessee	■		■				■	■				■	
Texas	■		■		■						■	■	
Utah			■										
Vermont			■	■	■	■	■	■			■		■
Virginia				■		■					■	■	
Washington	■	■	■	■	■	■	■	■	■		■	■	
West Virginia				■								■	
Wisconsin	■	■	■	■	■	■				■		■	■
Wyoming		■				■					■	■	
# States	24	15	31	20	21	36	16	13	3	6	35	37	15

144 1991–1992 GREEN INDEX

STATUS OF 50 STATE POLICIES

State	WATER QUALITY								AGRICULTURE				
	Issue NPDES Permit 27	Regulate Federal Sites 28	Pre-trtmt Program 29	Protect Ground-Water 30	Under-Ground Tanks 31	Ground-Water Toxics 32	Wetland Protec-tion 33	Phos-phate Ban 34	Pesti-cide Permits 35	Certify Organic Food 36	Assist Organic Mrktg 37	Assist Sust'ble Farming 38	Bio-tech-nology 39
Alabama	■	■	■										
Alaska						■							
Arizona				■	■	■			■				
Arkansas	■	■	■										
California	■	■		■	■	■			■		■		
Colorado	■			■	■	■				■	■		
Connecticut	■			■	■	■	■						
Delaware	■			■			■						
Florida	■			■	■	■	■				■		
Georgia	■	■	■	■		■		■					
Hawaii	■	■	■	■	■				■				■
Idaho				■		■							
Illinois	■	■		■	■	■							
Indiana	■	■		■	■			■					
Iowa	■	■	■	■	■						■		
Kansas	■	■		■	■						■		
Kentucky	■	■		■	■								
Louisiana						■							
Maine				■	■	■	■			■	■	■	
Maryland	■		■	■	■	■	■						
Massachusetts				■	■	■			■		■		
Michigan	■	■	■	■	■	■	■	■					■
Minnesota	■	■	■	■	■	■	■			■	■	■	■
Mississippi	■	■	■	■	■								
Missouri	■	■	■	■							■		
Montana	■	■			■	■				■	■		
Nebraska	■	■	■	■	■						■		
Nevada	■	■	■	■									
New Hampshire						■	■			■	■		
New Jersey	■			■	■	■	■						
New Mexico				■	■						■		
New York	■	■		■	■	■	■	■	■		■	■	■
North Carolina	■	■	■	■	■	■	■				■		■
North Dakota	■			■	■		■						
Ohio	■	■	■							■	■		
Oklahoma				■	■	■							
Oregon	■	■	■	■	■	■							■
Pennsylvania	■	■	■				■	■					
Rhode Island	■	■	■	■		■	■					■	■
South Carolina	■	■	■										
South Dakota					■	■							
Tennessee	■		■			■							
Texas					■	■			■	■	■		
Utah	■	■	■	■	■								
Vermont	■			■	■	■	■				■	■	
Virginia	■	■		■	■	■	■						
Washington	■		■	■	■	■			■		■		
West Virginia	■	■	■								■		
Wisconsin	■	■	■	■	■	■	■	■				■	
Wyoming	■	■		■	■	■							
# States	38	30	26	38	37	29	16	11	8	8	21	6	7

STATUS OF 50 STATE POLICIES

State	Least Cost Energy 40	Stop Global Warming 41	Local Auto Tests 42	State Auto Tests 43	Certify Auto Tests 44	Seat Belt Law 45	Mass Transit Funds 46	Growth Mgmt Plan 47	Coastal Zone Mgmt 48	Indoor Pollution 49	Workplace Safety 50	# in State	Rank
Alabama							■				■	10	47
Alaska			■		■					■	■	9	48
Arizona	■		■				■					13	38
Arkansas							■				■	9	48
California	■	■	■	■	■	■	■		■	■	■	38	1
Colorado			■		■	■		■		■	■	19	23
Connecticut	■	■	■	■	■	■	■			■	■	32	4
Delaware	■		■			■		■			■	17	30
Florida	■		■			■	■	■		■	■	25	15
Georgia			■			■	■				■	16	31
Hawaii						■	■	■		■	■	19	23
Idaho			■			■	■			■	■	13	38
Illinois	■		■		■	■					■	22	19
Indiana			■		■	■						20	22
Iowa		■				■	■				■	23	18
Kansas						■					■	18	28
Kentucky			■									16	31
Louisiana			■			■	■				■	19	23
Maine	■		■	■			■	■	■	■	■	33	2
Maryland	■		■			■	■		■			26	14
Massachusetts	■	■	■	■	■		■				■	27	13
Michigan			■		■	■	■			■	■	28	10
Minnesota		■	■			■	■			■		31	6
Mississippi							■				■	15	34
Missouri		■	■			■	■			■	■	22	19
Montana						■				■	■	13	38
Nebraska										■	■	16	31
Nevada	■		■		■	■				■		12	44
New Hampshire	■	■	■				■				■	19	23
New Jersey		■	■	■	■	■		■		■	■	31	6
New Mexico			■				■			■	■	14	36
New York	■		■		■	■				■	■	32	4
North Carolina			■			■	■		■		■	24	16
North Dakota							■			■	■	12	44
Ohio			■			■	■				■	24	16
Oklahoma			■			■	■				■	13	38
Oregon	■	■	■		■		■	■		■	■	33	2
Pennsylvania			■		■	■					■	21	21
Rhode Island	■	■	■	■		■	■	■		■	■	31	6
South Carolina						■	■					15	34
South Dakota							■				■	5	50
Tennessee			■			■	■					14	36
Texas	■		■			■					■	18	28
Utah						■			■			13	38
Vermont	■	■	■	■				■				28	10
Virginia			■			■			■			19	23
Washington	■	■	■		■	■	■			■	■	28	10
West Virginia											■	11	46
Wisconsin	■		■			■	■			■	■	29	9
Wyoming						■	■					13	38
# States	17	12	37	6	17	35	33	9	5	24	35		

RENEW AMERICA SCORE FOR 17 POLICIES

State	Forest Manage-Ment 1989	Waste Recycling 1989	Drinking Water Policy 1989	Food Safety Policy 1989	Growth Manage-Ment 1989	Surface Water 1988	Pesticide Control 1988	Land Use Plans 1988	Indoor Pollution 1988	Highway Safety 1988	Energy Pollution 1988	Air Pollution 1987
Alabama	4	2	2	6	2	4	2	5	4	2	4	3
Alaska	3	3	3	5	3	3	2	2	7	2	5	7
Arizona	3	1	6	6	4	4	6	7	4	1	3	7
Arkansas	3	2	1	6	1	1	3	3	4	2	4	1
California	9	7	8	9	9	5	10	8	5	7	9	10
Colorado	3	3	5	4	5	5	2	7	5	6	4	4
Connecticut	3	9	6	5	7	6	8	8	8	6	7	9
Delaware	4	4	4	5	5	4	2	6	7	6	7	1
Florida	6	8	4	6	8	5	6	9	9	4	8	7
Georgia	5	4	5	7	6	8	2	4	3	4	6	4
Hawaii	6	2	5	4	5	5	8	7	2	9	7	4
Idaho	9	3	5	5	3	4	2	3	5	5	6	2
Illinois	5	8	5	4	6	4	5	5	5	6	4	7
Indiana	6	2	2	2	3	4	4	6	7	3	4	6
Iowa	3	8	7	10	6	8	5	3	6	6	6	5
Kansas	4	3	5	5	3	6	4	3	5	3	4	2
Kentucky	3	3	2	4	3	5	4	3	3	4	4	7
Louisiana	2	2	1	3	2	2	5	6	2	2	3	5
Maine	3	5	10	4	7	5	7	6	6	4	8	3
Maryland	7	6	6	6	7	6	3	8	2	10	6	3
Massachusetts	8	7	9	5	8	5	9	9	6	6	10	6
Michigan	4	3	5	5	6	5	6	7	6	6	8	8
Minnesota	8	8	6	8	8	6	7	5	6	6	8	5
Mississippi	4	1	4	6	1	4	3	4	1	1	4	1
Missouri	6	5	5	5	4	5	3	3	3	4	5	5
Montana	5	2	3	6	2	6	4	4	3	5	7	2
Nebraska	3	4	5	5	3	8	3	6	4	5	5	4
Nevada	5	4	1	1	3	4	2	5	2	2	4	2
New Hampshire	5	4	3	5	5	4	8	7	9	3	7	6
New Jersey	5	8	9	4	8	6	5	9	10	7	7	9
New Mexico	4	3	2	4	3	4	2	4	5	2	5	1
New York	4	8	3	5	8	5	8	8	9	6	7	5
North Carolina	5	3	8	6	7	10	5	8	4	5	8	8
North Dakota	3	2	4	6	4	5	5	4	4	4	6	1
Ohio	5	6	2	5	6	5	6	6	5	4	4	8
Oklahoma	2	3	5	4	3	3	2	1	3	5	5	5
Oregon	9	10	5	5	10	7	6	10	5	6	8	6
Pennsylvania	6	8	3	4	7	4	2	4	8	8	5	8
Rhode Island	5	8	4	4	7	5	6	6	7	5	8	6
South Carolina	5	1	6	8	4	7	3	5	4	2	3	6
South Dakota	3	2	2	4	2	6	2	4	3	5	7	1
Tennessee	2	2	1	4	2	5	2	3	3	2	5	3
Texas	3	3	4	7	4	1	9	3	2	2	2	7
Utah	2	2	2	3	3	5	2	6	5	5	5	3
Vermont	4	7	5	4	7	6	6	8	5	4	7	3
Virginia	6	4	7	6	5	8	2	5	6	8	5	8
Washington	10	5	3	6	6	4	5	6	6	6	5	8
West Virginia	3	3	6	2	1	6	4	3	3	5	3	2
Wisconsin	6	8	7	8	8	7	7	7	8	7	9	9
Wyoming	3	4	3	3	2	6	1	3	2	2	1	1

RENEW AMERICA SCORE FOR 17 STATES

State	Soil Conservation 1987	Groundwater Control 1987	Hazardous Waste 1987	Solid Waste Mgmt 1987	Energy Conservation 1987	SUMMARY OF 17 RENEW AMERICA POLICIES			SUMMARY OF 50 GREEN INDEX POLICIES			COMPOSITE SCORE FOR 67 POLICIES	
						Total Points	% of 170	Rank	Total Points	% of 50	Rank	Average Percent	Rank
Alabama	3	2	3	3	2	53	31.2	46	10	20.0	47	25.60	47
Alaska	3	3	2	2	1	56	32.9	45	9	18.0	48	25.45	48
Arizona	3	7	5	2	3	72	42.4	32	13	26.0	38	34.20	35
Arkansas	3	2	5	3	4	48	28.2	48	9	18.0	48	23.10	50
California	3	7	9	9	10	134	78.8	1	38	76.0	1	77.40	1
Colorado	6	4	3	4	3	75	44.1	30	19	38.0	23	41.05	26
Connecticut	6	9	4	9	7	117	68.8	5	32	64.0	4	66.40	5
Delaware	8	6	3	4	2	78	45.9	29	17	34.0	30	39.95	28
Florida	4	9	8	6	7	114	67.1	7	25	50.0	15	58.55	12
Georgia	5	7	4	3	3	80	47.1	24	16	32.0	31	39.55	30
Hawaii	4	3	2	2	4	79	46.5	26	19	38.0	23	42.25	25
Idaho	1	6	1	2	6	68	40.0	34	13	26.0	38	33.00	37
Illinois	9	5	7	7	6	97	57.1	15	22	44.0	19	50.55	18
Indiana	5	4	6	7	8	79	46.5	28	20	40.0	22	43.25	24
Iowa	10	5	5	7	7	107	62.9	11	23	46.0	18	54.45	17
Kansas	5	8	8	4	2	74	43.5	31	18	36.0	28	39.75	29
Kentucky	3	1	6	8	3	66	38.8	35	16	32.0	31	35.40	33
Louisiana	3	3	7	2	1	52	30.6	47	19	38.0	23	34.30	34
Maine	6	7	6	6	8	101	59.4	13	33	66.0	2	62.70	9
Maryland	8	7	6	6	4	101	59.4	14	26	52.0	14	55.70	14
Massachusetts	4	8	9	6	8	123	72.4	4	27	54.0	13	63.20	8
Michigan	7	8	9	8	3	107	62.9	12	28	56.0	10	59.45	10
Minnesota	6	5	9	9	4	114	67.1	8	31	62.0	6	64.55	7
Mississippi	3	2	4	2	2	47	27.6	49	15	30.0	34	28.80	43
Missouri	6	7	8	1	4	79	46.5	27	22	44.0	19	45.25	23
Montana	5	6	3	1	6	70	41.2	33	13	26.0	38	33.60	36
Nebraska	6	6	2	6	7	82	48.2	23	16	32.0	31	40.10	27
Nevada	6	4	2	2	7	56	32.9	43	12	24.0	44	28.45	44
New Hampshire	5	5	7	5	4	92	54.1	18	19	38.0	23	46.05	22
New Jersey	6	7	10	10	5	125	73.5	3	31	62.0	6	67.75	2
New Mexico	2	8	5	1	6	61	35.9	40	14	28.0	36	31.95	39
New York	5	10	8	8	7	113	66.5	9	32	64.0	4	65.25	6
North Carolina	7	8	6	6	7	111	65.3	10	24	48.0	16	56.65	13
North Dakota	3	4	2	3	3	61	35.9	39	12	24.0	44	29.95	41
Ohio	8	4	5	5	4	88	51.8	22	24	48.0	16	49.90	19
Oklahoma	5	5	4	7	3	65	38.2	37	13	26.0	38	32.10	38
Oregon	2	7	5	7	8	116	68.2	6	33	66.0	2	67.10	4
Pennsylvania	6	5	5	3	5	91	53.5	20	21	42.0	21	47.75	20
Rhode Island	4	6	4	7	3	95	55.9	16	31	62.0	6	58.95	11
South Carolina	5	7	5	2	6	79	46.5	25	15	30.0	34	38.25	31
South Dakota	8	6	2	2	4	63	37.1	38	5	10.0	50	23.55	49
Tennessee	3	4	7	5	7	60	35.3	41	14	28.0	36	31.65	40
Texas	2	2	5	3	7	66	38.8	36	18	36.0	28	37.40	32
Utah	4	3	2	1	3	57	33.5	42	13	26.0	38	29.75	42
Vermont	3	5	6	4	7	91	53.5	19	28	56.0	10	54.75	15
Virginia	7	6	2	3	7	95	55.9	17	19	38.0	23	46.95	21
Washington	1	6	5	5	3	91	53.5	21	28	56.0	10	54.75	15
West Virginia	5	2	4	1	1	56	32.9	44	11	22.0	46	27.45	45
Wisconsin	8	8	7	8	9	131	77.1	2	29	58.0	9	67.55	3
Wyoming	3	8	1	2	1	46	27.1	50	13	26.0	38	26.55	46

SPENDING ON ENVIRONMENTAL AND NATURAL RESOURCE PROGRAMS

State	AIR QUAL. CONTROL $ Per Capita	Rank	WATER RES. & POLLUTION $ Per Capita	Rank	HAZ. & SOLID WASTE $ Per Capita	Rank	FISH, WILDLIFE & FORESTRY $ Per Capita	Rank	SPENDING ON ALL ENVIR. PROGRAMS Total in $1,000	$ Per Capita	Rank	% Total State Budget	Rank	COMPOSITE SCORE FOR SPENDING Score	Rank
Alabama	0.48	45	3.24	42	0.52	45	8.53	26	64,907	15.73	42	1.02	41	241	46
Alaska	3.03	2	14.33	18	5.23	8	195.67	1	131,684	256.69	2	4.00	4	35	2
Arizona	0.81	31	4.97	35	1.35	29	4.12	42	46,613	13.45	45	0.96	43	225	42
Arkansas	0.39	47	3.78	38	0.73	39	12.31	19	44,189	18.24	39	1.15	39	221	40
California	2.26	5	25.49	5	6.26	4	15.84	11	1,486,124	52.76	8	2.60	9	42	3
Colorado	1.96	7	5.01	34	1.18	32	13.08	18	76,150	23.15	34	1.65	24	149	24
Connecticut	2.64	3	5.02	33	4.42	13	7.05	36	61,996	19.13	38	0.77	46	169	32
Delaware	2.10	6	14.45	17	7.58	2	17.27	10	33,170	50.26	9	1.80	19	63	7
Florida	0.58	37	20.28	9	4.31	14	9.83	23	465,591	37.62	13	2.51	11	107	13
Georgia	0.55	40	1.61	48	0.55	43	10.50	21	93,344	14.58	44	1.07	40	236	45
Hawaii	1.58	12	10.61	20	3.29	17	4.27	41	27,832	25.46	29	0.85	44	163	27
Idaho	0.78	34	22.10	6	1.83	24	33.77	5	61,442	61.50	6	4.22	3	78	8
Illinois	2.38	4	21.08	8	4.58	12	1.47	49	392,844	34.03	18	2.26	14	105	12
Indiana	0.85	26	3.32	41	1.16	33	2.65	47	52,766	9.46	49	0.68	47	243	47
Iowa	0.38	48	16.38	14	0.33	50	7.23	35	88,065	31.07	22	1.44	32	201	35
Kansas	0.84	29	9.44	21	1.11	34	3.75	44	47,817	19.23	37	1.23	37	202	36
Kentucky	1.16	16	6.73	26	1.08	35	6.32	40	120,289	32.33	20	1.64	25	162	26
Louisiana	0.99	19	21.89	7	1.18	31	8.53	27	193,836	43.85	11	2.64	7	102	11
Maine	0.55	39	3.78	39	7.93	1	15.18	12	39,332	32.61	19	1.88	16	126	18
Maryland	0.99	20	8.57	23	2.38	22	6.63	39	150,091	32.32	21	1.60	26	151	25
Massachusetts	0.83	30	28.70	3	5.15	9	2.94	45	237,936	40.53	12	1.56	27	126	18
Michigan	0.84	28	11.01	19	1.36	28	7.29	34	221,425	23.81	32	1.42	33	174	33
Minnesota	0.78	33	4.56	36	4.76	10	18.11	8	126,236	29.32	28	1.46	31	146	23
Mississippi	0.50	43	1.96	46	0.42	48	13.58	17	54,154	20.61	35	1.40	34	223	41
Missouri	0.47	46	8.34	24	0.58	42	9.22	24	119,907	23.33	33	1.73	21	190	34
Montana	1.48	13	26.72	4	7.57	3	37.63	4	69,560	86.52	3	4.29	2	29	1
Nebraska	0.34	49	4.29	37	0.63	41	7.72	31	27,988	17.48	40	1.29	36	234	44
Nevada	0.52	42	18.68	11	0.47	46	14.15	13	36,487	34.42	17	2.57	10	139	22
New Hampshire	0.88	25	15.86	15	5.57	6	8.00	29	33,588	30.62	23	2.41	12	110	14
New Jersey	1.68	9	58.29	2	3.78	15	2.19	48	523,874	67.86	5	3.61	5	84	9
New Mexico	0.99	18	6.92	25	3.73	16	10.05	22	44,782	29.66	27	1.48	29	137	21
New York	0.90	24	5.11	32	3.06	18	3.75	43	236,484	13.21	46	0.59	50	213	38
North Carolina	0.50	44	1.91	47	0.67	40	7.83	30	96,943	14.85	43	1.00	42	246	48
North Dakota	1.66	10	17.90	13	0.75	38	13.71	15	32,524	49.06	10	2.32	13	99	10
Ohio	1.02	17	2.49	45	2.10	23	2.90	46	125,669	11.56	48	0.65	48	227	43
Oklahoma	0.60	36	1.58	49	0.44	47	7.00	38	40,869	12.52	47	0.79	45	262	49
Oregon	3.87	1	6.30	28	4.66	11	40.28	3	186,438	68.02	4	3.03	6	53	5
Pennsylvania	0.95	22	5.54	30	2.88	20	7.70	32	288,766	24.01	31	1.49	28	163	27
Rhode Island	0.78	32	18.04	12	5.26	7	7.03	37	35,879	36.06	15	1.86	17	120	17
South Carolina	0.26	50	2.52	44	0.76	37	13.99	14	71,124	20.36	36	1.21	38	219	39
South Dakota	0.53	41	6.35	27	0.33	49	18.19	7	21,264	29.74	26	1.85	18	168	31
Tennessee	0.58	38	5.61	29	1.42	27	7.40	33	81,180	16.50	41	1.34	35	203	37
Texas	0.68	35	1.05	50	0.55	44	1.46	50	113,797	6.78	50	0.60	49	278	50
Utah	1.24	14	9.01	22	1.30	30	13.65	16	51,419	30.41	24	1.80	20	126	18
Vermont	1.60	11	3.72	40	2.60	21	17.45	9	20,222	36.37	14	1.94	15	110	15
Virginia	0.93	23	5.30	31	1.66	25	8.58	25	152,149	25.38	30	1.47	30	164	29
Washington	1.22	15	14.73	16	5.97	5	23.54	6	246,873	53.45	7	2.63	8	57	6
West Virginia	0.85	27	3.11	43	3.03	19	8.49	28	56,189	29.82	25	1.68	23	165	30
Wisconsin	0.96	21	19.78	10	1.46	26	11.47	20	167,779	34.54	16	1.70	22	115	16
Wyoming	1.89	8	145.11	1	0.77	36	46.78	2	128,051	271.87	1	7.73	1	49	4
U.S. Total	1.15		12.47		2.82		9.17		7,327,640	29.89					

SOURCES FOR STATE POLICY INDICATORS

RECYCLING PROGRAMS

1. Statewide law
State has a comprehensive recycling law with statewide plan of action with one or more provisions for stimulating recycling.
Source: "Recycling in the States," October 1990. Published by the National Solid Wastes Management Association, 1730 Rhode Island Avenue, NW, Washington, DC 20036 telephone (202) 659-4613.

2. Grants or loans
State law provides grants or loans to assist local implementation.
Source: Same as 1.

3. Specific goals
State law has specific waste reduction goals, although method of measuring waste is often unclear.
Source: Same as 1.

4. Mandatory action
State law requires mandatory recycling programs for municipalities.
Source: Same as 1.

5. Source separation
Separation of different recycled materials is required, usually through curbside collection.
Source: Same as 1.

6. Buy recycled goods
State agencies are allowed to spend 5 to 10 percent more for products made with recycled content.
Source: Same as 1.

7. Goals for buying
State sets goals for amount of recycled material that must be purchased by state agencies.
Source: Same as 1.

8. Offer tax aid
State gives tax incentives for recycling.
Source: Same as 1.

9. Bottle deposit law
Bottle recycling law promotes return of glass, aluminum, and plastic containers by levying deposit redeemable from retailers.
Source: "Coming Full Circle," Environmental Defense Fund, 1988, 1616 P Street, NW, Washington, DC, 20036; telephone (202) 387-3500. Also, Glass Packaging Institute, 1801 K Street, NW, Suite 1105-L, Washington, DC 20006; telephone (202) 887-4850.

10. Limit one-time diapers
State has law to discourage use of disposable diapers and/or to promote use of biodegradable or cloth diapers.
Source: Data from Center for Policy Alternatives, 1875 Connecticut Avenue, NW, Suite 710, Washington, DC 20009; telephone (202) 387-6030.

11. Newsprint reuse
By law, or under a voluntary agreement that requires reports to state officials, newspaper publishers must meet goals for using recycled newsprint.
Source: "Recycled Fiber Goals/Mandates for Newsprint," October 10, 1990. Published by American Paper Institute, 1250 Connecticut Avenue, NW, Washington, DC 20036; telephone (202) 463-2420.

LANDFILLS

12. Test groundwater
State has groundwater monitoring standards for municipal landfills.
Source: "Updated Review of Selected Provisions of State Solid Waste Management Regulations," July 1988. Published by Office of Solid Waste, U.S. Environmental Protection Agency, Washington.

13. Cleanup standards
Specific requirements for corrective action of leaking landfills are identified.
Source: Same as 12.

TOXIC WASTE

14. Superfund plan
State has authorized, active, and funded cleanup program for Superfund and state-identified hazardous waste sites.
Source: "An Analysis of State Superfund Programs," November 1989. Published by Environmental Law Institute, 1616 P Street, NW, Washington, DC 20036; telephone (202) 328-5150.

15. Citizen's right-to-sue
State Superfund statute or program allows citizens to sue toxic polluters.
Source: Same as 14.

16. Strict liability
State Superfund statute or program holds polluters to strict liability standards.
Source: Same as 14.

17. Right-To-Know
State promotes public access to information on toxic chemical usage and releases.
Source: "Working Notes on Community Right-To-Know," March 1990. Newsletter published by Working Group on Community Right-To-Know, 215 Pennsylvania Avenue, Washington, DC 20003; telephone (202) 546-9707. Data from Center for Policy Alternatives.

18. Aid for Right-To-Know
State has fees or other significant funding of Right-To-Know programs.
Source: "Community and Worker Right-To-Know News," February 8, 1991. Special supplement in newsletter published by Thompson Publishing Group, 1725 K Street, NW, Washington, DC 20006; telephone (202) 872-1766.

19. Worker protection
Members of state emergency response commission (SERC) and local emergency planning committee (LEPC) are protected from liability claims.
Source: Same as 18.

20. Toxic cuts law
State has law promoting cuts in toxic chemical production at its source, but it does not require facility plans or detailed reporting.
Source: Data from Center for Policy Alternatives, Washington, March 1991.

21. Plan and report cuts
Law includes requirements for facilities to plan and report on reductions, but allows use of traditional waste management strategies.
Source: Same as 20.

22. Focus: Reduce toxics
Law requires reduction plans and reporting, and does not count use of such waste management practices as incineration, end-of-pipe treatment, off-site recycling, and transfers of toxics to another medium.
Source: Same as 20.

AIR POLLUTION

23. Stop acid rain
State was one of first to take initiative to control sulfur dioxide and nitrogen oxide emissions which cause acid rain.
Source: "The State of the States, 1987," Renew America, 1400 16th Street, NW, Washington, DC 20036; telephone (202) 232-2252.

24. Control air toxics
State has air toxics control program in place, although its standards and enforcement may be weak.
Source: "NATICH Data Base: Report on State, Local, and EPA Air Toxic Activities," July 1989. Published by Office of Air Quality Planning and Standards, U.S. Environmental Protection Agency, Washington.

25. Air emission fees
State supplements its air pollution control program by collecting fees from holders of emission permits.
Source: "Air Permit and Emission Fees," April 1989. Published by State and Territorial Air Pollution Program Administrators and Association of Local Air Pollution Control Officials, 444 North Capitol Street, NW, Washington, DC 20001; telephone (202) 624-7864.

26. Ozone protection
State has law or plan to ban, recycle, or reduce consumption of chlorofluorocarbons (CFCs) in such products as refrigerants or foam packaging. CFCs destroy the ozone layer protecting the Earth from cancer-causing radiation.
Source: "Policy Alternatives on Environment," January 1991. Published by Center for Policy Alternatives, Washington.

WATER QUALITY

27. Issue NPDES permits
EPA has approved state program for issuing National Pollution Discharge Elimination System (NPDES) permits.
Source: "The State of the States, 1989, Drinking Water Focus Paper." Published by Renew America, Washington.

28. Regulate federal sites
   State has authority to regulate wastewater discharge from federal facilities.
   Source: Same as 27.

29. Pretreatment
   State has EPA-approved program for requiring pretreatment of wastewater sent to facilities with NPDES permits.
   Source: Same as 27.

30. Protect groundwater
   State has developed a plan for protecting groundwater from contamination, although implementation may be weak.
   Source: "Survey of State Groundwater Quality Protection Legislation Enacted from 1985 through 1987," October 1988. Published by Office of Groundwater Protection, U.S. Environmental Protection Agency. Also, "The State of the States, 1987," Renew America, Washington.

31. Underground tanks
   State law sets criteria for underground tanks, detection of leaks, or their cleanup.
   Source: Same as 30.

32. Groundwater toxics
   To protect groundwater, state uses specific numeric standards for a dozen or more hazardous chemicals.
   Source: "Groundwater Quality: State Activities to Guard Against Contaminants," February 1988. Published by U.S. General Accounting Office, Washington.

33. Wetland protection
   State has law protecting inland or freshwater wetlands.
   Source: "The State of the States, 1989," Renew America, Washington.

34. Phosphate ban
   To reduce nutrient load in state waters, state bans phosphate in laundry detergent.
   Source: Data as of May 1990, from Soap and Detergent Association, 475 Park Avenue South, New York, NY 10016; telephone (212) 725-1262.

AGRICULTURE

35. Pesticide spraying
   State requires a permit before pesticides may be sprayed.
   Source: "The State of the States, 1988: Focus Paper on Reducing Pesticide Contamination," Renew America, Washington.

36. Certify organic food
   State certifies "organic" crops or has regulation that defines "organic" food.
   Source: "Survey of Organic Crop Certification Programs and Policies," March 1989. Published by National Association of State Departments of Agriculture and Alberta Agriculture, 1616 H Street, NW, Washington, DC 20006; telephone (202) 628-1566.

37. Assist organic marketing
   State personnel or programs assist the marketing of organic foods.
   Source: Same as 36.

38. Assist sustainable farming
   State assists low-input or sustainable farming with its own grants.
   Source: Same as 36.

39. Biotechnology
   State regulates release of genetically produced or altered organisms into environment.
   Source: R. Steven Brown, "The State Role in Regulating Biotechnology," *Policy Studies Journal*, Fall 1988, and interview with the author at Council of State Governments, February 1990.

ENERGY AND TRANSIT

40. Least-cost energy
   State program makes utilities plan construction and conservation to minimize need for expensive, new power plants; program includes public hearing on plans.
   Source: "Least Cost Utility Planning," 1989. Published by the National Association of State Utility Consumer Advocates, 1101 14th Street, NW, Washington, DC 20005; telephone (202) 727-3908.

41. Stop global warming
   State law or policy promotes energy conservation and reduction of global warming gases, such as carbon dioxide and CFCs.
   Source: "Policy Alternatives on Environment," January 1991. Published by Center for Policy Alternatives, Washington.

42. Local auto tests
   Inspection of exhaust or emission system required in some localities in state.
   Source: "Inspection/Maintenance Program Implementation Summary," January 1991. Prepared by Environmental Department, Motor Vehicle Manufacturers Association of the U.S., 7430 Second Avenue, Detroit, MI 48202; telephone (313) 872-4311.

43. State auto tests
   Inspection of exhaust or emission system required statewide.
   Source: Same as 42.

44. Certify auto tests
   Certificate of compliance required.
   Source: Polk's Motor Vehicle Registration Manual, Volume II," 1989. Published by R.C. Polk Statistical Services Division, 431 Howard Street, Detroit, MI 48231; telephone (313) 961-9470.

45. Seat belt law
   State law requires use of safety belts.
   Source: "Factsheet," 1990. Published by Highway Users Federation for Safety and Mobility, 1776 Massachusetts Avenue, NW, Washington, DC 20036; telephone (202) 857-1231.

46. Mass transit funds
   State used part of its oil overcharge refund from U.S. Department of Energy for rideshares, vanpools, or similar programs.
   Source: "1989 Survey of State Involvement in Public Transportation," American Association of State Highway and Transportation Officials, 444 North Capitol Street, NW, Washington, DC 20001; telephone (202) 624-5800.

PLACE AND POLLUTION

47. Growth management plan
   State has law for growth management planning for entire state.
   Source: "The State of the States, 1989," Renew America, Washington.

48. Coastal zone management
   State has comprehensive coastal zone management law.
   Source: Same as 47.

49. Indoor pollution
State regulates smoking and other pollutants in at least 10 different types of locations.
Source: Data from "The State of the States, 1989," Renew America, published in "The 1990 Development Report Card," Corporation for Enterprise Development, 1725 K Street, NW, Washington, DC 20006; telephone (202) 293-7963.

50. Workplace safety
Federal jurisdiction over workplace safety prevails through the U.S. Occupational Health and Safety Administration (OSHA) or the state has its own program with tougher standards than those used by the federal government.
Source: "The Book of the States, 1988-1989," 1990. Published by Council of State Governments, 444 North Capitol Street, NW, Washington, DC 20001; telephone (202) 624-5460.

50 POLICY SUMMARY

50 policy score
Number of policies in place out of possible 50 and rank

RENEW AMERICA POLICY AREAS

Rating for 17 different environmental programs
Results from Renew America's analysis of various policies and programs between 1987 and 1989. Rating of 10 is best in each area; total of 170 possible points. Renew America prepared separate reports on each area, as well as a summary for each year.
Source: "The State of the States, 1989," Renew America, 1400 16th Street, NW, Washington, DC 20036; telephone (202) 232-2252. Also, reports for 1988 and 1987.

Composite policy score
Percent of possible totals (50 policies and 170 Renew America points), averaged together to produce each state's score. Ranking on score, with highest percent of possible policy points ranking 1.

STATE SPENDING

Funds for air quality control
Per-capita spending in fiscal 1988 for state programs to administer state clean air laws and federal Clean Air Act. Includes state, federal, and other funds (fines, licenses, etc.) that pass through state budgetary process.
Source: "Resource Guide to State Environmental Management," second edition, 1991. Published by Council of State Governments, P.O. Box 11910, Lexington, KY 40578; telephone (606) 231-1939.

Funds for water pollution
Per-capita spending in fiscal 1988 for state drinking water programs, water quality protection, and water resource conservation and development. Includes state, federal, and other funds (fines, licenses, etc.) that pass through state budgetary process. Excludes funds for coastal water and marine protection.
Source: "Resource Guide to State Environmental Management," 1991. Published by Council of State Governments, Lexington, KY.

STATE POLICY INITIATIVES 155

Funds for solid and hazardous waste
Per-capita spending in fiscal 1988 to monitor, manage, minimize, and regulate solid and hazardous wastes. Includes state, federal, and other funds (fines, licenses, etc.) that pass through state budgetary process. Excludes funds raised and spent by municipal and county governments for garbage or waste management.
Source: "Resource Guide to State Environmental Management," 1991. Published by Council of State Governments, Lexington, KY.

Funds for fish, wildlife, and forestry
Per-capita spending in fiscal 1988 to protect, manage, and enhance fish, wildlife, and forestry resources, and to enforce state fish and game laws. Includes state, federal, and other funds (fines, licenses, etc.) that pass through state budgetary process.
Source: "Resource Guide to State Environmental Management," 1991. Published by Council of State Governments, Lexington, KY.

Spending for all environmental programs
Total spending in fiscal 1988 for state programs addressing environmental and natural resources. Includes state, federal and other funds (fines, licenses, etc.) that pass through state budgetary process. Excludes funds raised and spent by municipal and county governments. Also, per-capita spending in 1988 and percent of total state budget spent on environmental programs, with ranking for both indicators.
Source: "Resource Guide to State Environmental Management," 1991. Published by Council of State Governments, Lexington, KY.

Index

Pages for tables of indicators are in **bold typeface**. Pages listed for states do not include references to these tables.

Acid rain 16, 18, 19-20, **24**, 27, 32, 44, 101, 118, 123, 135, 139, 140, **143**
Adirondack Mountains (NY) 20
Agriculture: regulations 97-100, 104, 136, 137, 138, **144**, **147**; reliance on chemicals 97-100; run-off 27, 32-34; sustainable farming practices 99-100, **144**; value of 31, 97, **106**, 119; *see also* farms
Air pollutants 15-26, **146**; carbon dioxide 16, 21, **24**, 44, 50, 100, 137; carbon monoxide 15, 16, 17, **22**, 140; end-of-stack controls 18, **23**; fees 140, **143**; global warming gases 16, 18-19, 21, **24**, 42, 43, 124; ground-level ozone or smog 9, 15, 16-17, **22**, 48, 49, 118, 140; nitrogen oxides 16, 20, 21, **24**, 44, 135; ozone-depleting chemicals **23**; sulfur dioxide 19-20, 21, **24**, 32, 44, 101, 135; toxic chemicals 7, 17-19, **23**; *see also* motor vehicles
Air quality control spending 134-135, 140, **148**
Alabama 1, 11, 31, 44, 65, 67-68, 83, 119, 120, 121, 135, 138, 139, 141
Alaska 2, 11, 18, 21, 28, 30, 34, 43, 46, 63, 65, 67, 68, 69, 70, 86, 87, 104, 119, 120, 121, 122, 135, 138, 139, 140
ALCOA (IA) 18
AMAX Magnesium (UT) 18, 140
American Association of State Highway and Transportation Officials 60, 153
American Cancer Society 93
American Cyanamid (LA) 29, 65
American Forest Council 114
American Lung Association 15
American Paper Institute 150
Ameripol-Synpol (TX) 17
Appalachian states 19, 34, 44
ARCO Chemical (TX) 87
Arizona 11, 17, 28, 34, 44, 48, 64, 98, 99, 119, 120, 135, 136, 139
Arkansas 9 (map), 11, 28, 31-32, 47, 48, 65, 67, 70, 83, 104, 138
Army Corps of Engineers 104

Asarco, Inc. (AZ) 64
Association of Local Air Pollution Control Officials 151
Atomic Energy Commission 66
Auburn Foundry (IN) 84
Automobiles *see* motor vehicles; mass transit
Automotive industry 18, 47-49, 87, 65, 122
Avtex Fiber (VA) 29

Barton, Joe (TX) 122
Bastian Plating Co. (IN) 84
Bates, Jim (CA) 120
Bethlehem Steel (MD) 28
Bhopal, India, pollution deaths 18
BioCycle magazine viii, 80, 81
Biomass energy 49, 50
Biotechnology 99, **144**
Birth defects 19, 28, 31, 32, 65, 67 (map), 70, **74**, 140
Boats 104, **109**
Boehlert, Sherwood (NY) 120
Boeing (WA) 86
Boggs, Lindy (LA) 122
Boise Cascade (ME) 18, 88
Bottle-deposit laws 137, 139, **142**
British Petroleum (OH) 19
Brown & Root (TX) 88
Brown, Jerry (CA) 50
Bryan, Richard (NV) 122
Burford, Anne Gorsuch 123
Bush, George 20, 21, 66-67, 122, 123, 134
Byrd, Robert (WV) 118

California 9, 11, 17, 18, 19, 21, 28, 33, 34, 43, 47, 48, 49, 50, 63, 64, 65, 67, 68, 69, 71, 85, 88, 99, 100, 101, 103, 118, 120, 121, 134, 135, 136, 139, 140, 141
Campbell, Tom (CA) 120
Cancer 9, 16, 17, 18, 19, 28, 34, 45, 64, 65, 68, 70, 83, 84-85, 86, **89**
Cancer-causing chemicals 10, 16, 17-19, **23**, 28, 29, 32, 34, 44, 67, **74**, 86, 101, 102, 123 Carbon emissions 21 (map), 43, 44, 48, **52**; *see also* air pollutants
Cargill 99

Center for Budget and Policy Priorities 95
Center for Policy Alternatives vii, 134, 136, 139, 140, 141, 149, 150, 151, 153
Champion International (NC) 31
Chem-Dyne Corporation (OH) 33
Chemical Products Corporation (TN) 67
Chemical Waste Management (AL) 68
Chemical industry 18, 19, 28, 29, 43, 47, 64-65, **73**, 88, 101, 103, 121, 122, 138, 140
Cheney, Dick 124
Chlorofluorocarbons (CFCs) 16, 18-19, 21, 136-137; *see also* ozone-depleting chemicals
Citizens Clearinghouse on Hazardous Waste 71
Citizens Fund 65, 78, 79
Clean Air Act 15, 17, **22**, 49, 117, 118, 119, 121, 122
Clean Water Act 31
Coal 20, 44, **51**, 101
Coast 32, 43, 102, 103, 104, **109**; coastal zone management 97, 103-104, **145**
Cochran, Thad (MS) 120
Collins, Cardiss (IL) 122
Colorado 11, 17, 21, 32, 45, 69, 70 (map), 71, 86, 100, 120, 141
Columbian Chemicals (MO) 28
Common Cause viii, 120, 133
ConAgra 99
Congressional voting records 118-124, **125-132**
Connecticut 11, 16, 18, 19, 20, 21, 28, 30, 47, 48, 65, 71, 102, 119, 120, 121, 135, 136, 139, 140
Conservation Foundation 124
Conservation Reserve Program 99-100, **106**
Conservation Technology Information Center 113
Corporation for Enterprise Development vii, 60, 154
Council of State Governments viii, 40, 80, 135, 153, 154, 155
Cranston, Alan (CA) 120
Cypus Miami Mining (AZ) 64

DPRA Inc. 79
Dannemeyer, William (CA) 121
Davol Company (RI) 18
Delaware 11, 17, 18, 28, 47, 65, 67, 68, 71, 85, 102, 119, 139
Democrats 119, 120
Diamond Shamrock Corporation (MD) 66
Diapers 139, **142**
Dingell, John D. (MI) 118
Dioxin 10, 19, 31, 32, 64, 71, 88, 101-102
Dow Chemical (LA, TX) 65
Drinking water, use of 28, 31, 34, **38**, 66, 140; violations 30, 33, 34, **38**; state policy **146**
Dupont (AL, LA, TN) 29, 65, 68, 99

Earth First 101
Eastman Kodak (NY, TN) 18, 29, 32, 67
Electricity: cost of 45, 46, **54**; from coal **54**, 123; from nuclear power 44-45, **53**, 120, 121; from oil or gas **54**; from renewable sources 48 (map), 49-50, **56**
Emelle landfill (AL) 67-68, 69

Emerson, Bill (MO) 120
Employee Benefit Research Institute 93, 96
Energy Conservation Coalition 42
Energy PACs 120, 121, 122, 123, **126-132**
Energy consumption and conservation 9, 21, 42, 43, 45, 46-47, 50, **52**, 101, 121, 136, 137, **145**, **147**
Energy from solid waste 49-50, **56**
Energy industry 16, 43, **51**, 120-122; dependency on 21, 43, 47, 50, **51**, 119, 120, 138, **146**
Energy sources, alternatives to 46; subsidies of 42, 46; *see also* biomass energy; geothermal energy; municipal waste energy; oceans; solar energy; wind
Environment and economic development 8, 9, 28, 123, 137-138
Environment and health 8, 10, 34, 70, 82, 83, 104, 137, 140; *see also* health problems
Environmental Action 46, 121, 124
Environmental Defense Fund 30, 149
Environmental Law Institute viii, 150
Environmental Protection Agency (EPA) 29, 63, 64, 88, 123-124; air pollution 15; enforcement practices 17-18, 34, 66, 67, 70, 71; water pollution regulations 28, 29, 30-32, 34, 70-71; *see also* Toxic Release Inventory
Environmental organizations, membership 104, 134, **111**
Environmental protection, state spending for 134-136, **148**; fee 135, 140
Everglades (FL) 33, 103, 122
Exxon (AL, AK, LA) 65, 68, 103
Exxon Valdez 43, 103, 122

Farm Belt states 9, 31, 34, 83, 86, 138; *see also* Midwest states; Great Lakes
Farms: average size 99, **105**; change in number 98, 99, **105**, 138; conservation tillage 99, 100, **106**; cropland erosion 98, **106**; cropland irrigated 32, 97, 98, **106**; planted in trees **107**; *see also* agriculture
Federal Trade Commission 134
Fertilizer use 30, 32, 33, 97, 98, 99 (map), **105**
Fields, Jack (TX) 122
Fish and fishing 27, 28, 30, 31, 32, 33, 102-103, **108**; licenses **108**; state spending for 135, **148**
Fishers and hunters 104, **109**; spending by 104, **109**
Florida 10, 11, 17, 19, 30, 33-34, 43, 46, 48, 49, 50, 63, 71, 88, 99, 103, 119, 122, 135, 136, 139, 140
Florio, Jim (NJ) 124
Food processing 29, 86, 88, 99
Food safety 97-98, 99, 100, **146**
Ford Motor (MI) 118
Forest products industry 49, 86, 100-102, 103, **107**, 120, 123, 138
Forests: ancient 101, 123; change in acreage **107**; erosion of land 100, 101, 102, 104; land in 9, 100, 102 (map), **107**, 137; management 100-101, **146**; ownership 101, **107**; state spending for 135, **148**
Formaldehyde 15, 28, 101
Fossil fuel production 42, 43, 48, **51**; waste 16, 20, 21, 29, 70; *see also* individual fuels
Foundation for Advancement of Industrial Research 84

Freeport McMoran (LA) 28
Fresh Kills landfill (NY) 69-70
Friends of the Earth 124

Garbage *see* solid waste
Garn, Jake (UT) 120
Gasoline use and pollution 33, 46-49, **54**, 120, 122
General Electric (AL, TN) 67, 68
General Motors (AL) 68
Georgia 10, 11, 17, 18, 20, 21, 31, 47, 48, 49, 67, 102, 119, 121, 135, 141
Georgia-Pacific 10, 101, 102
Geothermal energy 49, 50
Gilman, Benjamin (NY) 120
Global warming 16, 18, 21, 33, 42-43, 100, 137, **145**; *see also* carbon emissions
Gorton, Slade (WA) 123
Graham, Bob (FL) 119, 122
Gramm, Phil (TX) 122
Grant Thornton 84, 96
Great Lakes 31-32; states 30, 64; *see also* Farmbelt states
Great Northern Nekoosa Corp. (ME) 101
Greenhouse effect *see* global warming
Greenpeace 64-65, 118
Groundwater pollution 7, 9, 27, 28, 32-34, **38**, 43, 62, 66, 70, 97, 98, **106**; regulation 33, 34, 120, 135, 137, 138, 140, **144**, **147**; use 32, **37**, 140
Growth management planning 97, **145**, **146**
Gulf of Mexico 43, 103

Hall, Ralph M. (TX) 122
Hanford Nuclear Reservation (WA) 44, 68
Hatch, Orin (UT) 120
Hatfield, Mark (OR) 123
Hawaii 2, 8 (map), 11-12, 18, 47-49, 67, 69, 85-86, 99, 100, 104
Hazardous waste 10, 19, 33, 65-69, **75**; emergency response personnel **143**; facilities **75**; importing of 67, 68; off-site disposal 67, 68; on military bases 9, 68-69, **75**; on-site disposal 67, 68, **75**; regulation of 65-67, **147**; sites **76**, 82, 86, 140; spending to control 69 (map), **76**, 140-141, **148**; transport accidents 68, **75**; workers handling **91**
Health problems 8, 9, 19, 28, 34, 44, 70, 82, 83; *see also* birth defects; cancer; heart diseases; learning disabilities; miscarriages; nerve-damaging diseases; premature deaths; respiratory illnesses
Heart diseases 16, 19
Helms, Jesse (NC) 120
Herger, Wally (CA) 120
Hi Mill Manufacturing Company (MI) 66
Highway Users Federation 59, 153
Highways 48, 49, **55**, **146**; fatalities 47 (map), 48, **54**; *see also* motor vehicles
Hoagland, Peter (NE) 120
Homes: inadequate plumbing 34, 83, 87, **90**; indoor pollution **145**, **146**; weatherized 46, **52**
Humphrey, Gordon (NH) 120

Hunters, *see* fishers
Hydropower 49, 50

IBM (AL, CA) 19, 63
Idaho 12, 18, 32, 33, 46, 47, 64, 67 86, 100, 101, 119, 120, 121, 123, 135, 138, 139
Illinois 12, 21, 28, 31, 32, 34, 44, 45, 46, 48, 50, 64, 69, 99, 100, 104, 122, 140, 141
Impoundments and lagoons 33, 43, 63, 64, 65-66, 70, **76**; *see also* landfills
Incinerators 19, 50, 62, 64, 67, 70, 71 **77**
Indiana 12, 20, 21, 33, 50, 63-65, 68, 84, 104, 122-123, 135, 141
Indoor pollution **145**, **146**
Infant mortality rate 83, 86-87, **90**
Inland Steel (IN) 63
Institute for Southern Studies vii, 2
International Paper (ME) 10, 18
Iowa 9, 12, 31, 33, 46, 47, 83, 87, 97, 99, 100, 120, 137, 139

J & L Specialty Products Company (OH) 64
James River Company (ME) 32
Jefferson Proving Ground (IN) 68
Jeffords, James (VT) 49
Jobs: handling hazardous waste **91**; in industries with highest injury rates 44, 86, **91**; in industries with most toxic releases 85, **91**; with high risk of disabling diseases 85, 86 (map), 87, **91**; vehicle-related jobs 47, **55**; versus environment 123, 138
Johnston, J. Bennett (LA) 32, 121-122

Kaiser Aluminum (LA) 63
Kansas 12, 29, 32, 33, 43, 46, 47, 48, 50, 64, 83, 98, 100, 104
Kean, Thomas (NJ) 137
Kennecott Utah Copper (UT) 63
Kennelly, Barbara (CT) 121
Kentucky 10, 12, 20, 21, 34, 44, 45, 47, 65, 67, 83, 104, 119, 120, 121
Kerr-McGee Corporation (OK) 66
Kerry, John (MA) 120

Lakes, pollution of 19, 27, 31, 32, 34, **37**
Land: acres **109**; federal government ownership of **109**; in state parks and recreational areas **110**; state land-use planning **146**
Landfills: cleanup requirements 70-71, **142**; garbage 70, 71; groundwater testing 70, **142**; hazardous waste 65, 66, 67; number of 9, 69, 70-71, **77**, 82, 86; restrictions on items 137, 139, **142**; toxic waste 64
Leach, Jim (IA) 120
League of Conservation Voters viii, 118, 119, 120, 122, 124, 133
Learning disabilities 32, 70
Leiberman, Joseph (CT) 121
Lightfoot, Jim Ross (IA) 120
Lockheed Aeronautical Systems (TN) 67
Lott, Trent (MS) 120

Louisiana 7, 8 (map), 12, 18-19, 21, 28, 29, 33, 43, 63, 64, 65, 67, 70, 85, 102-103, 119, 120, 121-122, 140
Love Canal (NY) 66

Maine 10, 12, 18, 19, 20, 32, 34, 48, 49, 70, 71, 87, 88, 101, 104, 119, 120, 121, 134, 135, 136, 137, 139, 141
Marine Shale Processors (LA) 19
Markey, Ed (MA) 122
Maryland 12, 17, 28, 47, 48, 66, 68, 70 (map), 71, 85, 102, 119, 139, 140
Mass transit use 9, 42, 47, 48, 49, **55**, **145**
Massachusetts 12, 16, 18, 28, 29, 34, 45, 46-48, 49, 66, 71, 83, 87, 101, 102, 119, 120, 121, 122, 134, 136, 137, 139, 140, 141
Medicaid, state program 85, 87, **90**
Medical care: doctors per capita 86, 87, **89**; state spending for 83, 85, 86, **90**; underserved areas 34, **89**
Medical insurance, coverage 10, 83, 86, 87, **89**, **92**
Metals industry 18, 32, 64, 65, 66, 101
Michigan 10, 12, 19, 20, 32, 47, 48, 63, 64, 66, 71, 87, 118, 136, 139
Mid-Atlantic states 70, 103
Midwest states 20, 30, 32, 84, 85, 87, 104, 118, 136; *see also* Farmbelt states
Military, hazardous waste sites 9, 68-69, **75**
Mine Safety and Health Administration 83
Mining 9, 19, 34, 44, 64, 82-83, 86, 87, 118, 120, 135, 138
Minnesota 12, 31, 33, 48, 67, 71, 83, 87, 88, 99, 104, 120, 122, 135, 136, 137, 140, 141
Miscarriages 19, 28, 31, 85
Mississippi 10, 12-13, 29, 31, 33, 34, 47, 50, 86, 100, 101, 119, 120, 121, 138, 141
Mississippi River 28, 85, 103
Missouri 13, 21, 28, 63, 67, 100, 104, 119, 120, 139
Mobil Oil (NC) 43
Monsanto Company (ID, IL, MO, TX) 18, 28-29, 65, 99
Montana 13, 20, 28, 31, 43, 64-66, 70, 82, 100, 120, 135, 139
Motor Vehicle Manufacturers Association 25, 47, 59, 60, 153
Motor vehicles: density 17 (map), **22**, 42, 47, **55**; emissions **145**; fuel efficiency 47, **54**; pollution by 15-17, 19, 20, 21, 48, 49; regulation of 48, 49; seat belt law **145**; taxes 48, 49, **55**; use of 47, **55**
Municipal waste energy 49, 50, **56**

National Acid Precipitation Assessment Program 20
National Association of State Departments of Agriculture 152
National Association of State Park Directors 115
National Association of State Utility Consumer Advocates 153
National Audubon Society 26
National Environmental Law Center 141
National Fertilizer Development Center 112
National Forest Products Association 113
National Governors' Association vii, 134, 135
National Institute for Occupational Safety and Health 88, 94
National Oceanic and Atmospheric Administration 103
National Safe Work Institute 83
National Safety Council 83
National Solid Waste Management Association 149
National Steel (MI) 32
National Toxics Campaign 71
National Wildlife Federation 41, 104
Natural Resources Defense Council 18, 26, 29, 30, 123, 135
Natural gas production 33, 43, 46, 50, **51**
Natural resources 97; dependency on 9, 104, **110**, 119, 120, 138, 141 (map); state spending for 135, 136 (map), **148**
Nebraska 13, 32, 33, 44, 47, 67, 83, 97, 98, 100, 104, 119, 120, 121, 139
Nekoosa Papers (AR) 32
Nerve-damaging diseases 19, 31, 65; chemicals that cause 65, 67 (map), **74**
Nevada 13, 17, 20, 21, 28, 31, 34, 47, 50, 64, 70, 86, 98, 100, 104, 120, 121, 122, 138, 139, 140, 141
New England states 16, 18, 19, 21, 30, 32, 44, 46, 48-49, 70, 100, 101, 121
New Hampshire 13, 18, 30, 34, 71, 120, 136, 139-140
New Jersey 13, 16-18, 19, 21, 28, 30, 34, 45, 46, 47, 48, 49, 50, 64, 67, 68, 70, 71, 85, 119, 120, 124, 134, 135, 136, 137, 140
New Mexico 13, 20, 21, 28, 31, 32, 64, 67, 69, 70, 86, 98, 100, 121, 140
New York 13, 17, 18, 19, 20, 30, 32, 33, 45, 47, 48, 49, 64, 65, 67, 69-71, 88, 100, 102, 119, 120, 135, 136, 139, 140
Newspapers, recycled content 139, **142**
Nickles, Don (OK) 120-121
Nielson, Howard (UT) 120
Nitrates in wells 33, 98, **106**
North Carolina 13, 17, 19, 31, 34, 43, 47, 48, 65, 88, 99, 103, 120, 135-136, 140, 141
North Dakota 13, 20, 21, 28, 34, 44, 47, 67, 68, 97, 99, 100, 120, 138, 139
Northeast States for Coordinated Air Use Management 49
Northeast states 8-9, 19, 20, 21, 28, 87, 103, 136
Northwestern National Life Insurance Company 93, 94
Nuclear Information and Resource Service 58
Nuclear Regulatory Commission 45
Nuclear issues in Congress, voting records 120-122, **125**
Nuclear power plants: decommissioning 44, **53**; regulation 44-45, 120-122, 124; safety citations 44-45, **53**; waste 44, **53**, 68, 69
Nuclear weapons: testing 86; production 45

O'Neill, Tip (MA) 118
Occidental Chemical Corporation (FL) 63
Occidental Petroleum 99
Occupational deaths 9, 10, 44, 82, 86, 87, 88, **91**
Occupational disease and injury 83-84, 101
Occupational safety and health, state laws **145**
Occupational Safety and Health Administration 84, 88, 95

Occupational Safety and Health Law Center (WV) 83
Oceans, energy from 49, 50
Office of Technology Assessment 62-63, 64, 71
Ohio 13, 18-21, 29, 31, 32, 33, 44, 45, 47, 63, 64, 65, 71, 85, 104, 135
Oil 7, 21, 33, 43, 46, 47, 50, **51**, 65, 120, 121, 122; oil industry 16, 103; government subsidy of 46; imported oil 42;
Oil and gas injection wells 33, 43, **51**, 66
Oil and related spills 33, 43, **51**, 103, 120
Oil, Chemical and Atomic Workers International Union 87
Oklahoma 13, 21, 30, 33, 43, 48, 65-67, 71, 100, 104, 120-121, 135, 138
Oregon 1, 9, 13-14, 30, 45, 49, 65, 71, 85, 101, 104, 123, 135, 136, 139, 140, 141
Organic food promotion 98, 99, 100, **144**
Ozone-depleting chemicals 16, 18-19, **23**, 63, 64; laws to control 134, 136-137, **143**

PCBs 31, 32, 64, 68, 84-85
Pacific Northwest states 49, 101, 104, 123
Paper-pulp mills 10, 18, 29, 31, 32, 65, 101-102, 103, **108**, 135, 138
Parks, local and state funds for parks and recreation areas 104, **110**
Parks, state funds for 103 (map), **110**; visits to 104, **110**
Pashayan, Charles Jr. (CA) 120
Pennsylvania 14, 17, 20, 21, 44, 45, 46, 47, 49, 63, 64, 66, 67, 70, 83, 100
Pentagon, hazardous waste 68, 69
Pepper, Claude (FL) 119
Perdue Farms 88
Pesticides and herbicides 7, 9, 32, 33, 34, 97, 98, 99, 100 (map), **105**; regulation 98, 99, 138, **144, 146**
Petrochemical industry 8, 16, 64-65, 85, 103, 120, 121
Phillip Morris (AL) 68
Phillip's Petroleum 87, 88
Phosphate ban 32, 140, **144**
Pipelines violations 43-44, **51**
Places Rated Almanac 104, **116**
Policymakers, role of 8, 9, 117-124, 134-141
Political action committees 120, 121, 122, 123, **126-132**
Population density 104, **111**, 135
Poverty and environmental health 8, 9, 10, 34, 69, 82, 86, 137-138
Premature death rate 10, 83, 84 (map), 85, 86, 87, **89**
Public Citizen's Critical Mass Energy Project 49, 58, 59, 60, 61, 121, 133
Public Citizen's Health Research Group 94
Public Health Foundation 94
Pyro Mining Co. (KY) 83

Quality of life 9, 97, 104; in metropolitan areas 104, **111**
Quayle, Daniel 124

Race and environmental health 8, 10, 34, 69, 82, 83, 85, 86, 119
Racon Inc. (KS) 29
Radioactive Waste Campaign (NY) 69
Radioactive waste: generated 44-45, **53**, 66, 68, 69, 120; transported 45, **53**
Reagan, Ronald 117-118, 123, 134
Real estate developers 101, 103-104, 138
Recreational opportunities 31, 32, 101, 101, 104
Recycling programs 70, 71, **77**, 135, 137, 138, 139, 140, **142, 146**
Reilly, William 124
Renew America vii, 41, 57, 136, 151, 152, 153, 154
Renewable energy 46, 49-50, **56**, 119; *see also* energy sources
Republicans 119, 120
Resources for the Future 112
Respiratory illnesses 16, 18, 19, 20, 33, 71
Rexene Products (TX) 63
Rhode Island 14, 16, 18, 28, 30-31, 47, 65, 71, 85, 87, 119, 120, 121, 136
Right-to-know laws 137, 138, 140, **143**
Right-to-sue laws 137, **143**
Rivers and streams, pollution of 9, 19, 20, 27, 31, 32, 34, **37**, 70
Rocky Flats Plant (CO) 44, 69
Rocky Mountain states 9, 20, 32, 44, 48, 64, 86, 98, 100, 104, 119, 123, 138, 141
Ros-Lehtinen, Ileana (FL) 119
Royster Company (FL) 63
Ruckleshaus, William 123

Safe Drinking Water Act (SDWA) 34, **38**
Savannah River nuclear complex (SC) 44, 69
Scott Paper (AL, ME) 32, 49
Septic tanks 34, **37**, 103
Sewage systems, investment needs 28, 29, 30, 31, 34, **36**; toxic chemicals sent to 27-34, **35**; violating EPA standards 28, 30, **36**, 103
Sharp, Philip R. (IN) 122-123
Shays, Christopher (CT) 120
Sheldahl (MN) 88
Shell Oil (LA) 29, 65; (AL) 43
Shellfish waters 102-103, **108**
Sierra Club 49, 135
Sikorski, Gerry (MN) 122
Silicon Valley (CA) 69
Simpson, Alan (WY) 121
Smith, Peter (VT) 120
Smith, Virginia (NE) 120
Smog *see* air pollutants
Soap and Detergent Association 152
Solar energy 49, 50, **56**
Solid waste 62, 69-71, **77**; recycled 71, **77**; spending for **76**, 134-135, **148**; state management **147**
South Carolina 14, 45, 47, 65, 69, 71, 86-87
South Dakota 14, 18, 28, 34, 67, 97, 99, 100, 104, 138, 139, 140
Southern Regional Council 95, 96

Southern states 8, 9-10, 16, 18, 29, 34, 44, 47, 48, 65, 67, 70, 86-87, 99, 103, 119, 120, 135, 138, 141
Southwestern states 44, 100
State and Territorial Air Pollution Program Administrators 151
Strangeland, Arlan (MN) 120
Sununu, John 124
Superfund program 18, 63, 124; sites 32, 66-70, **76**, 86; state cleanup plan 138, 140, 141, **143**
Surface water, pollution of 20, 21, 27, 28, 30, 31, **35**, **37**, **38**, 66, 69, 70; protection of 29, 34, **146**; *see also* acid rain; coast; Great Lakes; oil spills; rivers; water

Tauzin, Billy (LA) 122
Tennessee 14, 17, 18, 19, 28-29, 34, 49, 65, 67, 69, 71, 104, 135, 138, 141
Tennessee Chemical Company (TN) 19
Texaco (LA, TX) 17, 65
Texas 7, 14, 16-17, 21, 28, 29, 33, 43, 44, 46, 48, 50, 63, 64, 65, 68, 87, 88, 100, 102, 119, 120, 122, 135, 136, 140
Texasgulf (NC) 32
Thomas, Craig (WY) 121
Thomas, Lee 123
Thompson Publishing Group 150
Tourism and travel spending 104, **110**
Toxic Release Inventory (TRI) 18-19, 28, 29, 63-65; compliance with 19, 63, 64
Toxic chemical releases 9, 10, **23**, **35**, 62-65, **72**, **73**, 101, 140; into air 7, 17-19, **23**; into ground 29, 33, **36**; into sewage systems 27-34, **35**; into surface water 27-28, 29, 30, **35**; off site 63-64, **72**; on site 63-64, **72**; regulations to control or reduce 7, 16, 63, 134, 137, 138, 140-141, **143**

U.S. Department of Energy hazardous waste sites 68-69
U.S. General Accounting Office 28, 32, 34, 71, 140
U.S. Forest Service 101
U.S. PIRG 141
U.S. Supreme Court 134
U.S. Travel Data Center 116
Underground storage tanks 33, 140, **144**
Unemployment 44, 87, **92**; insurance benefits 87, **91**; insurance coverage 85, **92**
Union Camp (TN) 67
Union Carbide (WV) 18; (TX) 7
Unions 82, 87, **92**
United Church of Christ 69
United States Steel (PA) 63
Unocal Chemical Division (AK) 63
Upjohn Company (MI) 63
Utah 14, 18, 32, 47, 50, 63, 64, 86, 119, 120, 138, 140
Utilities, electric 16, 19, 20, 21, 31, 44-46, 120; cogenerators 46; costs 45, 46; overproduction 44; regulation of 1, 45, 46

Vermont 14, 34, 49, 67, 70 (map), 71, 87, 104, 119, 120, 137, 139
Virginia 14, 17, 18, 28-30, 47, 65, 68, 70 (map), 71, 88, 121, 139, 140, 141
Vulcan Chemicals (KS) 29

W.R. Grace (MD) 28
Wallop, Malcolm (WY) 120-121, 122
Washington 9, 10, 14, 17, 18, 28, 30, 34, 45, 48, 49, 68, 71, 85, 86, 101, 103, 119, 120, 123, 135, 141
Water: consumption 31, **35**, 123; inland acreage 30, **109**; recreational uses of 27, 30, 31; *see also* acid rain; drinking water; groundwater; surface water; water pollutants
Water pollutants 27-34, 50; nitrates 33, 69, 98, **106**; oil and related spills 33, **51**, 103; pesticides 32, 33, 34, **38**, 98, **106**, 139-140, **144**; phosphates 32, 140, **144**; regulations of 27, 29, 30, 32, 33, 70-71; spending to control 28, 33, **37**, 134-135, **148**; toxic chemicals 27-34, **35**, 66, 103, 140
Watt, James 123
Waxman, Henry A. (CA) 118
Weatherized low-income homes 46, **52**
Weiss, Ted (NY) 120
Wells, use of 34, **37**, 137; nitrates in 69, 98, **106**; *see also* oil and gas injection wells
West Coast states 9, 85, 103, 136; *see also* Pacific Northwest states
West Virginia 14, 18, 20, 31, 34, 44, 65, 67, 70, 82, 83, 87, 118, 121, 138, 140, 141
Westinghouse (IN) 84-85
Wetlands 9, 27, 32, 34, 102-103, 104, **108**; protection 97, **144**; *see also* Everglades
Weyerhaeuser 10, 49, 101
Whirlpool (TN) 67
Wildlife 30, 31, 32, 49, 97, 100, 101, 102, 104, 123, 135; spending to protect 135, **148**
Wilson, Pete (CA) 120
Wind, energy from 49, 50
Wisconsin 10, 14, 19, 31, 32-33, 48, 64, 70, 83, 101, 104, 119, 120, 136, 139, 140
Worker's compensation 88; disability benefits 82, 86, 87, 88, **91**
Worker's rights, state laws 10, 83, 84, 86, 87, **92**
Working Group on Community Right-To-Know 25, 150
World Wildlife Fund 124
Wycon (WY) 29
Wyoming 14, 18, 20, 21, 28, 29, 32, 33, 34, 43, 44, 47, 49, 64, 65, 70, 86, 100, 119, 120, 121, 122, 124, 135, 138, 140

ALSO AVAILABLE FROM ISLAND PRESS

Ancient Forests of the Pacific Northwest
By Elliott A. Norse

Balancing on the Brink of Extinction: The Endangered Species Act and Lessons for the Future
Edited by Kathryn A. Kohm

Better Trout Habitat: A Guide to Stream Restoration and Management
By Christopher J. Hunter

Beyond 40 Percent: Record-Setting Recycling and Composting Programs
The Institute for Local Self-Reliance

The Challenge of Global Warming
Edited by Dean Edwin Abrahamson

Coastal Alert: Ecosystems, Energy, and Offshore Oil Drilling
By Dwight Holing

The Complete Guide to Environmental Careers
The CEIP Fund

Economics of Protected Areas
By John A. Dixon and Paul B. Sherman

Environmental Agenda for the Future
Edited by Robert Cahn

Environmental Disputes: Community Involvement in Conflict Resolution
By James E. Crowfoot and Julia M. Wondolleck

Forests and Forestry in China: Changing Patterns of Resource Development
By S. D. Richardson

The Global Citizen
By Donella Meadows

Hazardous Waste from Small Quantity Generators
By Seymour L. Schwartz and Wendy B. Pratt

Holistic Resource Management Workbook
By Allan Savory

In Praise of Nature
Edited and with essays by Stephanie Mills

The Living Ocean: Understanding and Protecting Marine Biodiversity
By Boyce Thorne-Miller and John G. Catena

Natural Resources for the 21st Century
Edited by R. Neil Sampson and Dwight Hair

The New York Environment Book
By Eric A. Goldstein and Mark A. Izeman

Overtapped Oasis: Reform or Revolution for Western Water
By Marc Reisner and Sarah Bates

Permaculture: A Practical Guide for a Sustainable Future
By Bill Mollison

Plastics: America's Packaging Dilemma
By Nancy Wolf and Ellen Feldman

The Poisoned Well: New Strategies for Groundwater Protection
Edited by Eric Jorgensen

Race to Save the Tropics: Ecology and Economics for a Sustainable Future
Edited by Robert Goodland

Recycling and Incineration: Evaluating the Choices
By Richard A. Denison and John Ruston

Reforming The Forest Service
By Randal O'Toole

The Rising Tide: Global Warming and World Sea Levels
By Lynne T. Edgerton

Saving the Tropical Forests
By Judith Gradwohl and Russell Greenberg

Trees, Why Do You Wait?
By Richard Critchfield

War on Waste: Can America Win Its Battle With Garbage?
By Louis Blumberg and Robert Gottlieb

Western Water Made Simple
From *High Country News*

Wetland Creation and Restoration: The Status of the Science
Edited by Mary E. Kentula and Jon A. Kusler

Wildlife and Habitats in Managed Landscapes
Edited by Jon E. Rodiek and Eric G. Bolen

For a complete catalog of Island Press publications, please write:
Island Press, Box 7, Covelo, CA 95428, or call: 1-800-828-1302

ISLAND PRESS BOARD OF DIRECTORS

PETER R. STEIN, CHAIR
Managing Partner, Lyme Timber Company
Board Member, Land Trust Alliance

DRUMMOND PIKE, SECRETARY
Executive Director
The Tides Foundation

SUSAN E. SECHLER, TREASURER
Director
Rural Economic Policy Program
Aspen Institute for Humanistic Studies

ROBERT E. BAENSCH
Director of Publishing
American Institute of Physics

PETER R. BORRELLI
Vice President of Land Preservation
Open Space Institute
Natural Resources Defense Council

CATHERINE M. CONOVER

GEORGE T. FRAMPTON, JR.
President
The Wilderness Society

PAIGE K. MACDONALD
Executive Vice President/Chief Operating Officer
World Wildlife Fund &
The Conservation Foundation

HENRY REATH
President
Collectors Reprints, Inc.

CHARLES C. SAVITT
President
Center for Resource Economics/Island Press

RICHARD TRUDELL
Executive Director
American Indian Lawyer Training Program